CULTURE, RELIGION

AND

PATIENT CARE

IN A

MULTI-ETHNIC SOCIETY

A Handbook for Professionals

'It is only through the identification of differences that the uniqueness of each person can be recognised, and individual needs of patients met. It is only through the identification of similarities that a common ground for humanity, understanding, and mutual respect among different cultures can be found, and the dream that "All men are brothers" as a Chinese saying goes, can become a reality.' (Huang 1989)

'Knowledge helps, but knowledge *alone* is not going to help anybody. If you do not use your head and your heart and your soul, you are not going to help a single human being.' (Kübler-Ross 1991)

'Nothing has changed except our attitudes, so everything has changed.' (De Mello 1983)

Alix Henley & Judith Schott

CULTURE, RELIGION
AND
PATIENT CARE
IN A
MULTI-ETHNIC SOCIETY

A Handbook for Professionals

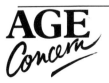 BOOKS

Note to readers

Writing anything about people's needs, beliefs and lifestyles is like walking a tightrope. So-called 'facts' that health professionals might perceive as 'helpful information' may be misleading or even offend. It is essential to avoid stereotypes and generalisations and to show the subtleties and variety that exist within each culture and community. It is important to help professionals think sensitively about providing care for patients and families whose culture they do not share. This is what we have tried to do.

Permission to reproduce material in any form must be sought from the publishers and from the authors, who will wish to ensure that the context in which the material is used is consistent with the philosophy and approach of this book.

Alix Henley and Judith Schott

© 1999 Alix Henley and Judith Schott

Published by Age Concern England
1268 London Road
London SW16 4ER

First published 1999
Reprinted 2001, 2002, 2003, 2004

Editor Gillian Clarke
Production Vinnette Marshall
Designed and typeset by GreenGate Publishing Services, Tonbridge, Kent
Cover design by Ben Schott
Printed and bound in Great Britain by Bell & Bain Ltd, Glasgow

A catalogue record for this book is available from the British Library.
ISBN 0–86242–231–0

Bulk orders
Age Concern England is pleased to offer customised editions of all its titles to UK companies, institutions or other organisations wishing to make a bulk purchase. For further information, please contact the Publishing Department at the address above. Tel: 0870 44 22 120. Fax: 0870 8000 100. E-mail:books@ace.org.uk.

CONTENTS

ABOUT THE AUTHORS

Alix Henley is a freelance writer, researcher and consultant. She specialises in matters to do with health and health care, and has a particular interest in communication between professionals and service users, and in equal opportunity issues. Her recent books include *Equality in Action: Introducing equal opportunities in voluntary organisations*, co-author Mee-Han Cheung-Judge (NCVO Publications, 1994), *When a Baby Dies: The experience of late miscarriage, stillbirth and neonatal death* with Nancy Kohner (Pandora, 1991) and *Miscarriage, Stillbirth and Neonatal Death: Guidelines for professionals* also with Nancy (UK Stillbirth and Neonatal Death Society, 1991). At present she lives in Switzerland.

Judith Schott is a freelance writer on health issues and trains health professionals, working under the name of PROSPECT. She has worked in and around the health service for over 30 years as a health professional, consumer representative, parent educator and researcher. Her particular interest is in devising and running experiential training for health professionals in order to support them in their work of providing sensitive and appropriate care. She runs workshops throughout the UK with staff at all levels, on a range of topics including cultural and religious aspects of care. She is co-author with Judith Priest of *Leading Antenatal Classes: A practical guide* (Butterworth Heinemann, 1996) and with AVERT of *AIDS and Childbirth* (1994). She lives in London.

Together, Alix and Judith have written *Culture, Religion and Childbearing in a Multiracial Society: A handbook for health professionals* (Butterworth Heinemann, 1996) and *Breaking the Barriers: A training package on equal access to maternity services* (Bloomsbury and Islington Health Authority, 1992).

ACKNOWLEDGEMENTS

We could not have written this book without the help of a great many people. We are indebted to all of them, especially to the people of different cultures and religions who trusted us enough to invite us into their homes and workplaces, allowed us to ask intimate questions about beliefs, customs and preferences, and then commented on what we wrote. Each one of them taught us a great deal and helped us to examine our own cultural assumptions. They bore with our ignorance, tolerated our occasional inadvertent insensitivity and prompted us to formulate questions we did not know we needed to ask. We are grateful to everyone for their patience, tolerance and encouragement, and for the constant reminder that, although there are many cultural and religious variations between people, fundamentally we all share many more similarities than differences. In particular, we thank:

Fenik Adham; Taslim Akhtar; Zeba Arif; Fiona Baker; Alan Barnett; Maryam Barnosh; Akgül Baylav; Rabbi van den Bergh; Mark Blake; Ydolina Bocanegra-Moser; Melanie Boshoff; Denise Brady, Librarian, St Christopher's Hospice; Alan Brash; the staff at the Brompton Branch and Interloan Section and the Royal Borough of Kensington and Chelsea Library Service; Auriol Burrows; John Carew; Thomas Chan; Mirai Chatterjee; Piki Chatterjee; Wai-Guen Cheong; Mee-Yan Cheung-Judge; Alice Clifton; Joy Conway; Irene Cooke; Alison Crombie; Daphne Crossfield; Lemuel Crossfield; Mrs Bernice B Dada; Dr Charles Daniels; Mary Dawkins; Sylvia Denton; Lakhtar Djellail; Peggy Dlamini-Grüniger; June Epstein; Catherine Ngozi Ezeigwe; Jacqueline Fitzgerald; Fok Hung-Sim; Donald Franklin; Milton Fruchtman; Rev Dr Jonathan Gibbs; Ros Greensmith; Jane Griffiths; Dr HK Gujral; Andrea Hafenbrack; Christopher Henley, of Henley Wright Repatriation Service; Dr Gill Hinshelwood; Antony J Hooker; Rashida Hunzai; Gillian Huteson; Shadia Ibrahim; The IQRA Trust; Suryakala Jacob; Neveen Jivan; Kusum Joshi; Vishwas Joshi; Mohammed H Kahin; Shivananda Kahn; Dr David Katz; Olapeju Kayode-Adedeji; Paula Keenan; Laila Kibria; Dr Nitin Lakhani, President of the UK Thalassaemia Society; Estriana Lewin; Anne Lister, Nurse Director of the North London Hospice; Dr Anna Livingstone; Dr Lyn Lyndpaintner; Neila Mahadevan MRCOG; Vishy Mahadevan FRCS; David Malyon; Gloria Malyon; Anjalee Marshall; Christine McDougal; Vanessa Morgan; Dr Virginia Murray; Dr MN Nandakumar; The Natural Death Centre; Joanna Nicholls; Mr and Mrs AO Oduwusi; Elizabeth Olajumoke Okuyiga; Lola Iyebode Oni; Patricia Pank; Bhanu Patel; Minat Patel; Costas Paul; Kem Kit

Poon; George Priest; Agnes Makonda Ridley; Elizabeth Riley, Civilian Coroner's Officer, Westminster Coroner's Court; Daniel Rosenfelder; Ruth Rosenfelder; Jacqueline Rothschild; Rabbi Walter Rothschild; Angeline Rothwell; Mary Rowley; Rev Patrick Ryall; Pauline Sandall; Carmen Schirling; Elizabeth Schischa; Vasugi Sellappah; Jane Shackman; Dr NK Shah; Dr RB Shah and members of the Swaminarayan Hindu Mission Neasden, North London; Dr Shastri; Debbie Shaw; Dr Maurice Sifman; members of the Sikh Educational and Cultural Association; Bhai Ram Singh; Mr Fauja Singh; Dr Kartar Surindar Singh; Dr Kulwant Singh; Dr Rajbinder Singh; Bibi Ranjit Kaur; Jenny Smith; Gillian Stellman; Hans-Peter Stoll; Meherun Suleman; Margaret Sullivan; Richard Taylor; Veronica Taylor; Ruth Teclu-Belay; Soo Tai; Esther Valentine; Rozmina Valimahomed; Ann Vaus; Anne Wadey; Margaret Wallace; Shirley Wan; Bridget Watson; Paul Weller; Sandy Wickenden; Pip Willcox; Allyson Williams; Richard Willis; Rabbi Jonathan Wittenberg; Wong Kuai-Peng and Suit Mui Wong; Audrey Yansen and Olashola Yemi-Akiniyi.

We are also grateful to the many health professionals throughout the UK who have attended PROSPECT Workshops on Culture, Religion and Childbearing. Their insights and reactions to our approach have also taught us a great deal. Despite all the help we have received, we may unwittingly have made mistakes or caused offence. We take full responsibility for this and we apologise.

We would also like to thank Richard Holloway of Age Concern whose support, flexibility and encouragement we have greatly valued.

Some of the material in this book is taken from our previous book *Culture, Religion and Childbearing in a Multiracial Society* (Butterworth Heinemann 1996), though much of it has been updated through interviews and additional research. The information and ideas we acquired when researching and writing the earlier book were crucial in the writing of this one. So we are grateful to the many people who helped us then and who shared their insights and knowledge with us. They include:

Jyoti Ahluwalia; Aisha Ahmed, Somali Women's Centre; Shanaz Akhtar; Iman Ali; Esther Amidu; Bridget Baker; Rajes Bala; Marti Biswas; Shelly Choudhery; Cherry Cunningham; Champa Desei; Frances Drain; Ros Finlay; Dr Yohannes Fassil; Carla Gavsey Jacobs; Dr AR Ghatrad; Supinder Ghatora; Jagdev Gilbert; Penny Gillinson; Gülçin Gökul; Mohamoud Omer Ibrahim; Saryu Joshi; Amran Mahmoud, Somali Women's Centre; the Health Aides at the Royal London Hospital; Ingred Mariott; Lesley Marks; Mary McCaffrey; Vicky McIntosh; Sabera Mirza; Nancy Ng; Bridget Okereke; Dora Opoku; Greta Ottway; Pauline Palmer; Regina Parry; Pushpa

Patel; Hansa Patel-Kanwal, The Naz Project; Maria Peppos; Rabbi Alan Plancey; Jackie Powell; Carla Rusconi; Agnes Sampare Kwateng; Shabnam Sharma; Aliya Sheikh; Rabbi Dr Nissan Shulman; Pastor Paul Sinclair; Joan Small; Sonia Stewart; Marie Webb; Moya de Wet; Dianne Williams Trottman; Saulan Yim; Tina Young; and Fawzia Zaidi.

We are grateful to Camden and Islington Health Authority London for permission to reproduce some of the material previously published in *Caring in a Multiracial Society* by Alix Henley. We are also grateful to Ros Morpeth and the National Extension College (NEC), Cambridge, for permission to reproduce some of the material by Alix Henley previously published in *Health Care in Multiracial Britain* (1985) (co-authored with Penny Mares and Carol Baxter), *Asian Names and Records* (1981), *Caring for Hindus and Their Families* (1983), *Caring for Muslims and Their Families* (1983), *Caring for Sikhs and Their Families* (1983) and *Caring For Everyone: Ensuring standards of care for black and ethnic minority patients* (1991). For more information about all NEC publications, contact NEC customer services, 18 Brooklands Avenue, Cambridge CB2 2HN.

Thanks are also due to both our families who have once again lived with the stresses of a book in preparation. Geoff and Jonathan Schott, who kept an eye on the medical literature for us and repeatedly brought us down to earth about the realities of working in the NHS . . . and Benjamin, who did not. Tana, Fia and Robbie Adelmann, who tolerated their mother's preoccupation with remarkable and increasing equanimity, and Fred who was supportive and encouraging throughout.

We especially want to thank Lotti Henley, Alix's mother. Without the many hours she spent bicycling all over London chasing articles and references for us, queuing at post offices, and acting as an efficient go-between between Judith in London and Alix in Switzerland, this book would never have seen the light of day. Her amazing and tireless practical support included dropping everything when emergencies arose and taking over a busy household and three children in Switzerland so that Alix could write. Her generous and thoughtful encouragement, her critical skills and suggestions as a reader and, above all, her unwavering belief in the importance of this book have been invaluable to us both. Thank you.

FOREWORD

by Christine Hancock

The delivery of health care does not happen in a vacuum. What nurses and other professionals demonstrate daily is that treating illness is not as simple as making a diagnosis and then prescribing a cure. You cannot isolate a person's health from the rest of their life – from their culture, upbringing or faith. Patients bring a lot more than their health problems to their local hospital or clinic.

One of the major challenges for health professionals in the twenty-first century is to provide high quality care that meets the need of a multi-ethnic society. Nurses have always put patients' needs at the centre of the care process, but now their needs are increasingly diverse. Our health services have always been stronger because of the rich diversity of people who choose to work in them, but sometimes all health professionals need help in understanding the beliefs and culture of the patients they care for.

This handbook provides that help, and also plugs an important gap in the materials available to support health professionals. It is much more than a set of guidelines on what you should do – it also shows you how you can do it, supporting the principles of good practice with some very practical ideas for identifying and meeting individual needs. In challenging our often stereotypical attitudes towards religious or cultural groups, the book covers new ground, encouraging health professionals to be humble enough to ask patients what we don't know, and flexible enough to change our practice.

This handbook is essential reading for all health professionals working with patients and their families from different cultural backgrounds. There are many patients whose needs are not currently being met; for them our health services seem distant, bureaucratic and inhuman. With the help of this handbook, I hope we can all work together at changing that.

Christine Hancock
General Secretary, Royal College of Nursing

FOREWORD

by Lola Oni

'All men are caught in an inescapable network of mutuality, tied in a single garment of destiny. Whatever affects one directly, affects all indirectly.'

[Martin Luther King Jr]

We all share a common humanity. We are born, we grow and we die, irrespective of who we are or what we become. But in between birth and death we are shaped by numerous experiences, some within our control but many forced on us by virtue of the family we by 'chance' are born into and the country, social class, social and cultural group we belong to.

Many of our attitudes, values, beliefs and ways of being are shaped by cultural experiences. These often leave an indelible mark that has a major effect on our perception of life and our reaction to situations, especially major life events such as ill-health. We can attempt to modify the impact of these experiences but it is impossible to eradicate the mark they have made on our subconscious.

Many would argue that an attempt to assimilate another culture results in internal conflict with possible loss of one's own identity, self-esteem and emotional, spiritual and mental well-being.

It stands to reason therefore that, in multicultural Britain, there needs to develop a commitment to developing a multicultural approach to the promotion of health care. Health and social care professionals need to create a climate that supports the principles on which the National Health Service was founded – that is, to provide care based on need, taking account of similarities and differences of individuals and groups within the total population.

Health and social care services are provided by individuals from diverse cultural backgrounds. One cannot assume that, by virtue of living in the UK, professionals from minority ethnic groups understand the culture of the majority population. One might argue that English people being cared for by a multicultural group of carers also have a right for their culture to be understood by those providing them with health and social care. This supports the truism that we are 'all caught up in a single garment'. All health, allied professionals and support staff need to provide services that meet the needs of a multicultural society.

The authors of this book are to be congratulated for having painstakingly researched their subject through literature and extensive interviews. It would be difficult to find another book that covers the subject in such detail and is written with such clarity. This is the most comprehensive book I have seen on the subject and will be of enormous benefit for professionals.

I believe the authors have set a precedent that will challenge others in future, when attempts are being made to address this very important subject. The approach is unique. Rather than providing the usual catalogue of 'thou shalt' and 'thou shalt not' in the management of 'minority ethnic groups', the book examines cultural values and practices of people in modern day Britain, a multicultural society that includes those of Anglo-Saxon origin. This book suggests that no culture is superior or inferior. No group has a monopoly on cultural beliefs, values and attitudes. No single cultural group has a right to have their needs met while others receive little consideration.

As a Nigerian who purports to know most of what is there to know about Yoruba culture, I was pleasantly surprised to find that Chapter 39 highlighted issues that I had not known about. This demonstrates that knowledge is not static and there may be deficits in one's knowledge even about one's own culture. All of us should be open to learning not just about other people's culture but even about our own.

Lola Oni
Nurse Director/Lecturer, Brent Sickle Cell and Thalassaemia Centre

FOREWORD

by Sally Greengross

Age Concern is delighted to publish this groundbreaking title that deals with the hitherto marginalised issue of meeting the health care needs of people of minority cultural and religious groups.

Although the book deals with the health care needs of people of all ages, it also focuses specifically on the needs of older people. We at Age Concern especially welcome this because the people who settled in the UK during the 1950s and 1960s are now approaching retirement age and their need for health care and social support is likely to increase.

Frank Dobson, the Minister of Health, recently wrote:

> 'No older person in hospital should go without the fundamental care that contributes to recovery – to be helped to eat and drink, to lie in a clean dry bed and to be treated with respect …' (HAS 2000 1998)

In a multicultural, multi-faith society it is essential that care is offered in a way that respects and accommodates everyone's cultural and religious needs. This comprehensive book offers both theoretical and practical approaches. It should promote a better understanding of individual needs and help to ensure that these are met. We wish the book every success and commend it to everyone who is involved in providing health care and social support.

Sally Greengross
Director General, Age Concern

'The label "multi-ethnic Britain" will, to many people, still signify just its ethnic minority communities. This, of course, is wrong. Multi-ethnic Britain means *all* of Britain and all of its people. Britain *is* multi-ethnic just as it *is* a parliamentary democracy.'
Sir Herman Ouseley, Chairman of Commission for Racial Equality, 1994

'The NHS must address the particular needs of the black and ethnic minorities living in this country, and take positive steps to eliminate discrimination.'
Chief Medical Officer, 1991

'As a registered nurse, midwife or health visitor, you are personally accountable for your practice and, in the exercise of your professional accountability, must … recognise and respect the uniqueness and dignity of each patient and client, and respond to their need for care, irrespective of their ethnic origin, religious beliefs, personal attributes, the nature of their health problem or any other factor.'
UKCC Code of Professional Conduct, 1992

INTRODUCTION

Britain, like most other countries, is a multi-ethnic, multicultural society. The major period of New Commonwealth immigration that followed the Second World War was part of a process that has gone on for many centuries. The legacies of industrialisation, European imperialism and colonialism, combined with modern mass media and transport, have made the movement and settlement of people a permanent feature of our world. In addition, continuing civil and international conflicts, particularly in those parts of the world where resources are scarce, lead to ever-increasing numbers of refugees. Over 90 per cent of the independent states in the world are now ethnically mixed, containing people of different origins, cultures and religions (Cheung-Judge 1993).

The needs of patients

Each of us, when we are ill, frail or dependent, needs care that is focused on *our* needs and on what is important to *us*. In our multi-ethnic, multicultural, multifaith society it is not possible, if it ever was, to assume what will be important to any patient. Nor is it acceptable to deliver standard, one-size-fits-all care. Health professionals and other professional carers need the skills, information and confidence to find out what each patient needs, and the support and flexibility to provide it.

At a time when professionals and services are under great pressure and resources are increasingly stretched, the demand for patient-centred care that takes into account different cultural, religious and personal needs may seem unrealistic. But what are the alternatives? Poor care, increased distress, anger and suspicion, wasted effort and resources, more complaints and litigation, and increased staff dissatisfaction and frustration.

Getting it right from the beginning is far better for both patient and professional, and far less wasteful for the system. This book provides practical information and guidelines to enable health and other professionals to identify and meet the needs of patients of all backgrounds and heritages sensitively and with confidence. It sets out the principles on which good care must be based in a multi-ethnic society. It also outlines ways of dealing with the conflicting needs and demands that are bound sometimes to arise in a diverse society. It encourages and supports good practice and reflection, and aims to reduce the anxiety and stress that committed professionals often feel when they are ill-prepared for the task in front of them.

Caring for older people

Our initial brief in writing this book was to focus particularly on the needs of older people. However, it soon became clear to us that the needs of older people who are ill or dependent are not significantly different from the needs of everybody else, though they are more likely to be overlooked. It is possible that older people will be more religious or more culturally conservative but this is certainly not inevitable. We have therefore broadened the scope of the book to include the care and support of adults of all ages.

The role of information

One of the aims of this book is to bring together information about the cultural and religious issues that surround patient care. However, 'facts' about a culture or a religion do not provide an answer. No set of 'facts' applies to any individual. Culture and religion are only two of many factors that may influence people's needs and wishes, and no culture or religion is static. None of us wants to be treated on the basis of stereotypes; we are all individuals. Good care is possible only when we find out from each person what their own wishes, needs and concerns are. As one patient told us,

'I want someone who thinks **with** me, not **for** me'.

We therefore do not want this book to be seen as providing a list of information that can simply be applied to people of certain cultural or religious groups. Our primary belief and message is that the answers lie with each individual patient and their family. At the same time, if health professionals are to identify and meet the needs of different religious and cultural groups, they need a framework of knowledge and ideas on which to base their thinking and their questions. They also need increased self-awareness so that they can understand and use the information sensitively and appropriately.

A note to readers in different countries

In this book we look at different cultures and religions primarily from the perspectives of Britain, the British health care system and traditional English culture. However, the issues we address apply to all multi-ethnic societies. The ideas and principles can be used to reflect on any system of health care in order to meet the needs of patients and families of different cultures and religions.

About this book

The book is divided into five parts. Certain ideas and themes are repeated in different parts of the book because we realise that most people will not read straight through from beginning to end.

Part One discusses the concepts of culture, 'race' and difference, and looks at inequalities in health and health care and the importance of equal access to care. It examines the situations and experiences of older black and minority ethnic people, and suggests ways in which these may be important in the provision of health care. Part One also includes opportunities for personal reflection, because our own beliefs and assumptions about people of different origins, cultures or creeds are likely to affect the care we give.

Part Two looks at aspects of patient care that may be affected by culture and religion. It includes opportunities for reflection as a basis for understanding, and practical suggestions for responding to other people's perspectives and needs.

Part Three focuses on the skills and awareness needed to communicate across cultural and language barriers, including ways of working well with professional interpreters. It also outlines different naming systems, how to address people correctly and how to keep safe, accurate manual and computerised records.

Part Four covers health issues that have specific relevance to certain cultural or religious minorities.

Part Five focuses on five traditional cultures and seven religions in relation to practices and values that may be important when people are ill. The content is based on what we have learned from meetings and discussions with British people of different cultural and religious heritages.

Caution! Some readers may be tempted to turn to Part Five first, to find out, for example, about Jews, Sikhs or Chinese people. We strongly urge you not to do this but to read and reflect on Parts One to Three first. Only by understanding our own culture-based beliefs and values can we avoid stereotyping and develop a sensitive and intelligent understanding of what the issues *might* be for people of other groups or communities. And only then can we usefully find out from each patient what she or he really needs.

Language and some definitions

Language has a subtle but very powerful influence on the way we view individuals and groups. Each of us is very sensitive to the terms used, particularly by others, to define us. Part of respecting people is respecting the way they define themselves and the labels they use. In this book we have tried to use terms that are acceptable to members of the communities we are talking about, but language and awareness are constantly developing, and in many cases there is no term that is universally accepted by every member of a particular group.

People's views of what is acceptable also change with time, whereas the words we have used here are fixed on the printed page and cannot change. We apologise if we have used words and phrases that are offensive or unacceptable to some of our readers. It is our intention to increase mutual respect and understanding, not in any way to diminish or insult people.

Definitions

BCE (Before the Common Era) is used as an alternative to BC, which has a specifically Christian reference point. (See also CE)

Black The term increasingly used by people of African-Caribbean, African and South Asian origin as well as others to underline the unity of their experience of discrimination on grounds of skin colour (Mares, Henley and Baxter 1985).

Black and minority ethnic groups Means the same as minority ethnic groups (see below) but may be more acceptable to many people who define themselves as black rather than as members of a minority ethnic group (Runnymede Trust 1994).

British A statement of nationality. Refers to everyone who is a British subject, whatever their heritage or ethnicity.

CE (Common Era) is used as an alternative to AD. (See also BCE)

English We use the term 'English' in this book when discussing the predominant culture in Britain. Health care in most of the British Isles is largely determined by English culture. We recognise that many people find the term 'English culture' uncomfortable and that it may offend people of Scottish, Welsh and Irish heritage. However, modern Britain is culturally very diverse and 'British culture' is the product of a huge range of cultural heritages (including English, Scottish, Welsh, Irish, African-Caribbean, Gujarati, Punjabi, Bangladeshi, Mirpuri, Jewish, Chinese, etc). Using the term 'British culture' to refer only to the traditional culture of white Britons excludes people who are perfectly British but not white and who have a different culture. This is inaccurate and unhelpful when we are discussing the legitimate rights and needs of Britons of a range of heritages.

Equal access Ensuring that an organisation's policies and practices do not result in any group receiving less favourable treatment on grounds that are not material; for example, 'race', colour, ethnic or national origin, creed, gender, marital status, class, disability or sexuality (Cheung-Judge and Henley 1994).

Ethnic group A social group with a distinctive language, values, religion, customs and attitudes (Hillier 1991). Also used in majority ethnic group (roughly speaking, the white British) and minority ethnic groups.

Health professional Used in this book to refer to everyone working in health care, whether in hospitals or in the community, who comes into direct contact with patients and their families or whose work influences the way care is given. This includes hospital doctors, general practitioners, health visitors, physiotherapists, social workers, chaplains, care assistants, receptionists and clerks, hospital and community managers and those commissioning services.

Hospital For grammatical simplicity we have used hospital to refer to all those institutions in which people who are ill, dependent or frail may be cared for.

Immigrant A person who was born in another country and has settled in Britain. Not their children, grandchildren or great-grandchildren.

Minority ethnic groups or communities Groups or communities that are distinguished in some way from the majority by, for example, their skin colour, their first language or their religion.

New Commonwealth The official term used to indicate Commonwealth countries whose populations are predominantly black; for example, India, Pakistan, Bangladesh, the West Indies, Nigeria, Ghana and Kenya.

Old Commonwealth The official term used to indicate Commonwealth countries whose populations are predominantly white; for example, Australia, New Zealand and Canada.

Racism Conscious or unconscious belief in the superiority of a particular 'race'. Acts of discrimination and unfair treatment, whether intentional or unintentional, based on this belief.

South Asian People born in India, Pakistan, Bangladesh and Sri Lanka – the Indian subcontinent – or descended from people born in those countries.

References

Cheung-Judge MY, Henley A (1994) *Equality in Action: Introducing equal opportunities in voluntary organisations.* NCVO Publications, London

de Mello A (1983) *Wellsprings.* Doubleday/Image, New York

HAS 2000 (1998) *'Not Because They are Old': An independent inquiry into the care of older people on acute wards in general hospitals.* Health Advisory Service 2000, London

Hillier S (1991) The health and health care of ethnic minority groups. In G Scambler (ed) *Sociology as Applied to Medicine.* Bailliere Tindall, London

Huang WWC (1989) Chinese perspectives on death and dying. In A Berger, P Badham et al (eds) *Perspectives on Death and Dying.* Charles Press, Philadelphia PA

Kübler-Ross E. (1991) *On Life after Death.* Celestial Arts, Los Angeles CA

Mares P, Henley A, Baxter C (1985) *Health Care in Multiracial Britain.* National Extension College, Cambridge

Runnymede Trust (1994) *Multi-ethnic Britain: Facts and trends.* Runnymede Trust, London

PART ONE
Culture, Difference and Health Care

●●●

1 Culture

When people are facing major difficulties and heightened physical and emotional stress – for example, at times of illness, dependency, death and bereavement – cultural patterns and ways of reacting and behaving often become particularly important. It is essential that the practical, emotional and spiritual care that are offered at these times take people's cultural needs into account.

What is culture?

Culture can most simply be defined as **how we do and view things in our group**. It is a shared set of values, assumptions, perceptions and conventions, based on a shared history and language, which enable members of a group or community to function together. Our culture vitally affects every aspect of our daily life, how we think and behave, and the judgements and decisions we make. It is like a set of lenses through which we look at the world and which defines both what we see and how we interpret it.

Like the air we breathe, our culture is all around us from the day of our birth. We acquire most of it unconsciously in early childhood. It is often hard to distinguish, even in ourselves, what is cultural from what is individual or personal (Hoecklin 1993, Trompenaars 1993, Hofstede 1991). As a result, many of us, especially those who are members of the majority culture, grow up unaware that we have a culture at all. We may not realise that what we regard as normal, universal values and ways of behaving are in fact cultural – 'normal' only to us. People who have grown up as members of a minority ethnic group, or who have lived and worked outside their own society, are generally far more aware of culture and its influence.

Visible and invisible aspects of culture

Some aspects of culture are visible or otherwise obvious (Trompenaars 1993, Hofstede 1991). These include, for example, clothes, written and spoken language, art and architecture, food, how homes are arranged, how hospitals are organised, and the ceremonial and public aspects of death and funerals. In looking at other cultures, these are the things that we notice are different.

The less obvious aspects of culture consist of the shared norms and values of the group, community or society. These are often invisible and unstated but they are absolutely fundamental and influence everything else. They define how people should behave, how things should be organised, and what is considered right and wrong, normal or abnormal, important or unimportant. In relation to this book they include, for example, ideas about the purpose of life and the meaning of illness and death; where, how and by whom people who are ill should be cared for; who should make decisions when someone is ill; what people who are dying should and should not be told; how and by whom bodies should be handled after death; how funerals are organised; and how grief is expressed.

Culture as part of 'human mental programming'

Hofstede (1991) sees culture as one layer of what he calls our 'human mental programming' (see Figure 1.1). **Culture** is not genetically inherited but is acquired during childhood when we are systematically taught the basic values and norms by which our family, society and community live.

The other two layers are:

- **human nature** – inherited, universal characteristics, needs and abilities that all human beings share, such as the need for food, safety and shelter, and the ability to feel emotions such as fear, grief, loss, love, anger and happiness. What gives rise to these emotions and how people express them is partly influenced by culture.
- **personality** – mental programmes, both inherited and learnt, that are unique to each person and are influenced by their individual life experiences; for example, childhood experience of death, previous experience of illness, experience of war or being a refugee.

None of us, therefore, is simply a package of culture. We are all affected by a myriad of different influences and, above all, each of us has our own unique personality. But the culture of the community in which we grew up is the predominant influence on the way each of us views the world, and on the way we behave. In some ways the effects of culture cannot be overestimated. At the same time it is important to bear in mind that culture is a framework, not a straitjacket. Within it there is a wide range of choices and options for each of us, a million ways in which we express our individuality and live our unique lives. We all have a culture, but our culture does not define us.

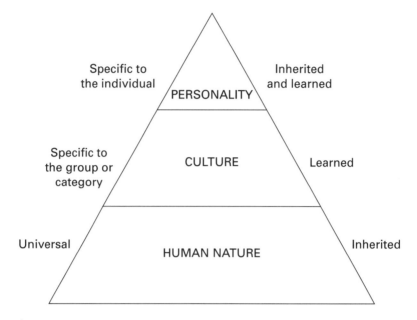

Figure 1.1 Three levels of uniqueness in human mental programming (Reproduced, with permission, from *Cultures and Organisations: Software of the mind* by Geert Hofstede, 1991, McGraw-Hill)

When working across cultures, therefore, we need both to be aware of the possibilities that may exist within a culture other than our own and to avoid assuming that any individual will conform to a particular 'cultural pattern'.

Diversity within cultures

Within every culture there is a range of norms, values and assumptions. We are not all the same and we do not all live the same way. But there is also a tendency for most people to be grouped around the middle, sharing key cultural values and characteristics, and for smaller numbers of people to differ to a lesser or greater extent, rather like the normal distribution of a bell curve in a statistical chart (see Figure 1.2) (Trompenaars 1993).

Within every culture there are also 'micro-cultures', influenced by, for example, social class and region of origin. Families as well as social, religious and professional and occupational groups also all have their own micro-cultures. So do organisations. Because cultures are always changing, people of different ages may also have certain different norms, values and attitudes, different micro-cultures. Each of us is therefore affected not only

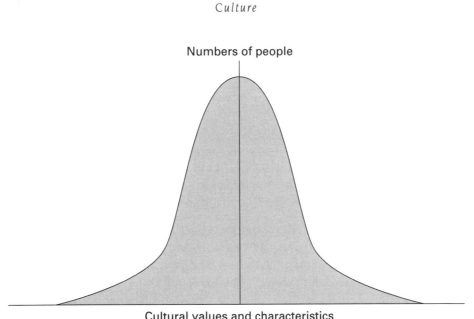

Numbers of people

Cultural values and characteristics

Figure 1.2 The distribution of cultural values and characteristics within a community

by the wider culture of our society or community but also by several micro-cultures within it.

Cultures and change

Cultures are not fixed or static. They change in response to new situations and pressures. Some change faster than others. Since the Industrial Revolution, for example, the pace of cultural change in western Europe and North America has been unprecedented. In 1982 Rack wrote of Britain:

'In the last twenty years the list of conventions that have been challenged, shibboleths abandoned, hierarchies dismantled, and moral restrictions lifted is a very long one indeed. Social inequality, acquisitive materialism, and the subordination of women have all come under fire. The public face of sexual morality has altered entirely, and the institution of marriage is under attack. Innovations in music and the other arts have been bewilderingly rapid. Dress and speech are no longer the insignia of class. Hair can be worn long, short, absent altogether or green and purple. The pace of social change is unparalleled, and appeals to tradition are greeted with derision.' (Rack 1991)

The speed of change has not diminished since then. Not everyone is happy about some of these changes, especially those that affect their family and personal lives. But cultural change is a powerful force, and it is difficult for individuals to withstand it.

Some societies change more slowly than others, either because they are not confronted by the same pressures to change or because their culture contains features that enable it to withstand such pressures. Societies that are strongly religious may be slower to change. Communities that are uprooted from their own society sometimes become more conservative, often as a response to fear of losing their identity or values in the face of external pressures. British expatriate communities, for example, are often more 'old-fashioned' than their contemporaries in Britain, retaining customs that seem outdated to those 'back home'. Similar patterns occurred among some South Asian communities in East Africa (Roberts 1977).

'Cultural differences are often viewed as obstacles within a physician–patient relationship. But cultural norms and values play an enormous role in maintaining the well-being of a cultural community. While it is true that some norms and values bring individuals into considerable conflict with the changing society in which they find themselves ... it is also true that such values tend to protect and maintain the mental and physical well-being of the cultural group.' (Masi 1992)

Change and individuals

For most people, the most radical force for change is moving away from their own society. They suddenly have to cope in an environment where little is familiar and almost everything is done differently. In this situation they are forced to make many practical changes simply to survive. At the same time, their identity – influenced by, for example, their culture, religion and life experience – is also under pressure. How far individuals change internally and externally in such a situation varies a great deal. It depends, for example, on whether they feel welcomed by and positive towards their new home, how much they are exposed to or sheltered from the new society, what responsibilities they have and how much these bring them into contact with the new society. It also depends on how different the values and customs of the new country are and on the social and economic pressures they experience. For most people it is important to retain their cultural values and practices but this does not take place in a social vacuum (Ahmad 1996). What is clear is that, for everyone, moving to a new country is a huge change with tremendous consequences that cannot be foreseen.

'Living in a foreign country is a constant assault on one's self esteem.'
Director, Centre for International Briefing, Farnham, UK

Younger people tend to embrace change more readily. This can cause difficulties in any family but perhaps particularly in more conservative communities and in families where parents or grandparents were born overseas. The younger generation, brought up in the UK, are part of two cultures and are influenced by both. Traditional values may be less important to them than to older people. Conversely, a small but growing number of young people are reclaiming their roots and, in some cases, the fundamentals of their religion. Strict religious observance may sometimes be much more important to them. Different value systems and beliefs within families often cause distress and conflict, especially when someone is ill, dependent or dying.

Culture as part of our identity

Just as we all have a **culture**, we are all members of an **ethnic group** (and sometimes of more than one). The term 'ethnic' is often misunderstood. An ethnic group is a social group that shares certain distinctive features, such as language, culture, physical appearance, religious affiliation, customs and values (Hillier 1991). In Britain, and especially in England, the **ethnic majority** is the white English. There are also a number of **minority ethnic groups** including, for example, Irish, African-Caribbeans and South Asians. In this book the term 'English' is used, rather than 'British', when discussing the majority culture. This is not intended to offend other groups but is deliberately chosen for precision: 'British' indicates legal status and nationality but not culture or ethnicity. We recognise that the English, the Scots, the Welsh and the Irish are different from each other even though they share aspects of cultural heritage.

All of us have many different identities. Our cultural or ethnic identity is only one of these; it does not capture everything about us (Pfeffer 1998). Depending on where we are and who we are with, different identities become more important. If we have children, we may be primarily parents when we are with them; the professional part of us often recedes. At work, we may become entirely professionals and forget that we even have children. With people who know us socially, within our religious community or with older family members, other identities may matter more.

Many people have multiple ethnic or cultural identities. An increasing number are of mixed heritage, with parents, grandparents or great-grandparents from different groups or communities. They operate effectively in two or more cultures, taking and adapting what they consider most valuable from each, and moving smoothly between them.

'I was born and brought up in North London. My parents both came from the West Indies when they were children. My father is African-Caribbean with one black parent and one white parent. My mother's family are Asian. In my family there has been intermarriage like this for several generations. I suppose I would describe myself as black but I get fed up with people assuming they know where I "come from". Some call me West Indian and I have also been called a Paki. Just as well my father brought me up to stand up for myself and not to put up with that sort of racist nonsense.'

Young black woman

Our sense of identity stems from many factors, including the culture(s) in which we grew up, our gender and sexual orientation, our position in the family, our occupation(s), our experiences and our personal situation.

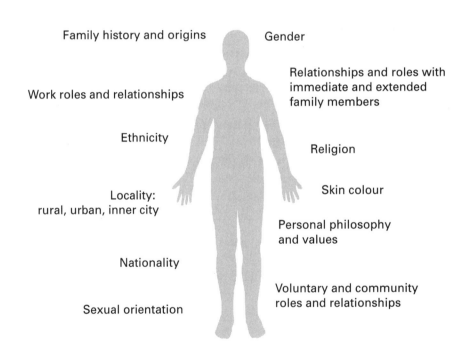

Family history and origins

Gender

Work roles and relationships

Relationships and roles with immediate and extended family members

Ethnicity

Religion

Locality: rural, urban, inner city

Skin colour

Personal philosophy and values

Nationality

Sexual orientation

Voluntary and community roles and relationships

Figure 1.3 Some of the influences that may contribute to your identities (Redrawn from an illustration by Helen Chown, and used by permission of Butterworth Heinemann, from *Culture, Religion and Childbearing in a Multiracial Society: A handbook for health professionals*)

Using Figure 1.3 as a starting point, you might like to make a list of your own identities, including the different relationships you have with different people, for example as parent, child, sibling, spouse, colleague, manager and so on:

- How do your different identities emerge in different situations?
- Which are most important to you?
- How do you feel when other people focus on one aspect of your identity (often the one most visible to them such as gender, age or skin colour) and ignore others that are equally or more important to you?

In the context of health care, focusing on the most visible or obvious part of a patient's identity, on their ethnicity, or even on their illness ('The bypass in bed 3') diminishes them and reduces our ability to understand and meet the full range of their physical, emotional and spiritual needs.

'What we think of a person influences how we will perceive him; how we perceive him influences how we will behave towards him; and how we behave towards him ultimately influences who he becomes.' (Kearl 1989)

2 Looking at culture and differences

Every culture seems normal to the people within it, though they may not like every aspect of it. But what makes sense and is acceptable to people in one culture may be odd or even abhorrent to people in another. It is not always obvious to outsiders how customs are interlinked, nor how they relate to the underlying value system. Part of treating individuals with respect involves a willingness to try to understand their culture and values positively.

In traditional South Asian culture marriages are arranged or guided. This is regarded as the best way to ensure a successful marriage and the stability of the whole extended family. Parents and older relatives are openly involved in selecting a suitable partner. They understand the young people involved and the kind of partner who will be most suitable for them. Although nowadays the young people usually have the final say, parents who do not arrange a marriage for their children may be strongly disapproved of for neglecting an important duty. Love is expected to grow in the years after the wedding within the family circle.

An English woman newly married to an Iraqi man went to stay with his family for the first time. The couple spent their time sitting and talking with family members, interspersed by the occasional meal. On the afternoon of the second day, the English woman felt that she needed some time alone and went to her room for two hours. The family was extremely upset and worried, and thought that they must have offended or angered her in some way. There is no word in Arabic for the concept of privacy.

Encountering another culture

Our own culture may only become noticeable when we come into contact with another culture. Take a moment to reflect on your own experience.

Think back to a time, maybe when you were a child, when you felt out of place. Perhaps you stayed with another family or started a new school:

- How did the 'culture' in which you found yourself differ from your own?
- How did you find out what the unwritten and unspoken rules were, what was acceptable or unacceptable?
- How did you feel?
- How did people behave towards you if you made a mistake?

What we notice about other cultures

In the situation outlined above, it is likely that there were more similarities than differences between your own culture and the culture into which you moved. But you were probably most aware of the differences. And the people you were with probably also noticed mainly what was different about you. You might have found it difficult to ask about the differences you observed for fear of increasing your vulnerability or causing offence. Because culture is so nebulous it is also sometimes difficult to know exactly what to ask.

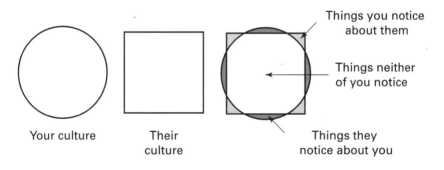

Figure 2.1 Working across cultures

Figure 2.1 shows what happens when people of one culture, symbolised by the square, look at a different culture, symbolised by the circle. Although most of the values and assumptions of the two cultures (indicated by the common unshaded area) are in fact shared, the people of each culture tend to notice what is different about the other. It is easy to focus on cultural and other differences and to ignore the large amount of common ground.

Not cultural facts but cultural possibilities

It is impossible to make any statement about a cultural group that can be usefully applied to all the individuals within it. Let us look at traditional British culture. It is clear that Scotland, Northern Ireland, Wales and England, as well as the regions in them, each has its own culture. To try to simplify the process, the exercise below focuses on English culture, recognising that this is still a huge oversimplification.

Consider, whatever your own cultural heritage, how you would answer the following questions about traditional English culture.

- What could you say about relationships between English men and women and about the structure of the family?
- How would you define the English diet, and style of dress?
- What are English attitudes to modesty, morality and sex?
- How would you describe English views on codes of behaviour and ways of expressing feelings?
- What are the attitudes of the English to health care and to doctors and nurses?
- How do the English view older people?
- How would you define English attitudes to death and dying?
- How do the English handle funerals and grieving?

Would you say these are the same throughout England and that they apply to all English people, regardless of age, social class and education?

You could say that the English are reserved, abnormally xenophobic, do not express their feelings openly, eat fish and chips, like custard, have a cup of tea at 4pm, are obsessed with sex and violence, behave badly at football matches and on the Costa del Sol, put old people in homes, are very concerned about their bowels, worry about catching chills, are embarrassed by displays of grief, avoid people who are dying or bereaved, and have small restrained funerals.

Some of these statements might be true for some English people some of the time, but, if your cultural heritage is English, how would you feel if someone assumed that they were all true of you **and then treated you** accordingly?

General information applied universally does not improve understanding. Lists of cultural traits give a false picture of uniformity and are always misleading. Any realistic description of a culture can describe only tendencies and possibilities, never facts. Within any culture there are always a huge number of variations, contradictions and contrasts. Even useful insights can be applied crudely and insensitively and can become a barrier rather than an aid. **If people believe that they 'know' about other cultures and religions they may take short cuts and act on assumptions, avoiding contact and communication with individuals rather than trying to build a relationship.**

'My family is Jewish but I'm not observant. When I was in hospital one of the nurses told me off for eating ham! She wasn't even Jewish. I was stunned.'
Male patient

'When people see me they simply see an 'Asian woman'. What I would like is to be seen as a normal human being with normal feelings, wants and needs. I may have different cultural perspectives but I still buy my knickers at Marks and Spencer's. Don't section me off and treat me differently. I don't want to be put in a separate category from white British people.'
South Asian health professional

General information about a patient's ethnic group or religion doesn't tell you anything reliable or specific about the real person in front of you or about their needs. But, provided it is reliable and respectful, it can be a framework within which, carefully and sensitively, to ask the right questions.

Attitudes towards other cultures

Us *and them*

We learn about our own culture from a very early age. Babies and young children are acute observers. We copy the things that adults say and do, and the way that they say and do them. If we behave in ways that do not fit in with the culture of our family or peers, they make their disapproval clear. So we are strongly encouraged to conform with accepted, often unspoken, norms of right and wrong behaviour, speech, dress, language and manners. A child from a religious family is taught an additional set of values and beliefs and learns what is acceptable to their particular religious group. Well before adolescence a child has internalised the perceptions and values of their culture and automatically views and does things in certain ways. Although many of us rebel against some of these values, especially as teenagers, they remain a subtle yet powerful influence throughout our lives.

As we learn what is acceptable within our own culture and/or religion, the foundations are laid for regarding difference with suspicion. If we are

taught that what we do and how we view things are 'correct' and 'right', we can be forgiven for assuming, however unconsciously, that people who do and view things differently are wrong and less deserving of our respect.

Difference or pathology?

'People fail to appreciate that our culture and traditions are of equal value and that they were evolved in response to the land and to the situation in which they arose.'
South Asian health professional

In societies where one ethnic group is dominant, the cultural practices and values of groups that differ from the majority norm are often regarded as wrong or even pathological. People whose needs and behaviour are unfamiliar may be seen as a problem, or treated as if they were strange or deviant. In the former Soviet Union, dissidents who expressed different political views from those of the ruling group were often put in psychiatric hospitals. Nobody should be labelled difficult just because of their culture, religion or appearance. Each person must be seen as an individual who deserves respect, and responsive and appropriate care. It is but a small step from 'cultural' to clinical pathology (Smaje 1995).

'In a Care of the Elderly unit, South Asian patients who wanted to eat with their fingers were viewed as having 'behavioural problems'. Some were identified as anorectic when they refused to eat because the nurses did not understand the significance of halal meat. Although the nurses meant well, they lacked insight and knowledge.' (Marr and Khadim 1993)

Assumptions and stereotyping

'White people don't see me; they see my colour and they automatically judge me negatively. But when I speak, you can almost see them having to change their minds as I sound very English and cultured.'
African-Caribbean woman

In the absence of personal contact and familiarity with people of different communities, we tend to rely on stereotypes. The further people are from our own experience, the more we do this. We don't usually stereotype members of our family and close friends. We do tend to stereotype people in groups that we don't belong to or like or that we know little about. But most stereotypes are negative, belittling and even hostile (Green, Kitzinger and Coupland 1990). They portray people as one-dimensional, leading us to distance ourselves and to treat them with less consideration and respect. Care based on stereotypes is bound to be inadequate and lacking in insight. When we are caring for people of communities other than our own, it is also easy to assume that something stereotypically cultural (and usually negative) is going on and to miss the real issues.

'A one year old baby daughter of South Asian parents was admitted to hospital with a fractured skull. At the case conference it was generally assumed that, because of the 'traditional South Asian preference for male children', the little girl must be unwanted and neglected. In fact she was the much-loved and long-awaited child of a rather slow mother who found it difficult to anticipate fully her daughter's activities and needs.' (Ahmed 1986)

'A Health Education Authority survey found that a high percentage of Bangladeshi and Pakistani women had never had a cervical smear test. It is often assumed that a low take-up of smear tests is inevitable among these communities because of religious prohibitions or modesty. In fact, the survey found that the main problem was that women did not know what a smear test was and/or had never been called for one. Embarrassment and fear (which could be seen as cultural) accounted for only about five per cent of those women who had not had a smear test.' (HEA 1994)

Stereotypes

To see how stereotypes can work, cover the shaded area below and try reading the lines one at a time. Notice your thoughts and assumptions, and observe how they change as you read:

Mrs Y is in renal failure,

she has three teenage children,

she likes cooking,

she speaks five languages,

she has an Open University degree in psychology,

she is a hospital cleaner,

she is a Gujarati Hindu.

Which of these statements tells you most about Mrs Y? None of them. They all offer you possibilities, but Mrs Y is no more defined by the fact that she is a Gujarati Hindu (possibly the thing you would notice first about her) than by the fact that she is in renal failure. All these facts about her are true. All of them affect her in some way (only she can tell you how) but she is more than the sum of all of them, and only by asking her will you find out what she needs.

The dangers of 'pattern recognition' and stereotyping

'We are trained to look for and recognise patterns in signs and symptoms in order to reach a diagnosis as fast as possible. Pattern recognition and prediction becomes a way of life, we do it automatically.'
Junior hospital doctor

You have been asked to admit or visit a number of new patients. You have very limited amount of information about each. Read the list below slowly, one line at a time. Notice your thoughts, assumptions and feelings in relation to each:

- a solicitor
- an Orthodox Jewish man
- a TV celebrity
- a consultant's wife
- Shameema Bibi
- a Jehovah's Witness
- a homeless man
- a lorry driver
- a woman of 86

Many people doing this exercise notice that they immediately form a view of what each person will be like. They find that they tend to focus on what it would be like for them to care for each patient, rather than on what the needs, feelings and views of the patient are likely to be.

When 'pattern recognition' is applied to people rather than to clinical signs and symptoms, it easily becomes stereotyping. This is especially likely if the patient is not of our own community or if we cannot communicate easily. If stereotypes remain at the forefront of our thinking, they can block our ability to understand and meet the patient's real needs. In addition, health professionals often feel under tremendous pressure to have all the answers and to know what to do. It may be easier to rely on stereotypes rather than take the risk of asking and feeling incompetent or vulnerable (see also Chapter 8 *Asking the patient*).

'Stereotyping – I find that the hardest thing. Don't judge me by the way I look or dress. Talk to me and try to understand **who** I am, not what I am.'
Sikh woman

First impressions

Judgements based on first impressions are powerful and difficult to reverse. We are particularly unlikely to change our minds if our first impression is negative, even in the face of subsequent contradictory information. We tend to select evidence to support our opinion and to ignore evidence that undermines it (Hicks 1993, Roberts 1985).

Visible characteristics, such as skin colour, gender, age, physical ability and appearance, form a crucial part of our first impressions. If we have negative stereotypes about people who are, for example, black or male or old or overweight or physically disabled or ugly, these contribute to our initial judgement. We then tend to behave towards the person on the basis of that judgement, setting up a circle of misunderstanding in which it is hard to adjust our assumptions.

'I was at a consultants' dinner at the hospital where my husband worked, and I sat next to a senior physician. Halfway through the meal he turned to me and asked in a rather patronising way, 'And what do you do, my dear?'. I said I also worked in the health service. 'You are a secretary or a receptionist,' he said. I began to answer but he cut me off; 'Then you must be a nurse'. 'Actually no,' I said, 'I'm a doctor.' 'In general practice are you?' he said, seeming slightly put out. 'Well, not really,' I replied. 'You work in a hospital? You are a registrar in geriatrics or psychiatry,' he said condescendingly. 'Actually, I'm a consultant thoracic surgeon,' I said. You should have seen his face!'
Fifty-year-old woman

Physical features reveal little of the huge variety of qualities and attributes that make up each human being. They convey nothing about a person's history and background, educational attainments, values, beliefs, experience, knowledge, skills or wishes. But they often affect the way people are treated.

Think back to a time when someone made an inaccurate and unflattering assumption or judgement about you.

- How did you feel?
- How did you react and behave?
- How did it affect your attitude to the person who made that assumption?
- How did you behave towards them afterwards?

Sources of inaccurate information

When we have little direct contact with individuals whose culture and lives differ from our own, we have to rely on what we learn from other people. Much of the information we get from the media, our colleagues and our families about cultures or groups other than our own is inaccurate. It tends to focus on differences and on negative characteristics (real or imagined), and to ignore positive characteristics and the things we share. In many cases such 'information' (intentionally or unintentionally) plays on our fears or boosts our sense of cultural superiority.

People who have frequently been misjudged on the basis of their appearance or 'group' often feel hurt, angry and defensive. They may begin to expect misjudgement and prejudice, especially from people in authority. With some patients and relatives you may have to undo the mistrust and suspicion caused by other people's prejudices and misjudgements.

Working across cultures

'Working across cultures feels a bit like driving a left-hand-drive car on the right-hand side of the road. Everything looks the same, the tasks we have to perform are exactly the same, but, at least at the beginning, we have to think consciously and very carefully about every single move. If we act automatically, we will cause an accident. With time and practice we get it right, but at the beginning it is exhausting, frustrating and confusing.'
Health professional

The reason that we operate so effectively and confidently within our own community is that we have a profound and detailed understanding of its culture with all its richness, variety, connections and contradictions. We automatically see people and their behaviour within our shared cultural context and can make appropriate assessments and interventions. We are able to go beyond generalisations and stereotypes and to understand each person as a rounded individual with their own needs and wishes.

It can be much harder hard to work with people whose culture we do not share. They may seem one-dimensional. Their behaviour may appear bizarre, contradictory, off-putting or frustrating.

'A West African woman who spoke no English refused to eat in hospital. Every time she was offered food she would shake her head and chant 'Ramadan–ramadan–ramadan.' The staff didn't understand that she was observing the Muslim fast of Ramadan and could therefore eat only during the

hours of darkness. They thought she was mad.'
English health professional

Learning about other cultures

'We do not see things as they are, but as we are.'

Immanuel Kant (1724–1804)

Culture is a double barrier of which our own culture is the first part. Judging people of other cultures on the basis of what seems 'normal' or 'appropriate' to us leads to misunderstandings, misjudgements and failures of care. We need, therefore, to become aware of what in ourselves is cultural so that we can step outside our cultural framework when necessary and care for other people in terms of their own needs. But this can be difficult: culture is so much part of who we are, how we understand the world and how we lead our lives. We may become aware of it only when we see it through the eyes of someone who finds it strange or different.

'Learning about a culture is like learning a language. The same words often mean different things. What does family mean? Responsibility? Respect? What does pain mean? What is a good life? These ideas probably exist in all cultures but they are not always thought of or expressed in the same way.'
West African health professional

Every culture is inherently logical and makes sense in its own terms. Every culture answers the age-old needs of a society. In an imperfect world, every culture contains a balance of advantages and disadvantages:

- In some cultures there is a high level of social control, in others relatively little. One advantage of greater social control is that crime rates are generally lower; one advantage of less social control is that individuals have greater freedom.
- In cultures where the extended family is strong, few people are ever lonely or unsupported, though everyone is expected to conform to certain, often inflexible, rules that present serious problems for some individuals.
- In cultures where the individual is paramount, many weaker members are lonely and unsupported. Often no one takes responsibility for them. On the other hand, stronger members enjoy greater freedom and fewer restrictions.

Our reaction to other people's cultures often tells us as much about our own culture as about theirs. If something in another culture seems illogical or bizarre, this is usually a sign that we do not understand it or its cultural setting.

A middle-aged Indian man with three children lamented the total lack of family love and morality in Britain. 'English people do not love or protect their daughters,' he said. 'All they think about is money. As soon as their daughters are 16 the parents let them go out and sleep around. Then when the girls get pregnant they are married off so the parents don't have to support them any more.'

Viewing a detail of culture in isolation from the overall culture in which it is rooted makes it almost as meaningless as an isolated letter of the alphabet (O'Neill 1992). We need to find out much more about the cultural, religious and social frameworks within which people live. Only then can we see them properly in their own right and not merely as human stereotypes.

'Till one can penetrate into the forest one cannot see one tree as being different from another.' (Modood 1990).

Wanting clarity and explanations

There is a tendency to want clear definitions of other cultures; to want to know what people do and why they do it. However, culture is not that straightforward. We cannot always explain our culture to other people's satisfaction. We all do certain things in certain ways because we always have, without necessarily knowing why. People may also hold onto a familiar practice or belief, not merely because it is familiar or traditional but because it is linked to other important elements of their culture. It is necessary to bear this in mind when discussing cultural issues with people of other communities and expecting them to give satisfyingly coherent and logical explanations.

Judy was asked if she would have a couple from China with their two children, who were in Britain on a sabbatical, to stay for Christmas. On Boxing Day the fathers took the children to the playground and the two women tidied up. The Chinese woman tentatively asked Judy a few questions: 'Why do you cut down a tree and bring it into the house? Is it a special kind of tree? Why? Why do you put lights on it and a doll on the top? Why did you put a prickly leaf on your pudding yesterday? Was it a special leaf? Why did you set fire to the pudding?' Judy found it difficult to explain these things in a way that made any sense to the other woman.

Most of us find it hard to deal with stereotypes or misunderstandings of our own culture. It is rather like an outsider criticising one's family. We may also feel threatened or offended when our values are scrutinised (Seelye 1993). Cross-cultural discussion always requires sensitivity and tact.

Not everything is culture

It is important not to assume that, simply because someone is of another culture, everything they do, say or think is due to their culture. People's social, economic and physical environments are equally significant, especially when it comes to health. Attributing everything to culture may enable other crucial issues to be side-stepped. For example, much research on health outcomes in black and minority ethnic groups assumes that their culture and biology, as well as, in some cases, language barriers, are the main causes of negative differences. It largely ignores the importance of socio-economic factors, including racism (Ahmad, Kernohan and Baker 1989). Because culture, language and biology are in some ways the 'responsibility' of the patient or at least can be located in the patient, society and the health service may be let off the hook. At the turn of the century, for example, high mortality rates in Glasgow were attributed to the 'racial stock' of the Irish immigrants even though mortality rates in Ireland were a lot lower. The poor social conditions of the Irish migrant workers were not mentioned (Sheldon and Parker 1992).

'Culture is important when we are tailoring care to individuals and planning services that will be genuinely accessible and acceptable, but we should not blame people's culture for inequalities in health that we know very well are related to poverty and other external factors.'
Health service researcher

Working well across cultures: a summary

Information about different cultures is useful only if it is relevant to the individual concerned, comes from reliable sources, is based on the assumption that all cultures have an intrinsic worth and are equally worthy of respect, and acknowledges the complexity and variety of the real world.

When working with someone whose culture differs from your own, it is always necessary to:

- be aware of your own cultural values and norms and how these may be affecting your thinking and judgements;
- notice any assumptions you are making about the other person and try to suspend them;
- listen with respect, set aside any defensiveness, and be willing to understand this person on their terms;
- ask them about their needs – they are the expert – and respond flexibly and sensitively;
- accept that cross-cultural encounters can be difficult and confusing for both sides.

The costs of cultural mismanagement

In international commercial markets the active acknowledgement of cultural differences is increasingly recognised as essential to competitiveness. Successful companies take cultural differences into account both in managing international subsidiaries and in marketing to people in different counties. Advertising that works brilliantly in one country may flop or cause offence in another. The same product may be given different names in different countries to avoid unfortunate connotations or the wrong impression. Even the ways in which meetings are run, decisions made, memos written and titles used in a company vary depending on the local culture. When failure to take cultural differences into account is seen to cost money, managers and staff become very culture-conscious (Hoecklin 1993, Trompenaars 1993, Hofstede 1991).

In relation to care for patients and their families, the financial costs of cultural mismanagement of health care are likely to be significant; the human costs far greater. The differences are that most of the costs do not show up on the balance sheet, and that most of them are borne by patients and their families rather than by the organisation or by individual health professionals and managers.

Direct costs to the health services include:

- wasted staff time;
- wasted tests, treatments and medication;
- staff frustration and loss of job satisfaction.

Costs to patients and families include:

- untreated or poorly treated conditions, or conditions treated only after they have become unnecessarily serious (these may then increase the direct costs of treatment to the NHS);
- increased morbidity and mortality;
- unnecessary pain, discomfort, anxiety, fear, hopelessness;
- wasted time and journeys;
- frustration, anger and grief when care has been inappropriate or inadequate;
- alienation and mistrust (NAHAT 1988).

To prevent the high human and financial costs of cultural mismanagement, health care institutions and individual health professionals must take responsibility for ensuring that the care provided is accessible and effective for people of all ethnic, cultural and religious groups.

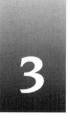

3 Culture, illness and health care

Culture and experience influence everyone's beliefs about health and illness. In a multicultural society, people may have different views about the causes and treatments of illness, when to seek treatment, whom to consult and what treatments are appropriate. **Health care is likely to be more effective when the beliefs, values and norms of both patient and professional are recognised and taken into account** (Boston 1993).

Many health professionals assume that when black and minority ethnic people have access to Western medical care they will gladly abandon the system they grew up with. But new ways are not automatically better. All of us need to see a good reason for changing before we give up something that works and makes sense to us. Currer, in a detailed study of the lives and health of Pathan (Pakistani) women in Bradford, found that most of them were keen to learn new ways of promoting health and dealing with illness, provided that these seemed a genuine improvement and made sense to them. But the decision had to be a rational one:

> 'It was not the women's ignorance but their intelligence that led to their refusal to adapt or abandon certain habits. They sought to understand the reason for such changes in terms that made sense to them. Not all those put forward by health workers did.' (Currer 1986)

Health beliefs

Different ways of thinking about the body influence the views of both health professionals and lay people. In cultures with a scientific orientation the body is often imagined as a machine. Problems are located in isolated organs or parts, which are then repaired or, possibly, replaced (Helman 1994). Medicine may be seen as an attacking force expressed through military metaphors: the 'battle' against disease and 'heroic surgery'. There are many other ways of thinking about health and illness. For example, the body may be seen as a single organism with physical, spiritual and emotional aspects, in which illness is caused by imbalances or blockages. The goal of health care then is to restore the balance by unblocking the flow of energy between them.

> 'Physicians should realise that, in order to understand and discuss illness and treatment, both they and their patient use explanatory models that are based on personal cultural values and beliefs. Respect for a patient's explanatory model does not necessarily imply agreement on the part of the physician; it merely means that the physician appreciates the impact of a deeply held belief on the care of that patient.' (Masi 1992)

Culture may also influence the following:

- What people regard as healthy and normal in terms of the way their body functions. In some cultures a daily bowel movement is regarded as an important sign of health. Some women with a heavy menstrual loss may worry about becoming weak and anaemic; others believe that a heavy loss is necessary to cleanse the body, and may worry if their flow is light.
- What people see as causing illness and how they present it. Most Western Europeans see physical illness as caused by some combination of bad luck, external factors, heredity and individual behaviour. In other societies people may consider other possibilities. These can include bad behaviour, divine purpose or divine punishment, family problems, emotional stress and sadness, or another person's ill-will or jealousy, often known as the evil eye.

> 'Here you see illness as mainly to do with germs and infection. At home the more important issue is why a person becomes ill. This has to do with their relationships with the outside world; germs and infection are merely the mechanism.'
> Ugandan doctor

- How people recognise and explain symptoms and show pain (see also Chapters 13 and 14). When presenting illness to health professionals, patients usually highlight the symptoms that seem most significant to them or which they assume will make most sense to the professional. In some cultures, pain and other physical symptoms are considered most important, others may focus more on emotional and psychological symptoms, and others on people's inability to carry out their daily tasks and responsibilities (Helman 1994, Currer 1986).
- How people respond to illness, and the behaviour they expect of themselves and of others when ill. In general, Western cultures regard taking control as important. People who do not expect or try to exert control

are often seen as weak. In some cultures, people may see themselves as having less control over their lives and their health. Powerful external factors, including the environment, society, spiritual or divine influences, or inherited characteristics, may be more significant. Control may be seen as an illusion or even as undesirable. One disadvantage of seeing one's life and one's body as amenable to control is that when people cannot control them, for example in the case of serious illness, they may be judged and judge themselves as failing (Helman 1994).

- What people regard as sensible methods of diagnosis and treatment. In the Western bio-medical system, biochemical and other physical tests are very important. Other practitioners may use, for example, a complex system of pulse taking or discussion about the patient's relationships and current circumstances. If illness is considered to have a spiritual explanation, moral and spiritual factors may be taken into account in choosing treatment. People may fast and pray to achieve a cure. Some cultures and some individuals use faith healing and spiritual healers. In systems that regard food as having a major influence on health and illness, practitioners often recommend dietary changes to maintain health.

At the same time, not everyone in a particular community has the same attitudes and assumptions regarding illness and health. **For example, there may be more similarities between the health beliefs or practices of different ethnic groups at the same socio-economic level than there are within the same ethnic group at different socio-economic levels** (Masi 1992).

Experience of different health care systems

People's expectations of health care are also influenced by their past experience. Even within Western allopathic medicine, which is often considered purely scientific and therefore impervious to culture, there are tremendous variations in culture and practice and therefore in what patients expect. For example, French people are more likely to attribute their physical symptoms to the liver; Germans to the heart. In much of Europe, low blood pressure is regarded as dangerous and requiring treatment. Drugs for low blood pressure account for the third largest percentage of all drugs prescribed in Germany. In the UK and the USA people with low blood pressure who are otherwise healthy are regarded as fortunate and may pay lower insurance premiums. In the USA, and increasingly in the UK, the fight against disease and death is often regarded as justifying any treatment, no matter how 'heroic' (Payer 1989). Choices of medication and the ways in which it is administered also vary in different societies (see also Chapter 14 *Patient adherence*).

In Britain, allopathic medicine has long been dominant; allopathic doctors are generally regarded as 'real doctors'. In continental Europe, homoeopathy and herbal medicine have always been part of mainstream care; they are not regarded as 'alternative' in any way. In most parts of the world, allopathic and local traditional medical systems exist side by side, all given equal status and respect (see also Chapter 31). People select a system and practitioner according to what they believe is most likely to help, and on the costs and accessibility of the different options.

Working with people of different cultures

Each of us tends to trust the system we have grown up with. We assume that practitioners in this system know what they are doing, and often mistrust those who do things differently. This can pose a real problem for people relying on an unfamiliar system. They may have little faith in the diagnostic methods and treatments recommended. They may prefer to find a practitioner who understands their culture and expectations, from whom they can get care that makes sense to them. When there is a language barrier, this can be particularly important.

'A research project in central London on the health care needs and expectations of Chinese families found several people who went to a private Chinese doctor to find out what was wrong with them in their own language and in terms that they understood. Since private prescriptions are very expensive they then went to their English-speaking GP for a second diagnosis (which they often could not understand) and a prescription for medication.' (Bloomsbury Health Authority 1984)

Concern about unfamiliar approaches and treatments and different styles of care may increase patients' fears and worries. If a patient expects an injection or tests and gets a counselling session, or vice versa, they may doubt the competence of the practitioner.

'I see a lot of foreign students and they often walk out looking so dejected. They have come to me with something they clearly regard as important and needing treatment, but which means nothing to me. Either I can't see the significance or it just doesn't add up to any disease process I can diagnose or treat.'
GP in south London

Try not to feel offended or hurt if patients or relatives react unfavourably, but to work at reaching some kind of shared understanding and approach.

'Basically it's a question of respecting how the patient sees their illness. We may not agree with them totally but we have to respect that they have views and also be open-minded enough to believe that their views may have validity.

Their views will certainly affect how they react to and comply with our advice and treatment. We need to show that we want to work with them, not against them.'
Health professional

The task of learning about a new health culture

When you started your training or your work, you entered a new world. What did you need to learn about:

- The way staff relate to: patients?
                          patients' relatives and friends?

- The way staff relate to each other: within the same discipline?
                                      across disciplines?
                                      within a hierarchy?
- How nurses view things?
- How doctors view things?
- The different cultures of different departments and units (eg an acute unit and a palliative care unit)?
- Language, medical terms, phrases and acronyms?
- Where you fitted in and what was expected of you?

How did you need to change? How did you feel during this learning process? Were there things that shocked or upset you initially? How did you feel? How did you behave?

Every health system has its own culture, its own language and its own accepted, if unspoken, ways of doing things. People who are new to a health care system have to learn what is available, how to get it, and the appropriate behaviour for each situation. In Britain, they have to learn the skills of a world organised largely according to white, middle-class English values, influenced by the army, Christianity and the poorhouse (Hart 1996). They are expected to conform to an unfamiliar set of rules and routines. Family members are suddenly outsiders, visiting on alien territory controlled by others (see also Chapter 17 *Relatives as 'visitors'*). Normal physical and emotional contact often becomes impossible because of a lack of privacy and space, as well as fear of breaking the rules. Instead, patients are attended in the most intimate ways by strangers, under the authority of strangers and judged by criteria of which they are often not aware (Helman 1994).

People who speak little or no English, as well as those who normally live in enclosed communities, can find it particularly stressful and alienating to adapt to health service culture. For patients and relatives who have been used to a more involved style of care, the separation and control imposed by most British hospitals may be difficult and confusing.

People who work within a strong institutional culture easily forget how different and strange it can be. Some health professionals react strongly and even angrily towards people who 'break the rules'. Often such people simply do not understand what is expected. Sometimes, however, the rules clash with their own cultural obligations and expectations (see, for example, Chapters 9, 17 and 18). When problems arise, it is most helpful to try to find out what lies behind them and together to work out ways in which the needs of the patient, the family and the institution can all be met.

The patient–professional relationship

The kind of relationship patients and families expect with health professionals varies a good deal. In many societies doctors must be treated with great respect. Below, an American journalist summarises humorously, but perhaps with some truth, the contrast between the attitudes of the British and American public to the medical profession:

'[The American attitude] A doctor is a necessary evil … a man in a white coat who gets you when you're down, overmedicates, operates at the drop of a chin-line and uses your misfortunes to pad his annual income. Watch him like a hawk. Ask plenty of questions and don't let him come near you with a wet cotton-swab unless:

1 it's a matter of life and death
2 you've had a second opinion
3 you've negotiated his fee.

'Remember that you can never win in any encounter with the medical profession. The rule is simple, and the odds are on their side. They get the money, but the results are never guaranteed.

'[The British attitude] Respect all medical men and women, dedicated servants of the community. Overworked healers with a sense of vocation, bleary-eyed with sleepless hours of service to mankind. Do not ask too many questions. Your case is paltry, and your life one tiny speck of light in the doctor's vast firmament. Anyway – being challenged or called to account or asked what is in a prescription seems to annoy him.' (Walmsley 1986)

The relationship between professional and patient in the British health system can puzzle people who are new to it. Some people may expect a more equal relationship with mutual personal responsibilities. Some may regard health professionals with respect and awe and may find it difficult to voice their questions or disagreement. Others may judge a health professional and their competence on personal rather than on professional grounds. In some countries the status of nurses and doctors is very different. In some countries it is rare for women to hold positions of authority (see also Chapter 17 *Relatives as 'visitors'*). People who have been used to paying for health care privately or through insurance schemes may be used to a more personalised and overtly respectful approach.

> Take a few minutes to think about the kind of relationship that you expect to have with your patients and their families.
>
> - What is it suitable for you and your patient to discuss? Is it the same in both directions?
> - What do you give advice to your patient about? What do they give advice to you about?
> - Are you equally involved in each other's personal lives?
> - Where does your involvement with your patient stop? Where does their involvement with you stop?
> - What are your obligations to your patient and their family? What are your patient's obligations to you and your family?
> - What kinds of demands is it reasonable for you to make of the patient? What kinds of demands is it reasonable for them to make of you?
> - Do you have authority over your patient? Do they have authority over you? How far does this authority go?
> - Are there certain times when you do not have obligations to your patient? When are they?
> - How long does your relationship usually last?
> - How do you both know all this?

Assumptions about what is right or wrong, acceptable or unacceptable, in the professional–patient relationship are unstated and usually unconscious. If the two sides bring different assumptions and expectations, it is easy for one or both to become anxious, offended, angry or frustrated and for them to lose trust in each other.

Popular and unpopular patients

Health professionals often find patients of communities other than their own anxiety-provoking and threatening. They may feel negative towards such patients and respond by distancing themselves, limiting themselves to routine physical care (Murphy and Macleod Clark 1993).

Take a few minutes to think about the kinds of patients you prefer to care for.

- Which kinds of patients do you find most rewarding and satisfying?
- Which kinds of patients do you prefer to spend time with?
- Which kinds of patients do you find most difficult and frustrating?
- Are there any kinds of patients whom you tend to avoid or to spend as little time with as possible?
- How does this affect the standard of care they receive?

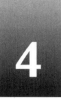

4 The needs and perspectives of older people

Most people in Britain and other industrialised countries die in old age. When older people are ill or dying, their particular needs and perspectives may require special consideration.

'Old age is no time to participate in social engineering.' (Karseras 1991)

A *unique generation*

People who are approaching the end of their lives now, have lived through an exceptional period of change, including two world wars and enormous economic, social and political upheavals. These have resulted in major population movements. Almost every country in the world is now ethnically mixed, containing people of different origins, cultures and religions. The proliferation of technology and the ever-increasing pace of social change have also made this generation very adaptable and flexible.

'My father fought in the German army against the British in the First World War.
I was a British army captain in the Second World War.'
Jewish man

'I remember the first car in our town. Now I have seen men on the moon.'
English elder

The lives of black and minority ethnic older people in Britain, especially those who were born in other countries, mirror these global changes. Their courage and achievements and the huge adaptations they have made in an often hostile society are largely unrecognised. Many, especially those who came to Britain as refugees, have experienced great losses and personal tragedies.

'Men and women prepared to cross oceans and continents in order to seek new occupational opportunities or a new way of life do not represent a random cross-section of humanity.' (Townsend, Davidson and Whitehead 1988)

At the same time, black and minority ethnic older people are an extremely diverse group of individuals with a wide range of experiences and values, and with very different needs.

The changing status of older people

The status and position of older people are changing in many parts of the world, particularly in the industrialised countries. They are increasingly seen as a burden rather than as a respected source of experience and wisdom. Advances in medicine and public health have increased their numbers; migration and urbanisation have led to the break-up of family units in which they played a dominant role; technological advances have often made their knowledge and skills irrelevant and reduced their power; exclusion from paid work has made them economically dependent; mass education and a cultural focus on youth have reduced the value of tradition (Blakemore and Boneham 1994).

'Young people have lost respect for their elders, and the days when we cared for them according to our religion and culture are gone.'
Sri Lankan woman

Ageism

'It would not be fair to characterise staff and services as generally "ageist" in their attitudes, but we did encounter examples of prejudiced attitudes towards older people and their care at almost every level of the service system – ward staff, training establishments, senior managers and representatives of the health authorities.' (HAS 2000 1998)

Ageism is the systematic stereotyping of and discrimination against people simply because they are old. It allows younger people to dissociate themselves from the undesirable process of ageing (Butler 1975). Ageism stereotypes older people's experience and knowledge as irrelevant and worthless, their intellectual powers as declining, and their habits and attitudes as inflexible. In fact, there is usually a huge difference between the personal experience of growing older – the normal physical processes of ageing – and the social experience of being treated by others as a completely different kind of person or as less worthy of respect and consideration simply because your body is changing. **Ageism has been** described as 'the daftest form of prejudice' since we all grow old (Eastham 1985).

> 'The only sure fact about older people is that they have lived for longer than those in younger generations. All other attributes vary between individuals.'
> (RCN 1996)

In contrast to the stereotype, many older people demonstrate great flexibility and adaptability. For example, the husband who takes over the total care of his wife; the grandmother who moves to Britain and adapts to a completely different way of life; the older refugee who runs language classes for the children in his community; the millions of older people who adapt to cope with physical limitations and other losses and changes. Because we stereotype the old as inflexible and reluctant to change, we often fail to see their flexibility or give them credit for it (Stevenson 1989).

> 'They see us as looking inwards and clinging together in an "unhealthy way" and "refusing to change". We see ourselves as having made the most tremendous adaptations and as pulled apart by life in this society. People can only change so much in their lives. If we change any more we shall lose our souls.'
> Vietnamese woman

Health service culture tends to reflect society's prejudices. Professionals caring for older people often have low status and little recognition. Medical training focuses on acute illness and still pays little attention to the common disabilities of old age or to illness in relation to older people. There is also evidence that some health professionals see older people as incapable, unintelligent, dependent and a nuisance. Older-sounding voices are often perceived as showing physical frailty and vulnerability and mental slowness, and as providing less accurate information (Fuller 1995, Redfern 1991). Older patients' basic practical needs – for warmth, physical comfort and food – are not always met; their social, emotional and spiritual needs even less (HAS 2000 1998).

> 'Nurses must believe in older people. This means to nurse not only with the head and the hands, but also with the heart and the spirit.' (Nazarko 1996)

Black and minority ethnic older people

Statistics

At the time of the 1991 Census, just under 17 per cent of the total population of Great Britain were aged over 65, compared with just over three per cent of the black and minority ethnic communities. However, 15 per cent of black and minority ethnic people were aged between 45 and 64. The numbers of black and minority ethnic older people will therefore increase significantly over the next few years and their age profiles will become more like that of the majority population (OPCS 1993).

People's health is fundamentally affected by the socio-economic and environmental context in which they live. 'One would thus expect many Black Britons to suffer the health disadvantages of the working class. They endure working class health inequality and then some more' (Grimsley and Bhat 1988). Studies confirm that older people and people approaching retirement age in black and minority ethnic groups are more likely to be in poor health than their white British peers (Blakemore and Boneham 1994, HEA 1994). Chronological age is not always the best indicator of who is elderly. Black and minority ethnic people may become 'old' at an earlier age (Bowling 1990).

In some minority communities, the expected ratio of women to men in the older age groups is reversed, reflecting their history. For example, there are more men than women over 75 in both the Pakistani and Bangladeshi communities. In the 55 to 75 age group there are more men than women in all the South Asian communities, and in the African-Caribbean and Irish communities (Bahl 1996, Tilki 1994). This has implications for patterns of family support and care at home.

Traditional expectations

'Britain is no country for old people.'
Jamaican woman

In most of the societies from which people have emigrated, the idea of social and religious duty to parents was strong. Younger people relied on older adults for emotional and practical support, and for guidance. In return, they would look after their seniors as they aged. Women generally accepted the care of older family members as part of their work. Although poverty, gender and past contribution to the family always affected their situation, most older people were respected and cared for (Blakemore and Boneham 1994). In many societies older people, especially men, controlled the family finances until they died.

'We like to think of our people caring for everyone within the family. Although that may have been universally true – and still holds true in most instances – that caring wasn't always spontaneous. It was a person's duty.'
Nigerian doctor (Creedon 1995)

Although there have often been changes in their 'home societies', many black and minority ethnic older people, like many of their white peers, look back to a time when the elderly were more likely to be respected for their wisdom and experience, and cared for (Blakemore and Boneham 1994). A study of black older people in Bristol found that although very few wanted to leave Britain, mainly because their families were here, many approached increasing age with considerable apprehension (Fenton 1987). Some, however, do choose to return to their country of birth.

'I don't want to die and be buried in a cold country.'
African-Caribbean elder

Family support

Black and minority ethnic families share the pressures and demands of modern life in Britain, often with additional pressures caused by racial discrimination (see Chapter 5). Nevertheless, many health and other professionals still believe that all minority ethnic families 'look after their own'; this belief often leads to different expectations and referral patterns. Despite a high level of need, many black and minority ethnic older people and those caring for them receive little or no help from community health and social services (Blakemore and Boneham 1994, Atkin, Cameron et al 1989).

'There is great pressure on us to assimilate and take on the values and behaviour of the majority. But at the same time there is an unspoken expectation that we should maintain some traditions like caring for elderly and sick relatives at home. When for personal or economic reasons it is hard for us to do this, we are judged and criticised in a way that the majority population are not.'
Black British woman

When family members do try to provide care there may, nevertheless, be practical or emotional problems. Sharing a home with parents or in-laws who have different backgrounds and expectations can lead to strains and breakdowns in relationships. Older people with traditional values may feel hurt if they are no longer seen as the head and centre of the household and are financially dependent (d'Ardenne and Mahtani 1989). Black and minority ethnic carers often lack information about what help is available or how to get it (see Chapter 16).

Isolation

Not all black and minority ethnic older people have families whose help they can call on. A study in Birmingham (Bhalla and Blakemore 1981) found that about 25 per cent of all older South Asians interviewed and 9 per cent of the African-Caribbeans had no close relatives in the UK. Many older people who do have families live alone, often at some distance from other relatives.

'My husband came from the same village in Poland. We met and married here after the [Second World] War. We had both lost everybody. But we made Polish friends here and we had a good life. Now he is dead and my children have moved away. They do not understand why the past is so important to me. They do not want to talk about it. I only have one Polish friend now and she cannot get out of her flat. The only person I can talk my own language to is myself. I am very lonely and frightened for the future.'
Polish widow

Social isolation is a serious problem for many older people. People who have lived almost entirely within their own cultural community may feel particularly vulnerable. Some have worked long hours all their lives and have had few opportunities to socialise (Modood, Beishon and Virdee 1994). Some speak little or no English, or may lose their English as they get older (see also Chapter 25 *Why do some people not speak English?*). Some feel threatened by racist violence and also by fears of public hostility and intolerance.

Poverty

Roughly one-third of all older people in the UK are very poor (Redfern 1991). Black and minority ethnic people are over-represented in this group (Blakemore and Boneham 1994) (see also Chapter 5 *The effects of racism*). Discrimination in employment, plus a decline in many of the industries to which they were recruited, have brought long-term unemployment and early retirement to many. Most have no income apart from the basic state pension. Some are dependent on Income Support because they have not worked long enough in Britain to accumulate the full pension entitlement, because they earned too little to contribute, because their employers did not make the necessary contributions, or because they had to return 'home' for long periods to deal with family and other problems (Amin 1992, Stevenson 1989). Some may have difficulty in providing the documentation needed to prove their entitlement to benefit; in many countries birth certificates were not issued until recently. People who came to Britain as refugees were unable to bring any money or savings with them and so had to depend on state benefits; many have found it impossible to find work and so have remained on or below the poverty line (Spencer 1994).

People who have spent their working lives on low incomes are unlikely to have savings to fall back on when they retire or become ill. In addition, many, especially African-Caribbeans and South Asians, have regularly sent money 'home' to support family members there (Modood, Berthoud et al 1997). Since 1980, families who have been allowed to bring 'elderly dependants' to live with them in Britain have had to declare that they 'will maintain and accommodate [their] dependants without recourse to public funds'. This causes major hardship for families already on a low income who have to support an additional dependent family member with no financial help or help with housing, even if an emergency arises (Amin 1992, Norman 1985). (NHS treatment is, however, free to anyone allowed to stay permanently in the UK, and, in emergencies, to visitors.)

Many black and ethnic minority older people, like many of their white peers, do not claim all the benefits to which they are entitled. Some are unwilling to be dependent on the state or do not want their privacy invaded (Walker 1990). Others do not know what they are entitled to or are unable to claim because of the complexity of the form, difficulties in providing the required documentation or language difficulties.

'For me, as a Muslim, it is important to live off what you have earned. It is wrong to be dependent on others, even the State. If I can manage, I prefer not to claim.'
Elderly man

Fears and worries

'What the elderly need is love and to feel they are still very important people. We have to make time to listen to them. And no one seems to have time any more.'
Nigerian woman (Creedon 1995)

Many older people in all communities face old age and increasing frailty with apprehension. Those who would traditionally look to their family for practical and emotional support worry that it will not be forthcoming when they need it. Some fear that their children have taken on what they see as the uncaring, selfish attitudes of the English towards older people (Fenton 1987). Many realise that, even with the best of intentions, their families cannot now provide for all their needs. **They often have a particular dread of hospital or residential care, fearing that British institutions do not yet understand or meet the needs of people with different lifestyles, habits, customs and beliefs** (Wassim 1991).

5 Racial discrimination in society

Racism: Conscious or unconscious belief in the superiority of a particular 'race'. Acts of discrimination and unfair treatment, whether intentional or unintentional, based on this belief (Mares, Henley and Baxter 1985).

'Races' and the origins of racism

There are no such things as different human races. All human beings come from a common genetic stock and share their genetic inheritance. The idea of separate and biologically distinct human 'races', each with a different genetic make-up that is linked to physical and behavioural characteristics, is false. It originated in Europe in the eighteenth century as part of an attempt to understand evolution and human variation (Godrej 1994, Senior and Bhopal 1994).

Although there are some variations in tissue type and disease patterns between populations originating in different areas of the world, most genetic variation occurs between individuals. There are more genetic differences within any one so-called racial group than between the averages of any two different 'racial' or national groups (Pinker 1994). The genes responsible for skin colour and other superficial physical features, the basis on which the Victorians divided people into so-called racial groups, are few and atypical. Around the world, genetic variation is gradual; populations merge into one another; there are no sharp dividing lines.

There is therefore no rational or scientific basis for dividing people into distinct 'races' or for regarding one 'race' as biologically or intellectually superior to another. Nevertheless, many people still act and talk as if separate 'races' with different characteristics exist as identifiable categories (Godrej 1994, McKenzie and Crowcroft 1994, Senior and Bhopal 1994, Sheldon and Parker 1992).

'There is no scientific validity for dividing up humanity into neat groupings on the basis of identifiable physical characteristics. While human variation is obvious for all to see, the existence of definable groups or races is more of a social construction than a scientific reality.' (Sheldon and Parker 1991)

Although the ideas of 'race' and of superior and inferior 'races' are only social constructs, they are powerful and potentially very destructive. They have been used to justify slavery and the Holocaust, as well as the colonisation and domination of Asian and African countries by Europeans. They still cause serious conflict all over the world.

'For 400 years the British systematically conquered territories in the four corners of the globe. These lands provided Britain with wealth, power and glory. Commerce and trade flourished as Britain and the other Imperial powers gained access to the natural resources of half the world. Through this accumulation of wealth and materials the momentum was gained for the industrial revolution which transformed agrarian Britain into the modern industrial country in which we now live...This occupation of other countries and enslavement of their peoples was justified by defining black people as inferior beings to whites.' (Klug and Gordon 1983)

Racism and prejudice

Skin colour and other 'racial' physical features have no meaning or status in themselves. But they become very important when societies give them meaning and status, assigning people to different 'racial groups' and then treating members of these groups better or worse. The circle is completed when, as a result of discrimination, people with different skin colour predominate in, for example, low-level and poorly paid jobs, among the unemployed, in poor housing and in deprived areas. Seeing black and minority ethnic people in undesirable situations confirms racist ideas and prejudices about their inferiority (Ahmad 1993).

'Colour is the greatest single factor which governs society's attitudes to members of minority groups and influences their own self-image, and it is inescapable.' (Rack 1991)

Although racism and racial prejudice, based on theories of racial difference and superiority, are very clearly a reality, 'race' is not. For this reason, the word 'race' is enclosed in quotation marks in this book.

Cultural racism

In addition to straightforward colour-based racism, certain groups in Britain are increasingly subjected to what has been called 'cultural racism'. This is based on the idea that white British culture is superior to other cultures. It is targeted particularly at ethnic groups that have distinctive cultural identities or community life and that are perceived by white people as assertively different and as not trying to 'fit in'. Such groups, for example South Asian Muslims, experience an additional layer of discrimination and prejudice (Modood, Beishon and Virdee 1994).

'In British society there is a hierarchy of cultures, and those of racial minority groups are ranked very low indeed.' (Ahmed 1986)

The effects of racism

Note Unless otherwise referenced, most of the information in this section is from E*thnic Minorities in Britain: Diversity and disadvantage*, the fourth Policy Studies Institute Survey (Modood, Berthoud et al 1997). Interested readers are recommended to refer to it for more detailed information and discussion. The terminology used here is based on that used in the 1991 Census and the fourth Policy Studies Institute Survey. Terms such as Indian, Pakistani and African-Caribbean refer to ethnic group and not to place of birth.

Racism in employment

In the post-war years, most black and minority ethnic people were restricted to manual work; almost everyone, even those with a degree or other higher level qualifications and experience, had to take jobs that were low paid, dirty and hard, often with shifts and night work, for which no white workers could be found. Many black and minority ethnic people, especially older people, have remained in these kinds of jobs.

In recent years, racial discrimination against people of Chinese, East African Asian and Indian heritage seems to have diminished, though not disappeared. However, there is still severe discrimination against people of African-Caribbean, Pakistani and Bangladeshi heritage. **Even when they have the same experience and qualifications,** there are major disparities in job levels, pay, working conditions and employment levels between African-Caribbean, Pakistani and Bangladeshi men and men in other groups. One response to the continued experience of discrimination has been to become self-employed.

Female employment follows a similar pattern. The main exception is African-Caribbean women, who are more likely to be in non-manual and supervisory positions (often in the public services) and who, as a group, earn more than African-Caribbean men. Forty per cent of African-Caribbean women in Britain work in hospitals and medical care.

Black and minority ethnic men have always been harder hit than white men by unemployment; current research confirms that this is still true for Pakistanis, Bangladeshis and African-Caribbeans. The low-paying industries that recruited black and minority ethnic men in the 1950s and '60s were often already declining; many, such as the textile industries, have almost disappeared. Jobs in inner city areas have also declined. Whatever the level of unemployment in a particular area, that for Pakistani, Bangladeshi and African-Caribbean men is always significantly higher, indicating that racism as well as structural factors are to blame. Rates of long-term unemployment are higher in all minority ethnic groups, but again highest in these three groups.

Income, poverty and standards of living

Black and minority ethnic people are almost twice as likely as white people to be in the poorest fifth of the population (Joseph Rowntree Foundation 1995). Pakistani, Bangladeshi, Indian and African-Caribbean households are particularly likely to be poor.

The single most important influence on a household's income is the availability of earnings from work. In 1994 half of all Pakistani and Bangladeshi households had no income from employment. Rates of unemployment among Pakistani and Bangladeshi men are very high (38 and 42 per cent respectively). For cultural reasons, women in these communities rarely go out to work. Those men who are in work in these communities tend to earn less. African-Caribbeans are also significantly more likely to have no income from employment, partly because of higher unemployment rates and partly because of the number of lone-parent households.

Pakistani and Bangladeshi families, though generally declining in size, also tend to contain more children than the average. Incomes that are already low must therefore be spread thinner to cover the needs of more people. Although the incomes of East African Asian and Indian households are roughly similar to those of white households, these households also often contain more people, particularly adults, and so again income must be stretched further.

Among the white population, pensioner households account for a high proportion of the low-income households. At present, the only minority group with a significant number of pensioner households is African-Caribbean.

Poverty and poor health are powerfully correlated: socio-economic status is as important a predictor of health for black and minority ethnic groups as it is for white groups (Modood, Berthoud et al 1997, Wilkinson 1997). Poverty also severely limits the kinds of home care and support that are possible when someone is ill or dying (see also Chapter 16 *Care at home*).

Racism, housing and homelessness

Black and minority ethnic people in all housing sectors are more likely to experience poor-quality housing and overcrowding (Sarre, Philips and Skellington 1989). Factors such as overcrowding, damp and lack of amenities may affect families' abilities to care for sick members at home.

It is estimated that black and minority ethnic households are four times as likely as white households to become homeless (NACAB 1991). Homeless people are often blamed for their situation, especially if they are black. But the reason most people are homeless is the general lack of affordable accommodation. Homeless people in temporary accommodation suffer overcrowding, lack of basic amenities (especially cooking facilities), lack of privacy and constant insecurity. Local authorities can move them at very short notice if cheaper accommodation is found (Schott and Henley 1992) (see also Chapter 35).

Racism and violence

'I came to Britain in the 1960s at the invitation of a London teaching hospital that was recruiting nurses. When I first came people would admire my long hair and my sari and ask how to put a sari on. Now there are many places I won't wear a sari because I get spat at and called a "dirty Paki".'
Tamil nurse

Racial hostility, based on skin colour and other visible differences such as dress, is a constant source of stress and anxiety for black and minority ethnic people in all communities. It ranges from unfriendliness and verbal abuse to physical harassment and violence, affecting people's daily lives and opportunities as well their emotional and physical well-being. Persistent experience of racism can also affect a person's self-image and generate a sense of inferiority. In some cases the constant stress of being devalued and rejected, and the endless series of large and small losses that result from racial discrimination, contribute to depression and other mental health problems (Fernando 1991).

'Even in the encapsulated world of purdah...racism touches these [Pathan women]. Awareness of public hostility towards them ran deep and it was to them incomprehensible. Apart from the rules of hospitality, to which they were themselves used, they could not see that they had caused any trouble that would warrant such reaction.' (Currer 1986)

The 1992 British Crime Survey estimated a national total of 130,000 racially motivated crimes against South Asians and African-Caribbeans in 1991: 89,000 against South Asians and 41,000 against African-Caribbeans. Most people, however, do not report such incidents to the police because they feel there is little point. Indeed, in a small number of cases police officers, either on or off duty, were the perpetrators.

Persistent racial abuse and hostility create a climate of cumulative fear and insecurity, which may lead people to restrict their activities severely:

- On one east London estate, 23 Bangladeshi and Somali families had suffered a total of 136 incidents of racial harassment in a six-month period.
- A study in Leeds found that half the black and minority ethnic people interviewed had been forced to change their lives in some way because of racial attacks. Some said they lived like prisoners in their own homes because they were too afraid to go out (Gordon 1990).
- A survey in Glasgow found that up to 90 per cent of South Asians and 16 per cent of Chinese residents had experienced racial abuse. Almost half the South Asian respondents had also been physically assaulted. Women bore the brunt of the harassment. Many said they stayed at home most of the time, only went out with husbands and friends, and avoided certain streets and times of day (Gordon 1990).
- Parents often keep children in, forbidding them to walk home from school alone or play in the park for fear of racist abuse or violence. Women keep the doors and windows locked when the men are at work (CRE 1993).

    'It's the children I'm frightened for. I don't want to teach them to be afraid all the time or to stay away from white people. But every time they go out of this house I'm frightened they won't come back. They're not even safe at school. And I don't like them to go out in the evenings. What kind of life is this for them? And what are they learning?'
    Ghanaian mother

Racial violence and harassment can be pictured as a pyramid, as shown in Figure 5.1.

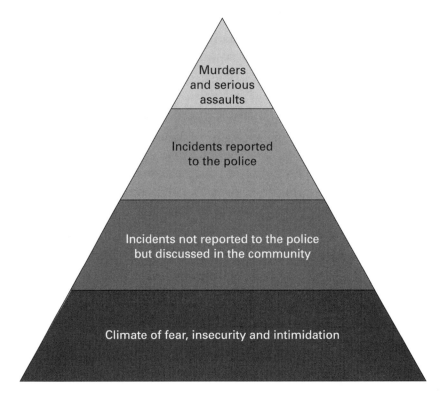

Figure 5.1 The racial violence pyramid (Reproduced, with permission, from *Multi-ethnic Britain: facts and trends*, 1994, Runnymede Trust)

- At the peak there are incidents of murder and very serious violence. It is estimated that, between 1992 and 1994, 15 people died in Britain as a result of what are believed to be racially motivated attacks. Petrol bomb and arson attacks on black and minority ethnic people's homes and workplaces as well as other serious crimes of violence are increasing in number. Such incidents are usually reported in the mainstream media, though in much less detail and depth than in the minority ethnic press.
- The next level contains incidents that are reported to the police but not usually covered in the mainstream press and so are unknown to most white people. They include physical violence and assault, verbal abuse and criminal damage. They are widely discussed within the black and minority ethnic communities.
- The next level contains incidents that are not reported to the police but are intensely distressing and have a long-term effect on the behaviour and consciousness of the victims, their families and friends.
- At the base of the pyramid there is a climate of fear, insecurity and intimidation that cramps the lives of almost all black and minority ethnic

people in our society. This compounds the effects of living in a society in which most black and minority ethnic people also see themselves disadvantaged and marginalised in key areas such as employment, politics and the criminal justice system. It also affects people's trust in institutions such as the health service and in the people who work in them. (After Runnymede Trust 1994, by permission.)

6 Racial discrimination, the law and implications for health services

What is the law on racial discrimination?

In the UK, legislation to prevent racial discrimination covers the provision of services such as health care, as well as employment, training and racial harassment. The 1976 Race Relations Act makes it illegal to discriminate against someone on 'racial grounds', ie because of their colour, 'race', nationality (including citizenship), ethnic or national origins.

The Race Relations Act forbids two kinds of discrimination, direct and indirect:

- **Direct discrimination** means treating someone less favourably on racial grounds than a person of a different racial group would be treated in the same circumstances.
- **Indirect discrimination** means imposing a requirement that applies equally to everyone (so it may appear fair) but the proportion of people of a particular racial group that can comply with it is considerably smaller than the proportion of people of other racial groups, and it cannot be objectively justified, and it is to the disadvantage of the person concerned.

It is the **effects** of any action on people that make it discriminatory under the law, not the motives of the individual(s) or of the organisation responsible for the action.

Direct, intentional racism in any form in health care is clearly unacceptable and should be treated by the employer as a disciplinary offence. However, indirect and unintentional discrimination are also illegal. Once discrimination of any kind has been identified, both the organisation and individuals have a legal responsibility to remedy it.

Liability for racial discrimination rests both with the person who does the discriminating and with any person who instructs them, or applies pressure on them, to discriminate. An employer is responsible for any racial discrimination by employees in the course of their work, unless the employer can show that they have taken practical steps to prevent discrimination. It is no defence for employers to plead ignorance of their employees' actions. It is also illegal to victimise a person in any way because they have asserted, or intend to assert, their rights under the Act (CRE 1992).

Discrimination in the provision of services

Under section 20 of the Race Relations Act it is illegal to discriminate on racial grounds in delivering any services to the public. It is illegal to discriminate, directly or indirectly:

- by refusing or deliberately omitting to provide services;
- by offering services of a lesser quality;
- by offering services in different ways or on different terms.

Direct discrimination in the provision of health services includes, for example:

- making racially prejudiced remarks;
- refusing to register clients who require an interpreter;
- taking the symptoms and worries of black and minority ethnic group patients less seriously than those of white patients, referring them for fewer diagnostic tests;
- asking only black people or people who do not speak English for passports to prove their right to free health care.

Indirect discrimination is more insidious and usually more difficult to identify. It occurs when **exactly the same services** are provided to everybody (so that they appear fair) but when for cultural, religious, linguistic or other reasons it is **not possible for members of one or more black and minority ethnic groups to benefit equally from them**. Both direct and indirect discrimination are sometimes built into routines and written protocols.

'The 1976 Race Relations Act...made visible the uncomfortable truth that "nice people" may be involved, through their routine professional practice, in generating discriminatory outcomes.' (Gerrish, Husband and Mackenzie 1996)

Examples of services that may discriminate indirectly against some members of black and minority ethnic groups include:

- Services that may be **unattractive or off-putting**. For example, if a hospital seems, through its information brochures, posters and notices, to be aimed only at white or English-speaking people; if certain staff or departments are known to be hostile to black and minority ethnic people or to people who do not speak English well; if an institution has an overtly Christian ethos and atmosphere in its publicity and in its services and routines.

- Services that may be **unacceptable**. For example, hospital menus that do not offer food that patients can eat; lack of suitable washing facilities in bathrooms and lavatories; no female doctors available for women who require them; no male nurses available for the practical care of male patients who feel strongly about this; hospital gowns that are immodest and humiliating; lack of space or privacy for people who wish to pray (see Part Two).

- Services that may be **useless**. For example, no trained interpreters for patients and family members who speak little or no English; important leaflets available only in English (see Part Three).

- Services that are **inflexible** and do not allow for cultural differences. For example, rules that only two visitors are allowed at a time; not permitting the extended family to be present at a death; failure to take account of families' cultural and religious needs when carrying out last offices; failure to issue certificates and release bodies as soon as possible for families when the funeral must be carried out within 24 hours (see Part Two).

- Care that is **based on stereotypes** about the characteristics or needs of certain groups. For example, assuming that people of African descent are more likely to be HIV positive and taking extra precautions with them rather than applying universal infection control precautions; offering limited choices of treatment to minority ethnic people because of prejudices or stereotypes about their preferences or what is 'best' or 'right' for them; failing to tell black and minority ethnic people about hospice care or other options, for the same reasons.

- **Lack of training** for professionals in the **skills and knowledge** they need to provide care for all patients and families, whatever their ethnic origin, culture, religion and personal preferences. Professionals who do not know about possible cultural and religious needs around the time of illness or death may fail to ask the right questions or may offer inappropriate care. They may lack the necessary skills to communicate well across cultures.

- **Lack of training** for professionals about particular aspects of **practical care** in a multi-ethnic population. For example, being able to: recognise jaundice and cyanosis in dark skins; care appropriately for black hair and skin; meet religious and cultural requirements in relation to washing and personal hygiene; deal with different naming systems, addressing people appropriately and filing their names correctly; give dietary advice that takes people's preferences and religious requirements into account; prescribe for people who observe religious dietary restrictions or who are fasting.

- **Lack of training** for staff about the reality and the effects of **racism** in society, how it operates within the health service, and how to recognise and combat it.

Institutional racism: what is it and how does it affect health care?

There is much evidence that black and minority ethnic people in Britain are likely to receive worse health care than the majority white population (Ahmad 1993, Mohammed 1991). The tangled combination of factors in an organisation that cause such discrimination are often referred to as institutional racism. Institutional racism has been defined as 'the collective failure of an organisation to provide an appropriate and professional service to people because of their colour, culture or ethnic origin' (Macpherson 1999). Institutional racism has three main planks:

- established organisational processes and systems;
- the culture of the organisation;
- individual attitudes and behaviour (Open College 1992).

These three form a powerful combination, creating and maintaining inequalities in access to health care.

Established organisational processes and systems

Much of the discrimination that occurs in an organisation is due to long-established policies, practices and procedures. Many of these are part of the 'unthinking operation of a system' (CRE 1983). To people who are used to them, they often seem to work well and to be non-discriminatory. But apparently neutral policies often fail to meet the needs of black and minority ethnic people. Institutional discrimination is perpetuated when, despite evidence that current provision is not meeting the needs of certain groups, an organisation continues to provide services that do not meet differing cultural and religious needs or maintains policies that have discriminatory effects.

'We must not view people of different cultures and ethnic groups as a problem. We must adapt our care to meet their needs. We are contracted to provide a

service. The service exists for the community, not for us health professionals. If we are not providing it then we are the problem.'
Director of midwifery education

Most of us automatically plan and provide services on the basis of our own experience and understanding of what is needed. It takes personal awareness, careful and wide-ranging consultation, and a flexible and open attitude to identify the changes that need to be made (see also Chapters 7 *Identifying and combating institutional racism* and 22 *Identifying local needs and issues*).

The culture of the organisation

The culture of an organisation consists of the values shared by most of its staff, its informal arrangements and the unstated beliefs (including the prejudices) that influence staff behaviour (Cheung-Judge and Henley 1994).

'The National Health Service is not a culturally neutral organisation.' (McIver 1994)

Health service culture includes ideas about the kinds of people the organisation really exists to serve. Care is generally geared to meet the needs of these kinds of people. Patients who do not fit these ideas or who have different needs and wishes are often marginalised, resented or simply ignored.

The colour-blind approach

Some professionals feel that it is wrong to take account of 'race' or culture, and may adopt a 'colour-blind' approach which they see as neutral. But, in reality, a colour-blind or culture-blind approach is also discriminatory. It maintains the status quo – provision based on the cultural preferences and historical needs of the white majority population – and neglects or marginalises the needs of black and minority ethnic communities (Mohammed 1991).

'It's difficult to say how many black patients we've had. We don't go round saying we've got two Asian patients today or whatever; that's discriminatory, it's something you shouldn't think about, they're just patients.'
Hospice deputy manager (Hill and Penso 1995)

Although a colour-blind approach is often well meant, the individual needs of black and minority ethnic people cannot be fully met if important factors such as culture and religion, as well as the experience of racism and marginalisation, are not taken into account.

'..the very notion of blindness about colour constitutes an ideological confusion at best, and denial at its very worst... "**I** don't think about colour, therefore **your** problems don't exist." If only it were so easy.' (Williams 1997)

Individual attitudes and behaviour

'In the 1994 Policy Studies Institute survey, a quarter of all the white people interviewed said they were prejudiced against South Asians and against Muslims, and 20 per cent against African-Caribbeans. Past research suggests that such questions usually produce an under-estimate of the level of actual prejudice.' (Modood, Berthoud et al 1997)

Wherever people have the power to make a decision affecting other people, they also have the power to discriminate, whether consciously or unconsciously. Health professionals are likely to share the attitudes and prejudices of wider society, and have enormous power in relation to patients and their families. If they are prejudiced or hostile towards black and minority ethnic patients, or feel that the needs and preferences of minority patients are not as important as those of white patients, this will affect the day-to-day decisions they make and the care they give.

Personal racism is often remarkably explicit. It includes racist comments and remarks, derogatory asides about patients to colleagues, sighs and gestures, off-hand treatment, inadequate explanations, rudeness, ignoring patients' requests, even shouting and swearing (Currer 1986, McNaught 1985). There is evidence that some black and minority ethnic people pay to see doctors privately because they have experienced racial and cultural prejudice, intolerance and dismissiveness in the NHS (Papadopoulos and Worral 1996).

'I see a lot of racism and prejudice among some of my white colleagues. The way they talk about their black patients, and the way they talk to them; if a patient is black they think she's stupid, never mind her education or experience or knowledge. And they don't feel that black patients have as much right to the service. A district nurse I know deliberately didn't tell a black family what they were entitled to. She said, "They all exploit the service if they can". My colleagues are pleasant to me now but I don't know what they say behind my back. And I wouldn't trust them to look after me if I was ill.'
African-Caribbean nurse

Personal racism also leads to more subtle differences in behaviour. For example, health professionals may offer less explanation to black and minority ethnic patients, or may take their symptoms and worries less seriously.

'I felt that the white patients were given more time and attention – probably the nurses felt more relaxed with them. But also I felt that some things were unfair. When I asked for more explanation about my operation the next day I think they thought I was being unreasonable, but I was frightened and I needed to know. And when I asked a nurse to draw the curtains at visiting time when there were a lot of male visitors on the ward, she got angry and said, "If you want purdah, don't come to hospital". But I haven't any choice.'
Muslim woman

Black and minority ethnic patients may even be offered different or less treatment or fewer diagnostic procedures.

'Research in the USA shows that, among heart patients who are already in the medical system, black people are less likely than whites to undergo a wide range of important medical procedures, even when other variables such as severity of disease, socio-economic status and payment method are controlled for. Where the indications for a procedure are very well defined, there are few differences. But wherever physicians exercise more discretion in recommending coronary procedures, substantial racial differences are found. Whether these differences reflect conscious racism, ineffective communication or some other factor is not clear. The result is the same: black patients are less likely to receive treatments that can often relieve symptoms and sometimes prolong their lives.' (Ayanian 1993)

Some health professionals regard people with different or unfamiliar needs and lifestyles as abnormal or a nuisance. Some consider black and minority ethnic patients as responsible for their own health problems because of their 'deviant' or 'unsatisfactory' culture, and feel that it is reasonable that the services provided may not meet their needs (Atkin 1992, McNaught 1985).

'The view of many health professionals is that nothing is wrong with the services provided. It is "those people", with "special diets", "strange religious practices", or "funny maternity habits", who have the problem.' (Parsons, Macfarlane and Golding 1993)

Discrimination in employment

It is illegal to discriminate, directly or indirectly, against a person on racial grounds in recruitment and selection, in the treatment of employees in their terms of employment, in access to opportunities for training, promotion, transfer or other benefits, or in dismissals or other detrimental acts, including racial harassment or abuse (CRE 1992).

Health service employment

Discrimination in employment in the health services has serious consequences:

- it causes personal distress and alienation to black and minority ethnic professionals who are denied the opportunity to use their skills and qualifications to the full (see also Chapter 7 *Combating racial abuse of staff*);
- it wastes resources by preventing many black and minority ethnic practitioners, teachers and researchers from achieving their full potential; and
- it prevents health services from becoming more flexible and responsive to the needs of minority group patients, and is a factor in the perpetuation of institutional racism.

Even in places with a large minority ethnic population and/or a high proportion of minority ethnic staff in junior positions, the senior professionals, managers, planners and teachers are still predominantly white. Almost inevitably, the services they provide, manage and plan are ethnocentric, reflecting their often unconscious cultural beliefs and values about what is normal, and their reservations about whether it is legitimate to change or adapt established services simply to meet the needs of 'immigrants'.

The NHS is the biggest employer in Europe and the largest employer of black and minority ethnic people in Britain (Ward 1993). The establishment and growth of the NHS would not have been possible without the active recruitment of professionals and other staff from overseas, especially from the Caribbean, West Africa and the Indian subcontinent. However, most black and minority ethnic professionals have been, and still are – regardless of their qualifications and experience – concentrated in the lower grades, the least popular specialities and hospitals, and on night shifts (Ward 1993, CRE 1983). In some cases, the discriminatory processes that prevent black and minority ethnic people's access to jobs and training have even been formalised.

'An investigation into the computer program that helped pick candidates for selection interviews at St George's Medical School found that the program had been set up to weight the scores of female candidates and those with a 'foreign' name. (Ethnic group was not marked on the application forms.) The program increased the scores of these candidates and so reduced their chances of being selected for interview. (Candidates with the lowest scores were more likely to be called for interview.)

'It was found that the person who had programmed the computer had been instructed to develop a program that would mimic as closely as possible the judgements of the human selectors. He observed their judgements over a number of years, created the program and then fine-tuned it. He found that, in order to reproduce the selectors' judgements as closely as possible, he had to give a negative weighting to members of black and ethnic minority groups and to women.

'St George's Medical school immediately discontinued the program and reviewed its selection and recruitment procedures.' (CRE 1987)

Recent research shows that there is still significant discrimination against black and minority ethnic doctors, nurses and others working in the health service: in medicine, racial discrimination has been found at all levels, from medical school applications, through the examination process to job applications. It also affects the manner in which complaints are made against doctors (Esmail and Carnall 1997). Black and minority ethnic nurses are disproportionately concentrated in the lower grades (Department of Health 1993). In a postal survey, over a quarter of black and South Asian nurses believed that they had been refused jobs because of their 'race' or colour, and similar percentages believed that they had been refused promotion or training on these grounds (Beishon, Virdee and Hagell 1995).

7 Achieving equal access to health care and challenging racism

Equal access to care

Equal access means ensuring that no one receives less favourable treatment because of their ethnicity, colour, creed, national origin, gender, marital status, class, disability or sexuality. It means that everyone has equal and full access to the health care that is available.

Equality is not the same as uniformity. Equal access does not mean **offering the same service** to everyone and assuming that each person will therefore **receive** the same service. It means **offering flexible, responsive services** in which differing needs are identified and accommodated so that each person **benefits** equally.

'Black people are increasingly unwilling to accept the role of passive recipients of those services which others consider it appropriate to offer. They are taxpayers and ratepayers, and they are entitled to expect relevant services, not as an afterthought or when additional resources are made available, but routinely.' (Connelly 1988)

Equal access to services cannot be achieved by ad hoc measures or by individuals working alone. It must be a policy of the organisation, understood and implemented by everyone, and backed up by training and practical support.

Poor take-up of services

If there is poor take-up of a particular service by members of minority communities, it is often assumed that they do not need them, possibly for cultural reasons. However, black and minority ethnic people have largely the same health care needs as white people. If people do not use services, the reasons are more likely to be:

- services are provided in a way that makes them unacceptable and inflexible;
- language barriers and poor general communication;
- negative experiences, not feeling welcome, fear of encountering hostility or racism;
- inadequate information about services, what they are and how to use them;
- fear that service providers will not understand or meet people's needs.

If black and minority ethnic patients and families are alienated or insulted by the treatment they receive, they are less likely to make full use of services when they need them or to benefit fully. They are certainly less likely to trust those caring for them.

How do services need to change?

The services that black and minority ethnic patients and families require are therefore not dramatically different from those of white consumers, nor are they mysterious. The four main areas where improvements are needed are:

- communication
- information
- the adaptation of services to meet religious and cultural needs, and
- the provision of acceptable food (McIver 1994).

Providing different services to different communities on the basis of narrow definitions of their cultures and traditions can simply reinforce stereotypes and is not usually necessary. In most cases, people do not need different services, only services that are organised and offered in a more flexible and responsive way.

'A study comparing Bangladeshi and English women's experiences of maternity care in Tower Hamlets found that the two groups had much the same wishes and complaints.

- **Both groups** wanted more privacy and more explanations during antenatal check-ups, shorter waiting times and a crèche in the antenatal clinic, better preparation for labour and childbirth, more help with looking after the baby, more home visits by community midwives and health visitors, and to be re-housed.
- **In addition**, the Bangladeshi women wanted an interpreter, women doctors, and staff who spoke Bengali. They also wanted to be able to eat with their fingers, to wear saris in hospital, and to observe their religious and cultural

requirements, such as saying prayers and resting after the birth, without being ridiculed.' (Grant 1987)

Where managers and professionals have made efforts to reach out to different groups and develop services in ways that genuinely meet their needs, take-up has often been dramatic (Godfrey 1997, McIver 1994). But unless this happens, members of black and minority communities are unlikely to benefit from services they urgently need and to which they are entitled.

'I had the naive idea that if someone needed help they would come forward. As they were not coming forward I assumed they did not have a problem. We need to help people access services.'
Continence project manager (Godfrey 1997)

Identifying and combating institutional racism

'Focusing attention on black people is not the same as meeting their needs.' (Stubbs 1993)

A great deal has been said and written over the past few decades about equal access, equal opportunities and institutional racism. Many people are fed up with hearing about the subject and think that everything necessary must have been done. But, in reality, remarkably little has changed.

Why is change so difficult?

Change in a complex, hierarchical institution is always slow and difficult, especially when the people in whose interests the change is required – in this case black and minority ethnic patients and their families – have little power and may even be resented. The status quo has a spurious authority and people dislike being asked to change the way they work. It is easier and less risky to go on running things the way they have always been run. Changes that improve provision for black and minority ethnic patients may be considered 'special provision' or 'bending over backwards' rather than part of the normal process of developing services to meet different needs and circumstances as they emerge. But:

'Health authorities are not being asked to do something extra or special. They are simply being asked to make up for existing deficiencies in their service.'
English health education officer

The battle against institutional racism (see Chapter 6) is often hard and time consuming:

- It can be difficult to see precisely how the discrimination is occurring, even when the effects are visible.
- Many of the processes involved are well established and seem neutral.
- The negative emotions and fears aroused by discussion of racism can stop people listening properly and thinking clearly.
- People are often reluctant to see that their own actions, even though unconsciously, may be contributing to discrimination.
- Many people dislike change, especially if they are afraid that it will disadvantage them or make them vulnerable.
- If the culture of the organisation discourages flexibility or is not patient-centred, it can be particularly hard for individual staff to push through changes that will meet patients' needs.
- When the people who are responsible for making the changes are already under extreme pressure running things as they are, it is very difficult for them to take on extra tasks and battles (Cheung-Judge and Henley 1994, Open College 1992).

Careful thought and planning are needed to explain and dismantle discriminatory practices. Good communication is essential: everyone must understand the legal, moral and organisational reasons for change and know what they are trying to achieve. People need practical training as well as information. They also need safe opportunities to talk through their fears and doubts and what the changes will mean for them. When individuals and teams succeed in improving services, their achievements should be acknowledged and celebrated. Mistakes and failures should be accepted and seen as part of the learning process, but this can be difficult if the culture of the organisation discourages risk and if people who make genuine efforts that go wrong are blamed and humiliated. Strong leadership and active support from the top of the organisation are essential (Cheung-Judge and Henley 1994).

Taking individual action against discrimination

The institution and its managers have a major responsibility to tackle racial discrimination but, in order to achieve real and lasting change, action needs to be taken by everyone. Individual efforts make a major difference in day-to-day situations and have a ripple effect. It is up to each one of us to take action and ensure that we are not colluding with discrimination. Start by reviewing attitudes and practices where you work:

- Is there a policy on equal access to services?
- If yes, how is it communicated and put into action? Does it work?
- How aware are you and your colleagues of the possible needs of different minority groups?
- How well do you and your colleagues identify and meet the differing needs of patients and their families?
- What training and information have you received on:
  - the law in relation to racial discrimination?
  - institutional racism and equal access to health services?
  - possible cultural and religious variations in relation to health care needs?
  - health care issues that specifically affect minority groups?
- Is there an equal opportunities in employment policy?
- If yes, how is it communicated? Does it work?
- Is there a policy to deal with racial harassment of staff?
- If yes, how is it communicated? Does it work?

Why are people racially prejudiced?

Discriminatory attitudes and beliefs are a mixture of misinformation and lack of information. Nobody is born with racist attitudes and beliefs. No child acquires racist or other misinformation by his or her own free choice. Prejudices and racist myths and attitudes are passed down the generations and handed on to children, often by the people they most love and trust. Once prejudices are formed, people go on to interpret what they see and hear in the light of those prejudices and so reinforce them. Prejudices and racist beliefs damage white people as well as black, dividing and isolating people from each other on the basis of false information, distorting their understanding of reality, and creating fear, resentment, guilt and hatred.

The situation is not hopeless. People can learn and change, even though the process of learning and changing is often painful. People will usually change their minds about deeply held convictions if:

- **they are not being blamed for having been misinformed;**
- the new idea is presented in a way that makes sense to them;
- they trust the person giving it.

Take some time to think about the following. You may find it helpful to jot down your thoughts and feelings as they surface.

Think back to your childhood.

- What is your earliest memory of hearing about people whose skin colour was different from your own?
- What is your earliest memory of seeing a person with a skin colour different from your own?
- What do you remember about the responses of the people around you?
- How would you like it to have been different?

Recognising that racism exists and how it can affect every aspect of many people's lives and relationships as well as their health can be very painful. We may feel guilty, anxious, powerless and frustrated. We may become overwhelmed by the fear of causing offence or making things worse (McIver 1994). Although each of us is responsible for our own behaviour and for anything we do that perpetuates racism, we are not to blame for historical acts of racism or for racism in our society or social institutions. Guilt-induced paralysis will not help us tackle racism.

How to tackle racism and racial inequality

Tackling racism is difficult and stressful. Many people feel uncertain where to begin. Below are some guidelines. Think through the implications of each for your practice. You may like to discuss them with your colleagues.

Challenge racist remarks and behaviour

'People say it's only harmless fun, but I think they forget that racism isn't about what you intend – it's about the way you make another person feel. I feel very offended when people make racist jokes. I flinch inside.'
South Asian health professional

Many racist remarks and incidents of racist behaviour are inadvertent or unconscious. Others are conscious and intentional. Either way they cause offence and can be very damaging. To assess whether something is offensive, ask yourself whether you would make the same remark, ask an equivalent question or behave in the same way towards a person whom you consider to be the same as yourself. If the answer is no, the remark, question or action is likely to be racist.

Challenging prejudice and discrimination is not easy. Many of us have painful memories of times when we have failed to act in the face of racism, or when we have not achieved as much as we wanted. It is helpful to think about why challenging racism is difficult, and how to do it more effectively, without blaming ourselves or becoming discouraged. It takes time to develop approaches that work, but any action that we take, however small, to counteract discrimination is important and positive.

- Begin by noticing how and when you and other people generalise, make assumptions or act differently towards people because of the group they 'belong' to.
- Then decide to stop and not to collude with other people when they do these things.
- Finally, challenge people firmly and politely when they make assumptions or generalisations or discriminate against patients or colleagues.

Racial discrimination and abuse are unprofessional and unacceptable in the health services. Each of us has a right to our own attitudes but we do not have a right to behave unacceptably or to express our prejudices at work. We have a responsibility to be equally welcoming and responsive to everyone, whatever their colour, religion or ethnic group. If necessary, or if the discriminatory behaviour continues, you may wish to complain to your own manager or to the personnel department. Your employer's equal opportunities policy should support you.

Find out about racism

Solutions begin with understanding the other person's position. Racism has separated black and white people to such an extent that many white health professionals are unaware of the black experience of discrimination and alienation and the effect it can have on people. If you are white, find out more about the reality of racism. Start by reading black and minority ethnic newspapers and magazines. When it seems appropriate, ask black colleagues and patients if they would be prepared to talk about their experiences of racism with you. Most black people have experienced the denial or trivialisation of racism, and have become used to keeping their feelings to themselves. Make it clear that you respect and want to hear their experiences and views. They are the experts on racism and its consequences. Listen with complete respect, do not argue or try to explain anything. Try to accept expressions of anger, resentment and pain without becoming defensive (Levy 1985).

Respect and support black and minority ethnic colleagues

Recognise the special contribution that black and minority ethnic colleagues can make in helping to care for patients whose culture or religion they share, and in helping all staff better understand the needs of such patients. At the same time, black and minority ethnic staff should not be pushed into caring only for people whose backgrounds they share. If there is a language barrier, they should not be routinely used as interpreters rather than as professionals in their own right. Both these are exploitative, undervalue the contribution of black and minority ethnic professionals, and may damage their career progress by limiting the breadth of their experience.

It is also important not to assume that all black and minority ethnic professionals are linguistic or cultural experts simply because of their membership of a minority group. Some, as a result of experiences of racism, may have suppressed or denied their ethnic identity. They may respond to requests for advice and help with hostility or anxiety. A few may be reluctant to identify themselves with a client group against whom their colleagues are clearly prejudiced. Such reactions are understandable. Clear demonstration that black and minority ethnic colleagues are respected and valued in their own right as people and professionals may help to overcome these problems (Tilki, Papadopoulos and Alleyne 1994).

Listen to and support colleagues who experience racial harassment. When appropriate, make it clear to the perpetrators that their behaviour is unacceptable (see also below).

Focus on the actions of institutions rather than individuals, and on outcomes rather than intentions. Make it clear that you realise that people may be acting in good faith but may be unconsciously perpetuating discriminatory practices because of systems set up by the institution. If there are clear disparities in health outcomes or in service use, target these areas and focus on ways to improve results rather than looking for people to blame (Editorial 1999).

Develop a vision of what genuinely equal access services would be like

Take time to work out, with your colleagues, a vision of what care would be like if it were equally accessible and effective for people of all ethnic groups (see also Part Two). Incorporate equal access into the standards you set for your own practice, your ward, department, clinic, unit or team. Make sure that you and your colleagues have the information, training and support you need to deliver such a service.

Push for policies on equal access and equal opportunities throughout your organisation, and for action to implement them. Although individuals can make a difference, it is everybody's responsibility to work towards equality: 'disparities caused unwittingly by organisations can only be eradicated through organisational change' (Editorial 1999). This change must be led and supported by senior management.

> 'Making services more appropriate to the needs of black and ethnic minority patients is not discriminatory, nor is it giving them extra privilege. It is a more effective allocation of resources on the basis of need.' (Baxter 1987)

Become a really effective agent of change

Because you will meet reluctance, hostility and inertia, you need to think strategically about how best to achieve real and lasting change and about the skills and information you need. For example, although aggressive campaigning is effective in politics, it can be counter-productive within an organisation, and can strengthen people's fear and resistance. You need good communication skills and a very clear understanding of the issues in order to argue persuasively and to get people to rethink their attitudes and practices. It is also important in achieving change to listen to other people's arguments with respect even if you do not agree with them (see also Chapter 23 *Listening with complete respect*) (Cheung-Judge and Henley 1994).

Recognise the positive influence you can have as a role model for junior and other staff in challenging discrimination and providing care that meets the needs of all patients.

Organise strong support for yourself both at and outside work. Ensure that you have somewhere to go to let off steam. Be reasonable about what you can achieve in the short term. Celebrate your successes.

Combating racial abuse of staff

Black and minority ethnic health professionals frequently experience racial abuse and other types of racial harassment. One survey found that roughly two-thirds of black and minority ethnic nurses had experienced racial harassment from patients and their families, and more than one-third from colleagues. In a very few cases, white nurses had experienced abuse from black and minority ethnic patients and families (Modood, Berthoud et al 1997).

In many cases it is assumed that staff will tolerate and forgive racial hostility and abuse as part of professional behaviour. Racist abuse from people who are ill and in pain, elderly or mentally ill is often excused on the grounds that normal standards of behaviour no longer apply. Although a few people are genuinely not in control of their behaviour, it is unacceptable as a general policy to excuse abuse on these grounds. Such a policy amounts to collusion with racism.

Racial harassment and abuse towards staff, like physical violence, are unacceptable. Continued experience of racial abuse and hostility is bound to affect black professionals' self-esteem, their relationships with patients, relatives and colleagues, their trust in their managers and the organisation, and their commitment to their work.

All organisations need a clear policy on dealing with racial abuse and hostility towards staff members, whether from patients, families or colleagues. This must be supported by a clear statement which states that rudeness and racist behaviour of any kind will not be tolerated and patients or visitors who are rude or abusive to staff may be refused care or offered limited care. The statement should be widely publicised, for example in patient information booklets, on posters in wards and in public areas. All staff need to understand the reason for the statement and to be able to explain it to patients, families and others when necessary. Health professionals and other staff should be encouraged to report incidents of racist abuse to their managers.

When racist abuse and hostility occur, the people affected and their manager need to discuss together how it should be dealt with. In most cases the perpetrator should be told that their behaviour is unacceptable, the reasons explained if necessary, as well as the action that will be taken if it happens again. In a few cases it may be decided that no action will be taken. This, however, should not be the norm, and should not be confused with ignoring the incident.

Whatever action is taken with regard to the perpetrator, the affected health professional must be supported and their needs discussed and met as far as possible. White colleagues should be encouraged openly to support black and minority ethnic colleagues who experience abuse. Managers need training in dealing sensitively and supportively with such incidents.

References

Ahmad WIU (1996) Family obligations and social change among Asian communities. In WIU Ahmad and K Atkin (eds) *'Race' and Community Care*. Open University Press, Buckingham, pp 51–72

Ahmad WIU (1993) Making black people sick: 'race' ideology and health research. In WIU Ahmad (ed) *'Race' and Health in Contemporary Britain*. Open University Press, Buckingham

Ahmad WIU, Kernohan EEM, Baker MR (1989) Influence of ethnicity and unemployment on the perceived health of a sample of general practice attenders. *Community Medicine* 11 (2): 148–56

Ahmed S (1986) Cultural racism in work with Asian women and girls. In S Ahmed, J Cheetham and J Small (eds) *Social Work with Black Children and their Families*. B T Batsford, London

Amin K (1992) *Poverty in Black and White*. Child Poverty Action Group, London

Atkin K (1992) Black carers – the forgotten people. *Nursing the Elderly* Apr: 8–9

Atkin K, Cameron E, Badger F, Evers H (1989) Asian elders' knowledge and future use of community social and health services. *New Community* 15 (3): 439–46

Ayanian JZ (1993) Heart disease in black and white. *New England Journal of Medicine* 329 (9): 656–7

Bahl V (1996) Cancer and ethnic minorities: the Department of Health's perspective. *British Journal of Cancer* 74 (Suppl 29): S2–S10

Barker J (1984) *Black and Asian Old People in Britain*. Age Concern England, London

Baxter C (1987) Steps to sensitising the service. *Health Service Journal* 4 Jun: 642–3

Beishon S, Virdee S, Hagell A (1995) *Nursing in a Multi-ethnic NHS*. Policy Studies Institute, London

Bhalla A, Blakemore K (1981) *Elders of Minority Ethnic Groups* [out of print]. AFFOR (All Faiths For One Race), Birmingham

Blakemore K, Boneham M (1994) *Age, Race and Ethnicity: A comparative approach.* Open University Press, Buckingham

Bloomsbury Health Authority (1984) *The Health Care Needs of Chinese People in Bloomsbury Health District: The report of a survey.* Bloomsbury Health Authority, London

Boston P (1993) Culture and cancer: the relevance of cultural orientation within cancer education programmes. *European Journal of Cancer Care* 2: 72–6

Bowling B (1990) *Elderly People from Ethnic Minorities: A report on four projects.* Age Concern/Institute of Gerontology, London

Butler RN (1975) *Why Survive being Old in America?* Harper & Row, New York

Cheung-Judge MY, Henley A (1994) *Equality in Action: Introducing equal opportunities in voluntary organisations.* NCVO Publications, London

Connelly N (1988) *Care in the Multiracial Community.* Policy Studies Institute, London

CRE (1993) *The Sorrow in my Heart: Sixteen Asian women speak about depression.* Commission for Racial Equality, London

CRE (1992) *Race Relations Code of Practice in Primary Health Care.* Commission for Racial Equality, London

CRE (1987) *Report of a Formal Investigation into St George's Hospital Medical School.* Commission for Racial Equality, London

CRE (1983) *Ethnic Minority Hospital Staff.* Commission for Racial Equality, London

Creedon J (1995) Vanishing cream for the mind. *New Internationalist* 264: 12–14

Currer C (1986) *Health Concepts and Illness Behaviour: The care of Pathan mothers in Bradford* (unpublished PhD thesis). Department of Sociology, University of Warwick, Warwick

d'Ardenne P, Mahtani A (1989) *Transcultural Counselling in Action.* Sage, London

Department of Health (1993) *Ethnic Minority Staff in the NHS: A programme of action.* HMSO, London

Eastham EA (1985) The ageing notion: a problem for society or created by society? *Health Visitor* 58: 352–4

Editorial (1999) Something borrowed from the blues? *British Medical Journal* 318: 616–17

Esmail A, Carnall D (1997) Tackling racism in the NHS. *British Medical Journal* 314: 618–19

Fenton S (1987) Ethnic minority populations in the United Kingdom. In A Squires (ed) *Multicultural Health Care and Rehabilitation of Older People.* Edward Arnold, London, pp 3–16

Fernando S (1991) *Mental Health, Race and Culture.* Macmillan, London

Fuller D (1995) Challenging ageism through our speech. *Nursing Times* **91** (21): 29–31

Gerrish K, Husband C, Mackenzie J (1996) *Nursing for a Multi-ethnic Society.* Open University Press, Buckingham

Godfrey K (1997) Incontinence in ethnic groups. *Nurse Prescriber* Jun: 42

Godrej D (1994) Race: unlocking prejudice. *New Internationalist* Oct: 4–7

Gordon P (1990) *Racial Violence and Harassment*, revised edn. Runnymede Trust, London

Grant J (1987) Getting it right. *Medicine and Society* **13** (2): 21–5

Green J, Kitzinger JV, Coupland VA (1990) Stereotypes of childbearing women: a look at some evidence. *Midwifery* **6**: 125–32

Grimsley M, Bhat A (1988) Health. In A Bhat et al (ed) *Britain's Black Population: A new perspective.* Gower, London

Hart C (1996) Working against the odds. *Nursing Times* **92** (43): 44–5

HAS 2000 (1998) *'Not Because They are Old': An independent inquiry into the care of older people on acute wards in general hospitals.* Health Advisory Service 2000, London

HEA (1994) *Health and Lifestyles: Black and minority ethnic groups in England.* Health Education Authority, London

Helman C (1994) *Culture, Health and Illness*, 3rd edn. Wright, Bristol

Hicks C (1993) Effects of psychological prejudices on communication and social interaction. *British Journal of Midwifery* **1** (1): 10–16

Hill D, Penso D (1995) *Opening Doors: Improving access to hospice and specialist palliative care services by members of the black and ethnic minority communities.* National Council for Hospice and Specialist Palliative Care Services, London

Hillier S (1991) The health and health care of ethnic minority groups. In G Scambler (ed) *Sociology as Applied to Medicine.* Bailliere Tindall, London

Hoecklin LA (1993) *Managing Cultural Differences for Competitive Advantage.* The *Economist* Intelligence Unit, London

Hofstede G (1991) *Cultures and Organisations – Software of the mind.* McGraw-Hill, London

Joseph Rowntree Foundation (1995) *Income and Wealth.* Joseph Rowntree Foundation, York

Karseras PA (1991) Health care for minorities. 2. Improving services. *Care of the Elderly* Nov: 468–70

Kearl MC (1989) *Endings: A sociology of death and dying.* Open University, Buckingham

Klug F, Gordon P (1983) *Different Worlds: Racism and discrimination in Britain.* Runnymede Trust, London

Levy DR (1985) White doctors and black patients: influence of race on the doctor patient relationship. *Pediatrics* 75 (4): 639–43

Macpherson W (1999) *Stephen Lawrence Inquiry.* Stationery Office, London

Mares P, Henley A, Baxter C (1985) *Health Care in Multiracial Britain.* National Extension College, Cambridge

Marr J, Kadim N (1993) Meeting the needs of ethnic patients. *Nursing Standard* 8 (3): 31–3

Masi R (1992) Communication: cross-cultural applications of the physician's art. *Canadian Family Physician* May: 1159–65

McIver S (1994) *Obtaining the Views of Black Users of Health Services.* King's Fund, London

McKenzie KJ, Crowcroft NS (1994) Race, ethnicity, culture and science. *British Medical Journal* 309: 286

McNaught A (1985) *Race and Health Care in the United Kingdom.* Health Education Council, London

Modood T (1990) Colour, class and culture: the three Cs of race. *Equal Opportunities Review* 30: 31–3

Modood T, Beishon S, Virdee S (1994) *Changing Ethnic Identities.* Policy Studies Institute, London

Modood T, Berthoud R, Lakey J, Nazroo J, Smith P, Virdee S, Beishon S (1997) *Ethnic Minorities in Britain: Diversity and disadvantage.* Policy Studies Institute, London

Mohammed S (1991) Improving health services for black populations. *Share Newsletter* 1: 1–3

Murphy K, Macleod Clark J (1993) Nurses' experience of caring for ethnic minority clients. *Journal of Advanced Nursing* 18: 442–50

NACAB (1991) *Barriers to Benefit: Black claimants and Social Security.* National Association of Citizens Advice Bureaux, London

NAHAT (1988) *Action Not Words: A strategy to improve health services for black and ethnic minority groups.* National Association of Health Authorities and Trusts, Birmingham

Nazarko L (1996) Power to the people. *Nursing Times* **92** (41): 48–9

Norman A (1985) *Triple Jeopardy: Growing old in a second homeland.* Centre for Policy on Ageing (Age Concern England), London

O'Neill A (1992) Cultural issues in palliative care. *European Journal of Palliative Care* **2** (3): 127–31

OPCS (1993) 1991 *Census: Ethnic group and country of birth – Great Britain* (CEN 91 TM EGCB). Office of Population Censuses and Surveys, London

Open College (1992) *Managing in Diversity: Understanding discrimination.* Open College, Manchester

Papadopoulos I, Worral L (1996) *An Examination of the Primary Health Care Needs of the Greek and Greek Cypriot Women.* Greek and Greek Cypriot Women of Enfield, London

Parsons L, Macfarlane A, Golding J (1993) Pregnancy, birth and maternity care. In WIU Ahmad (ed) *'Race' and Health in Contemporary Britain.* Open University Press, Buckingham

Payer L (1989) *Medicine and Culture: Varieties of treatment in the United States, England, West Germany and France.* Victor Gollancz, London

Pfeffer N (1998) Theories of race, ethnicity and culture. *British Medical Journal* **317**: 1391–84

Pinker S (1994) *The Language Instinct.* Penguin, London

Rack P (1991) *Race, Culture and Mental Disorder*, 2nd edn. Routledge, London

RCN (1996) *The Value and Skills of Nurses Working with Older People.* Royal College of Nursing, London

Redfern S (1991) The elderly person: the challenge of an aged society. In S Redfern (ed) *Nursing Elderly People*, 2nd edn. Churchill Livingstone, London

Roberts C (1985) *The Interview Game and How it's Played.* BBC Publications, London

Roberts C (1977) *Asians in Kenya and Tanzania with Reference to Immigration to Britain* [out of print]. National Centre for Industrial Language Training, Southall, Middlesex

Runnymede Trust (1994) *Multi-ethnic Britain: Facts and trends*. Runnymede Trust, London

Sarre P, Philips D, Skellington R (1989) *Ethnic Minority Housing: Explanations and policy*. Avebury, Aldershot

Schott J, Henley A (1992) *Breaking the Barriers: A training package on equal access to maternity services*. Obstetric Hospital, University College London Hospitals NHS Trust, London

Seelye HN (1993) *Teaching Culture: Strategies for intercultural communication*. National Textbook Co, Lincolnwood, Illinois

Senior PA, Bhopal R (1994) Ethnicity as a variable in epidemiological research. *British Medical Journal* **309**: 327–30

Sheldon T, Parker H (1992) The use of 'ethnicity' and 'race' in health research: a cautionary note. In WIU Ahmad (ed) *The Politics of 'Race' and Health*. Race Relations Research Unit, University of Bradford, Bradford, pp 53–80

Sheldon T, Parker H (1991) Ethnicity and race – a cautionary note. *Share Newsletter* 1: 3–4; King's Fund, London

Smaje C (1995) *Health, 'Race' and Ethnicity: Making sense of the evidence*. King's Fund, London

Spencer S (1994) *Strangers and Citizens: A positive approach to migrants and refugees*. Institute for Public Policy Research/Rivers Oram, London

Stevenson O (1989) *Age and Vulnerability: A guide to better care*. Edward Arnold, London

Stubbs P (1993) 'Ethnically sensitive' or 'anti-racist'? Models for health research and service delivery. In WIU Ahmad (ed) *'Race' and Health in Contemporary Britain*. Open University Press, Buckingham

Tilki M (1994) Ethnic Irish older people. *British Journal of Nursing* **3** (17): 909–13

Tilki M, Papadopoulos I, Alleyne J (1994) Learning from colleagues of different cultures. *British Journal of Nursing* **3** (21): 1118–24

Townsend P, Davidson N, Whitehead M (eds) (1988) *Inequalities in Health*. Penguin, London

Trompenaars F (1993) *Riding the Waves of Culture – Understanding cultural diversity in business*. Nicholas Brealey, London

Walker A (1990) The benefits of old age? In E McEwen (ed) *Age: The unrecognised discrimination*. Age Concern England, London, pp 59–70

Walmsley J (1986) *Brit-think, Ameri-think: A transatlantic survival guide*. Harrap, Edinburgh

Ward L (1993) Race equality and employment in the National Health Service. In WIU Ahmad (ed) *'Race' and Health in Contemporary Britain*. Open University Press, Buckingham

Wassim D (1991) Walthamstow Asian elderly concern: an example of a self-help group. In A Squires (ed) *Multicultural Health Care and Rehabilitation of Older People*. Edward Arnold, London, pp 55–8

Wilkinson RG (1997) Health inequalities: relative or absolute material standards? *British Medical Journal* **314**: 591–5

Williams PJ (1997) *Seeing a Colour-blind Future: The 1997 Reith Lectures*. Virago, London

PART TWO
Providing Care in a Multi-ethnic Society

Introduction: preparing to meet people's needs

Serious illness or advancing age inevitably brings loss of autonomy, dignity and independence. A person who becomes ill or dependent is forced to make tremendous practical and emotional adjustments. It is unreasonable and unrealistic to expect them to abandon their culture and religion as well. Indeed, for their own emotional stability and mental health it is important that they do not (Rack 1991, Furnham and Bochner 1986).

> 'Culture is not like a coat. You cannot take off your own culture when you leave your country and put on someone else's. Culture is woven into each of us as into a piece of cloth. If we pull out and discard the vital threads of culture, the whole cloth falls apart.'
> English researcher

Reducing the stress of the unfamiliar and the strange is also important from a medical point of view. Stress can impair healing and lower pain thresholds (Melzak and Wall 1996, Kiecolt-Glaser, Marucha et al 1995). It is therefore important to recognise and try to minimise the added stress likely to be experienced when patients are cared for by people who do not share or understand their culture or, in some cases, their language. Everything possible should be done to help individuals continue to maintain their normal way of doing things, based on their personal, cultural and religious values.

Note In this book the term 'English' is used rather than 'British' when discussing the majority culture (see Chapter 1 *Culture as part of our identity*).

Collecting facts

Once we have accepted the importance of culture and religion, it is tempting to try to solve the problem by learning a few facts about different communities and then applying them. However, this approach has serious flaws. It assumes that people can be neatly and predictably divided into groups, and that we can then predict individual needs on the basis of group membership. It encourages us to stereotype individuals and to ignore the huge range of differences that exist within any 'group' or 'community' (see also Chapter 2).

> 'Africa consists of approximately 11½ million square miles inhabited by about 630 million people – roughly 12 per cent of the world's population – who speak over 1,000 languages. Africa contains 52 independent countries, many of which are further divided into smaller regions with different languages, tribal groupings and religions. Yet we often talk about Africans as if they are a single uniform group, and "African culture" as though it was homogeneous.'
> Lecturer

If you are a member of a minority group, you will probably know what it feels like to be categorised. If you are a member of the majority, think for a moment what it would be like to be labelled 'European' and to have nurses and doctors assume that they know what food you prefer, your religious and spiritual needs, how your family works, and what your requirements and wishes are when you are ill, and do not need to ask you.

A *new way of thinking and working*

None of us likes to be categorised or have assumptions made about us. Categorisations and assumptions do not help health professionals meet people's individual needs. This section of the book offers a different approach. It offers you an opportunity to consider different important aspects of daily life and clinical care, and, in relation to each:

- reflect on your own assumptions and values;
- consider possible variations in people's needs and values;
- identify the implications of these variations for your day-to-day practice.

Reflections Whether we are aware of them or not, our own attitudes and beliefs profoundly affect the way we perceive and react to other people, particularly those whose lifestyles or beliefs differ from our own. Before we can hear and respond positively to others, we need to identify what we feel and believe and how this affects our judgements and attitudes. The reflections in this book are intended to help you with this process and to give you opportunities to think things through, away from the time constraints and pressures of daily work.

The reflections can be used to best advantage in discussion with a trusted friend or colleague, if possible someone of a background different from your own. You will need time and privacy. Take equal turns to listen to each other with complete attention and respect. Agree that everything you say will be in complete confidence so that you can both say what you really think and feel. Listen without interrupting, and discuss respectfully and without arguing. Pay attention to the **differences** between you as well as to the similarities. Although it is often easier to listen to someone who shares our views, it is the differences from which we can often learn the most.

If it is not realistic for you to set up such a dialogue, you can still gain a great deal from thinking through the reflections on your own. Be sure to articulate your thoughts clearly to yourself – do not be satisfied with a general sense of your reaction. You may find it helpful to write things down and also to discuss the ideas less formally with colleagues and friends at a convenient time.

8 Identifying people's needs and beliefs

People who are ill, frail or approaching death often have similar feelings and concerns. But each is also an individual with different needs that may be influenced by a range of factors, including their culture, spiritual and religious beliefs, family background and personal experience. When these are very different from our own, it is easy to feel uncertain and inadequate about how to give the best care.

Provided it is accurate, general information about different cultures and religions is useful in highlighting those things that **may** be important. But it tells us little about the individual in front of us. To find out what **this person** needs, we must combine sound general information with open, respectful questions. We must also be committed to trying to respond flexibly and constructively (Alladin 1992).

Asking the patient

'The patient teaches, the care-giver learns.'
Canadian nurse lecturer

The only person who can tell you what will or will not be right for them is the patient. If we really want to find out, we have to ask. This can be surprisingly hard, especially for those of us trained in the tradition of the 'all-knowing professional expert' who should always know what to do and have all the answers. Although we may accept intellectually the idea of patient-centred care – asking about and responding to patient's needs and wishes – old messages can be powerful. Asking may feel like failure, not being a 'good enough' health professional. It also affects the balance of power between you.

'The view that it is enough … to go armed with details of people's culture also suggests a top–down approach … This approach assumes that the health professional has knowledge (including knowledge about people's way of life) and that this knowledge allows the health professional to meet clients' needs. A different approach, starting with the client, would place the professional in the humbler position of learning from the client.' (Foster 1988)

- What messages did you absorb during your training or education about asking people about their needs and wishes?
- How do you really feel about asking patients what they want and need?
- How does asking change the relationship between you? How do you feel about this?
- How readily do you ask?
- If you tend not to ask, what gets in the way?
- How easy do you find it to listen to, and act on, the answers you get?

Even when we ask, we are bound to get things wrong now and then (though less often than if we don't ask!). We may overestimate or underestimate the importance of something. We may find it hard to frame the right questions. Our most tactful and respectful enquiries may be misunderstood, give offence or not produce the necessary answers. Asking requires courage, but unless we take the risk we will never find out what people really need.

Asking effective questions

Simply asking does not always elicit a useful response.

Imagine that you are taken to hospital in Mogadishu, the capital of Somalia. A health professional asks you, with the best of intentions, 'What do you need while you are in hospital?'.

- What would you say?
- How might you feel?
- What assumptions are you making about the system of care in Mogadishu?
- On what do you base these assumptions?

To give a useful answer to this question, you need to know quite a lot about the system of care in Mogadishu; for example, what sort of treatment you will be given, what the facilities are, what the food is like, when visitors can come and what role they are expected to play, how soon you will be expected to go home. Only then can you begin to decide what is important to you.

When people have to make decisions in an unfamiliar situation, it is often helpful to explain what usually happens, and why, so that they can work out what will or will not suit them. They may sometimes want to consult other people, for example family members, friends or religious leaders, before deciding.

Table 8.1 lists aspects of daily life and clinical care that may be influenced by culture and religion, and which you might like to bear in mind when discussing people's needs. It is not a checklist to be plodded through routinely, but a framework to help your own thinking. The areas listed may be relevant to anyone, whatever their situation, background and spiritual beliefs, not only to people of minority cultures or religions. Each person will have different priorities. With their agreement, record in the notes anything specially important for your colleagues.

Good places to begin discussion

There is a skill to timing and framing questions sensitively and appropriately. Certain topics are more likely to offer useful starting points for discussion. For example, when a person gives their religion, you could ask if they have any special requirements (such as privacy to pray at certain times) (see Chapter 10 *Practical matters*). Another useful starting point for most people, whatever their culture or religion, is dietary needs and preferences. The answers to these questions often indicate other issues to discuss. The way the patient and their family dress may also indicate possible cultural or religious needs and useful questions.

'It is tempting to see the admission procedure as the filling of a form, whereas it should be the using of that form to get to know the person better and to allow the person to express something of [their] individuality as well as [their] needs. It is also the time to show that the patient is going to be given choices and given back some control.' (Phillips 1991)

Do you need to explain why you are asking?

Try to build up a respectful and trusting relationship before you start asking questions about things that may be sensitive. 'Routine' questions are often intrusive and embarrassing, especially to people for whom modesty is a cultural or religious requirement (see Chapter 12). Some people may perceive certain questions as racist or as questioning their right to be in the UK (see also Chapters 13 *Different expectations and concerns* and *23 Mutual mistrust*). Some people are cautious or defensive about discussing with outsiders their culture, religion and other things that matter to them; they may have been misunderstood, distorted or criticised in the past. Some people

Table 8.1 Aspects of daily living and medical care

Daily life	Clinical care
Personal history and heritage	History and examination
	Investigations and treatment
Family structure	Symptom control
Family relationships	
Attitudes towards elders	Informed consent
Naming systems, forms of address	Confidentiality
	Telling the truth
Religious beliefs and practices	Giving bad news
Prayer	
Rituals and ceremonies	Place of care/place of death
Role of religious leaders	Role of relatives in caring
Religious festivals	The needs of relatives and close friends
Concepts of good and bad luck	
Spiritual beliefs and needs	Attitudes to death and dying
	Care around the time of death
Food	Expressing emotions
Fasting	
	Resuscitation
Clothing	Euthanasia
Modesty and privacy	Organ donation
Body space, politeness	Sudden death
Jewellery	
Make-up	Care of the body
Washing and elimination	Preparing the body for the funeral
Skin and hair care	Visiting the body
Concepts of cleanliness and pollution	Post mortems
	Referral to the coroner
	Taking the body home
	Patient's property
	Certificates and registering the death
	Repatriating the body
	Funerals
	Bereavement and grieving
	Attitudes to Western medicine
	Other medical systems

may be irritated or sceptical because they have been asked many times about their needs and nothing has ever been done to meet them.

Understanding the answers: our own assumptions and values

When people express very different values or wishes from our own, it can be hard to respond positively and respectfully. It is useful to consider the basis of our assumptions about what is 'normal' or 'reasonable', because on most issues we judge other people in relation to ourselves.

Consider **washing**, for example, and how we regard people with different habits. At one end of the spectrum below are people who shower or bathe three times a day and those who wash before each of five daily prayers. At the other end are people who wash once a week or less.

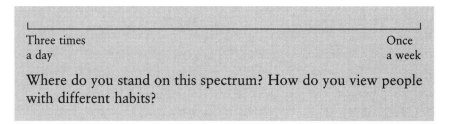

Three times
a day

Once
a week

Where do you stand on this spectrum? How do you view people with different habits?

Many people consider that those who wash less frequently than they do are dirty, and those who wash more often are obsessional. Such judgements are often unconscious and rarely rational, but they can powerfully affect our attitudes towards people whose habits and beliefs differ from our own (see Chapter 2). You may find it helpful to look again at Table 8.1 above and consider your own values and assumptions in relation to each.

Managing negative reactions

Occasionally people's choices and behaviour arouse strong negative reactions in us. It can be hard to accept values that are completely opposed to our own. It is also difficult when people's lifestyles and decisions conflict with what we consider healthy or safe, or even legal. How do we continue to provide responsive and responsible care, and at the same time deal with our own views and feelings?

Each of us finds certain things particularly threatening or hard to deal with. Our reactions are influenced by our own culture, heritage and religious or spiritual beliefs. It may upset us to work with families in which women are subservient and all decisions are taken by men. Some health professionals find it hard when relatives pressure them not to tell a patient the truth. Others are horrified and angry at the possibility of a patient refusing a life-saving intervention such as a blood transfusion.

> 'The idea that I might have to stand by and watch a patient die unnecessarily from a haemorrhage because they refused a blood transfusion is horrific. I don't know how I'd cope. I just hope it never happens.'
> Health professional

Health professionals are responsible for providing respectful care, for meeting patients' personal, cultural and religious needs, for informing and educating on health issues, and for enabling patients to make their own choices. They also have a duty to respect the choices that patients make. We are all entitled to hold personal views, but not to impose them. The indiscriminate expression of feelings such as anger, distress, shock, disapproval or horror, even if justified, usually makes things worse.

Separating out our professional responsibility and personal beliefs is hard, especially when our thinking is clouded by strong emotion. We need to find ways of dealing with negative feelings constructively and safely and to choose carefully where, when and with whom we do this.

- It is inappropriate and always unhelpful to let off steam anywhere near the patient or family involved.
- It is also unwise to let off steam with someone who shares the patient's heritage or values, because this can cause anger and conflict and ruin relationships.

> 'I get fed up when colleagues complain to me about Jewish patients. They seem to think that because I am Jewish I am a good person to talk to. But all that happens is that I feel embarrassed, helpless, defensive and resentful. Sometimes they are just prejudiced and stereotyping but, even when their complaints are justified, nobody benefits.'
> Jewish nurse

Be aware that you may not always know about a person's history, heritage or religious beliefs. Err on the side of caution when choosing whom to talk to.

- Make sure that you are not judging a whole group by the attitudes of a few. Every society has its strengths and weaknesses; every society contains different kinds of people, good and bad, easy and difficult. If you don't understand, it is usually better to ask questions than to make judgements or negative remarks.

- In general, avoid letting off steam to other people who are caring for the same patient. You risk generating additional negative feelings towards that patient or their family.
- Avoid people whom you know are prejudiced and negative. Your story is likely to increase their prejudice and is unlikely to help you deal constructively with your feelings. Later on, you may feel that you have made things worse.
- Instead, find someone whom you can trust and who can take time to listen to you in private.

Finding a good listener

The best listener in this situation is someone who understands that:

- they just need to listen with relaxed interest and to remain supportive and objective;
- their own opinions and experiences are not necessarily helpful;
- you need to have your feelings acknowledged and that you need to let off steam to someone;
- what you say and how you say it is not necessarily rational, and afterwards you may take a different view;
- everything you say must remain completely confidential.

Reflecting

Once you have had a chance to express your feelings to a good listener, you are more likely to be able to think clearly and to sort out your professional role and responsibilities. You can then work out how to handle similar situations in future. In doing so it may be helpful to reflect on the following:

- Your own accepted practice and belief, and the validity of established routines and advice. Can you be sure that you are right and the patient is not?

  'They wanted to put the body on the floor and stay with it until it was collected later that day. I was shocked by this, but when I thought about it, there really wasn't a good reason why they shouldn't. It's just not what we normally do or consider right. But it isn't wrong either. So we found a room in the mortuary that they could use.'
  English staff nurse

- The fact that people are unlikely to change their values and beliefs, especially when they feel criticised or under pressure.

- The possibility that your cultural or organisational values and practices are also causing conflict and distress to patients and their families. We are often unaware of the profound effects of our 'normal' practices and routines (see the rest of Part Two).

In the end, health professionals have to accept and accommodate other people's beliefs and decisions, provided they are within the law. It may help to understand the context and origins of other people's beliefs and practices, though sometimes we cannot find out. Occasionally nothing helps. All we can do is deal with our feelings away from the patient or family and make a conscious effort not to stereotype or react negatively towards people of that 'group' in the future. It can also be helpful to have regular time aside with colleagues or your supervisor to talk about troubling or upsetting incidents and to gain mutual support and different perspectives.

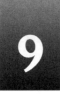

9 Family history, cultural heritage, names and family relationships

Family history and cultural heritage

Our family history and our cultural heritage – the circumstances in which we were brought up, our parents' way of life, values and beliefs – shape much of who we are, what we believe and how we live. We are also to some extent affected by the lives and values of our grandparents and even of our great-grandparents.

> Take a moment to reflect on your own family history and cultural heritage and how they have influenced you.
>
> - How have your birthplace and upbringing shaped your current attitudes and beliefs?
> - How much of your parents' values and beliefs do you share? What have you rejected or adapted?
> - If you or your parents were born outside the UK, how has this influenced you?
> - If your grandparents were born and live(d) outside the UK, how has this influenced you?
> - What aspects of your family history and cultural heritage are most important to you? Are there times when they become particularly important?

Implications for care

Unless we have a long-term relationship with a patient, we usually meet them only at a time of crisis. We see a snapshot, a stressful moment in an often long and complex life. Learning something about a patient's family history and cultural heritage can help us understand them better and offer more appropriate support and care.

This is especially important with people whose life experience and culture are very different from our own. Rather than simply assuming that they will be comfortable with our systems and routines, we can help them maintain their customary ways of doing things as far as possible. We may also come to understand and sympathise with behaviour that we might otherwise ignore, or dismiss as irrational or downright difficult.

> 'My mother lived through pogroms in Poland in her childhood before emigrating to Manchester where I was born and brought up. Towards the end of her life she became increasingly confused and would sometimes wake with a start from her afternoon nap and call out in a terrified whisper, "Quickly, quickly, draw the blinds, the Cossacks are coming to get us!"'
> Jewish man

Names

Most of us feel strongly about our name. It is part of our identity, often reflecting our family history or religion. It is important that people get our name right and that they pronounce and spell it correctly.

- How do you feel about your personal name(s) and your family name?
- Who chose your personal name(s) and why?
- Does your name reflect your origins or religion?
- How do you feel when people pronounce your name incorrectly or change or shorten it?
- How do you feel when someone you do not know addresses you by your personal name?

Politeness The way people address each other indicates their relationship. In English culture using personal names usually implies a degree of informality and intimacy. Title plus family name is more formal. Expectations vary between age groups. Even in English culture, a younger person (including a health professional) who addresses an older person by their personal name may be considered disrespectful rather than friendly and may cause offence. Terms such as 'duck', 'love' and 'sweetie' are also usually inappropriate.

Beatrice Matthews waited for some time in a packed Outpatients Department. At last a young nurse called out 'Beatrice'. Mrs Matthews was so affronted by being addressed in this way by a complete stranger barely out of her teens that she did not reply and the nurse went away. Hours later she was the only person left in the waiting room and someone asked her what she was doing there. By this time, the doctors had gone so she left without being seen.

In most minority cultures it is important to show respect for older people and parents by addressing them formally. Personal names may be used only by relatives and close friends. Other people may always use formal address or a phrase indicating the relationship, such as Aunty or Older Brother, even though they have known each other well for decades. In South Asian Muslim communities, a man's first name is often a religious name and is never used alone. In some Nigerian families, first names are not used to address or refer to older family members.

It is clearly very important to find out how each patient would like to be addressed and to indicate this in their notes. In general, it is most accept-able to use Mr or Mrs plus the full name or the last name until you have been able to check. (However, with people of Nigerian heritage including the first name may cause offence.) (For more about different naming sys-tems and how to record and use names correctly, see Chapter 30.)

Assumptions In Britain people commonly talk about Christian names and surnames. The assumption that everyone is Christian and has a surname is also reflected in many forms and databases. This is both inappropriate and can lead to confusion (see Chapter 30).

Families, relationships and roles

Although the idea and the underlying principles of the family are universal, what is meant by 'the family' varies enormously from culture to culture and within cultures. The late twentieth century saw tremendous changes in the family in Britain and there are now great variations. The roles of men and women are generally less differentiated. Many women are more autonomous and independent. Long-term unemployment has removed from many men the traditional role of breadwinner. Most adult women now work outside the home. In some families women are the main earners and are less able to care for ill or frail family members. The number of single-parent families is increasing. As more people re-marry or form second long-term relationships, more complex families are forming (see Chapter 2 *Not cultural facts but cultural possibilities*).

'When I came here from Ireland I found the strangest thing was all the divorce. My husband's parents had split up and both re-married and had more children of their own. And they were all part of his family and they all seemed to get on quite well. I was astonished!'
Irish woman

Despite these changes, many people in Britain still view the nuclear family – a married couple with children – as the norm against which they judge other families. Many English people have little contact with any relatives outside their nuclear family. Most feel that a married couple should be financially and emotionally independent of their parents and other relatives. Marriage does not usually create an alliance between two families; the husband's and wife's parents may never really get to know each other. Older people often expect, and are expected, to be independent for as long as possible.

In order to make an appropriate assessment of each patient's needs and to plan and provide care, it is necessary to understand their family situation, including the responsibilities and expectations of different members.

Take a moment to reflect on your own views about families.

- How important is your family to you? Every day? When major life events occur?
- What do you think of as a family? How many people? How many generations?
- Which do you think is the most important relationship in the family?
- In your family do men and women have different roles and responsibilities?
- Who do you feel has the right to give advice to whom in a family?
- Whom would you turn to if you were seriously ill? How would you expect them to respond?
- Do you feel closer to your family or to some of your friends?
- At what age or stage in their lives do you feel that people should stand on their own feet and be independent of their families?
- Whom should a person involve in decisions about their marriage or relationship?
- Who has ultimate authority over you?
- Does your reputation affect your family? Does this influence your behaviour?
- Do you expect to live with your children when you are old?

Different families

Ideas about how families should function and how they should support and care for sick or frail members vary from culture to culture. For example:

Family involvement In many communities the normal family is extended rather than nuclear. A large number of relatives may be concerned about the patient and actively involved in their care. Parents, for example, may be very closely involved with their adult children all their lives, in a way that many Westerners find strange. This has implications for confidentiality and patient autonomy (see Chapters 15 *Maintaining patient confidentiality* and 17 *Working together*).

> 'My son is 35 and has been very sick. I always go with him to the hospital. He prefers it and I want to be there. The last doctor was very rude and told me to leave. He said I was a problem for my son, my son is an adult and I should let him lead his own life. He said I had no right to be there. I was shocked. Does he not understand the way a mother feels?'
> Greek Cypriot woman

In many cultures people always turn to family members for practical help, support and advice. Some may feel that they would lose face or be considered strange or disloyal if they asked for outside help, even from health professionals. Some see health professionals as having responsibility for practical and physical things, but not as people with whom to discuss feelings.

> 'I have my own feelings and they are private. I don't want to discuss them with other people, especially strangers. It's not the way I was brought up.'
> Elderly Swedish woman

Sometimes the people closest to the patient are not members of their legal family. They need the same sensitive care and recognition as blood relations. (In this book the words family and friends are used to mean all those people who are close to the patient.)

Decision making In some cultures each person is seen as an autonomous individual who makes their own decisions; in others, each individual is part of a family group. It is expected that decisions will be made by the whole family, taking their joint perspectives into account.

> 'After some years abroad, I discussed my next steps with my family in Pakistan. We argued fiercely and I suddenly blurted out, "Look, it's **my** life, I will do what I think is right for me". They were shocked and horrified. My eldest brother asked for how long it had been "my life". When had I started to make such egoistic decisions? They were very hurt. There were several difficult discussions

after that. And the remark, "It's my life" is still used in our family, part jokingly, part sarcastically and part incredulously.'
Pakistani engineer

Authority In many cultures there is a hierarchy of authority in the family. Older people, and especially men, have great authority in the family and may make all major decisions. Younger women may be expected to defer to older women. Again this can have implications for decision making, consent and confidentiality.

In such families the person who makes many of the decisions may not be the person who carries them out. The daughter-in-law married to a younger son may be the primary 'hands on' care giver for ageing parents, but decisions about their care may be taken by the oldest son even if he has little first-hand knowledge of the situation (Van Steenberg, Ansak and Chin-Hansen 1993). Health professionals may need to work sensitively with both.

In families where the oldest man is head and has always made all the decisions and dealt with the finances, serious problems may arise if he becomes ill or incapacitated. Family members may be unsure how to react and what steps to take if he is confused or demented and behaves strangely or irrationally (Patel, Mirza et al 1998).

Men and women In some communities men and women have clearly differentiated roles and may lead largely segregated lives. Some people are unused to dealing with strangers of the opposite sex or to receiving intimate care or treatment from them (see also Chapter 12 *Modesty*).

Women in conservative families who rarely leave their homes may find being in or visiting hospital or other residential care particularly difficult. If their husband dies, they may have great difficulty in dealing alone with certifying the death, making funeral arrangements, and financial and other practical matters. If there are no male relatives who can help, special help and support may be needed.

In the West, monogamy is generally regarded as the only acceptable form of marriage. Polygamy is often seen as degrading to women. Under Islamic law, men can take up to four wives under certain conditions (see Chapter 44 *Polygamy*). In certain areas of Africa, polygamy is common among people of all religions. In cultures where polygamy is accepted, there are often recognised advantages for women. Wives usually support each other, especially at times of illness and difficulty. The first wife is regarded as senior; existing wives must normally agree before their husband can marry again.

Reputation In some cultures the behaviour of any one member affects the reputation and prospects of the whole extended family. Codes of correct behaviour may be strictly enforced for the sake of all the family members. Discreet behaviour and modesty may be particularly expected of women (see also Chapter 12 *Modesty*).

Public behaviour varies between and within cultures. In some cultures it is traditional for men to do all the talking outside the home. In some cultures it is considered that all private matters should be kept within the family. Some families are very formal in public and so can appear silent and unsupportive. In some cultures it is customary for everyone to be physically affectionate in public, in others public affection is shown only by family members of the same sex, in others not at all.

Care for older people and people who are ill In many communities older people are traditionally looked after entirely within their family. Everyone is expected to show them respect and to defer to them even when they become ill and frail. Families in Britain may feel an obligation to provide all the support for dependent older members, even where this is not possible. Some may feel extremely anxious about the care of their relative away from home. Some older people may feel ashamed and publicly humiliated because they are not being cared for by their own family (see also Chapters 4 *Black and minority ethnic older people* and 16 *Care at home*).

Acceptable behaviour when people are ill and the amount of sympathy and support they receive also vary between cultures and between families.

'If somebody's sick back home he's allowed to tell everybody, to express his illness; everybody will feel sorry for him, even if it's quite a small thing; everybody will come round and look after him and sympathise. But here you're encouraged to get better, stand on your own feet, put on a brave face, even if you've had major heart surgery. Doctors and nurses are not much liked at home. They are often seen as cruel and unfeeling and too direct. Sometimes I wonder if it is because many of them are trained by Westerners and their training doesn't fit in with our culture.'
Eritrean nurse

Family conflict Every family system has its strengths and its tensions. Family difficulties, unhappiness and conflict occur in all cultures, though how they are expressed and dealt with may differ. Differences in values and religious beliefs often cause distress and strife in families, especially when a member is seriously ill or dying. Friction may be more likely when some family members hold more traditional views or are more conservative than others, or when families contain members of different religions and heritages.

Health professionals often see people in crisis; it can be difficult to sort out how different a person's current behaviour is from what is accepted within their community, what their strengths are, and what support is available to them. **When working across cultures, there is also a danger that negative stereotypical images about people's family organisation and behaviour, derived from moments of stress and difficulty, will become the basis for everyday 'knowledge' about their community** (Arnold 1992).

10 Religious beliefs and practices

'For many members of the ethnic minorities, their faith, and their personal identity through their faith, and the reaction of the rest of society to that faith and to them as belonging to it are of the utmost importance. Indeed, for many, identity through faith will be more important from day to day than identity through national origins.' (CRE 1991)

The influence of religion on people's lives varies a good deal and cannot be predicted. Religion may provide essential meaning, spiritual support and moral guidance throughout a person's life, it may influence practical aspects of their daily life, or it may be only a mark of community membership. In the health service, however, a patient's religion is often noted and then disregarded; an important opportunity to find out more about their individual religious and spiritual needs and wishes is lost.

Asking a person's religion, and knowing something about the beliefs and practices of different religions (see, for example, the chapters on religions in Part Five), are good foundations for identifying possible needs, but they are only starting points. One 'Church of England' patient could be deeply religious, want to see the chaplain and to receive communion; another might have been christened but not attended church since childhood. A Jew who is not at all religious may reply 'Jewish' purely in order not to be identified as Christian. A Jain may reply 'Hindu' because they know that few people in Britain have heard of Jainism. A patient who gives no religion may nevertheless have strong moral and ethical values, a sustaining spiritual dimension to their lives, and possibly a firm belief in an afterlife. The only way to find out what is important to each person in terms of religious practice and what they will need in order to be comfortable is to ask (see also Chapter 23 *Listening with complete respect*).

Religious beliefs, values and decisions

Most people with a strong religious faith have a set of beliefs and values that are woven into the fabric of their lives. These influence their views and reactions, and the meaning that they ascribe to what happens to them. People's beliefs also determine their priorities and underlie many of their decisions.

> Consider the following statements of belief.
>
> - This life is a preparation and a test, however hard it may sometimes be, for eternal life in the next world.
> - Everything that happens is God's* will and part of His plan. It is our duty to accept it and to trust Him.
> - You've only got one life and there's nothing more. When you die that's the end.
> - This is just one life in a cycle of many, during which we work through the consequences of our past and determine our future.
> - There are evil spiritual influences in the world and we need to take steps to protect ourselves and those we love from them. There are also good spiritual influences whose power and protection we can call on.
>
> Think about how each of these beliefs might affect your attitude to life in general. How might each of them affect your attitude to:
>
> - serious illness?
> - the causes of illness?
> - symptom control?
> - continuing treatment when there is little hope of recovery?
> - dying?

A strong religious faith can be a great source of comfort and strength when life is difficult. It can give meaning to hardship, suffering and tragedy. It can give people purpose, courage and hope. For many religious people, faith and acceptance of the power of God's will, sometimes called fatalism, helps them get on with their lives and cope with things as they happen (Donovan 1986).

---

* We have used the English word God in most of this book. People of different faiths and speaking different languages will each use their own word (see also Part Five).

'My mother-in-law was 102. She felt that the time had come to die and go to God. She was quite ready, she spent her time reading the Bible and praying. She was happy and she radiated faith and love.'
Polish woman

But religious beliefs do not always help, and people's feelings about them may be complicated. People who make choices that are against the precepts of their religion may suffer guilt later or may feel that they have brought punishment or illness on themselves. Sometimes people feel guilty if they cannot accept what has happened to them when their religion tells them that they should. Although adversity turns some people towards religion, it leads others to question their beliefs and to lose their faith. Health professionals can often help most simply by listening supportively to people who want to talk about religious or spiritual beliefs and conflicts (see also Chapter 23 *Listening with complete respect*).

For some people, the experience of emigration or of belonging to a religious minority deepens their religious faith or leads them to rediscover the meaning and importance of their religious roots; others become less religious. Some people find that important life events, such as a death or a birth, lead them back to their religion; they may also find they have strong feelings about how things should be done. A Hindu who never went to the temple may want a religious funeral; a secular Jew may believe strongly in the religious requirement to preserve life at all costs. People's attitudes may change in times of crisis and serious illness.

'My father rejected his Jewish heritage and described himself as a humanist. He was practical and pragmatic rather than emotional or sentimental. Just before his death he wanted to plan his funeral. He asked for a mainly secular ceremony which we expected, but much to our surprise he also asked for some Jewish rituals and prayers to be included.'
English woman

Sometimes different members of a family have different religious beliefs and wishes. This may cause great distress, especially to more devout members who worry about what will happen to those who are less devout and may feel responsible or betrayed. Older people are often more religious. However, this cannot be taken for granted. Many young black and minority ethnic people return to their religion as they grow older, often reinterpreting and redefining what they were taught so that they can make sense of their lives (Patel, Naik and Humphries 1998). Others may turn to a new faith or denomination, perhaps one that stresses pride and self-esteem in a society that often rejects them and puts them down.

Understanding different religions

Many of the fundamental values of the different world religions are similar: belief in the sanctity of life and that life has a spiritual dimension and a greater purpose; belief in the spirit or soul and the value of prayer or meditation; the importance of truth and honesty, of doing right, and of fulfilling one's family responsibilities. All religions have their own festivals and histories, times for celebration, reflection and prayer. Most have rituals for birth, death and marriage. People of different religions may do different things for similar reasons: a Catholic might make a novena of masses for the recovery of a loved one, a Hindu might make a special fast.

There are also many differences in belief and practice, some of which affect a patient's needs. Some religions provide detailed rules, which may cover aspects of daily life such as diet, behaviour between men and women, prayer, modesty, the wearing of religious symbols, contraception or euthanasia. Others have a looser framework of values, principles and practices within which people make their own decisions. There are also different denominations within most religions, each of which has certain different beliefs, requirements and traditions. Most Christians expect health professionals to be aware of this and usually give their denomination (eg Methodist, Catholic, Seventh Day Adventist). People of other religions may not.

People of the same religion or denomination whose families originated in different parts of the world may have different practices and preferences. A Bosnian and a Somali may both be Muslims, but their religious attitudes and practices may vary a good deal. Hindus whose families originated in north-west India and in Sri Lanka may have different religious beliefs and practices. A Progressive Jew may be more religious than someone who is nominally Orthodox but chooses not to attend synagogue regularly (Wood 1998). Most important of all, individuals vary, within communities and within families. Muslims, Hindus, Buddhists, Sikhs and Jews are no more homogeneous than Christians.

Exploring our own attitudes to different religions

Religion deals with sacred matters and is a highly sensitive issue. Most people are reluctant to open themselves, their beliefs and practices to possible criticism or ridicule. Religious faith is sometimes expressed through signs and symbols that can be misinterpreted.

'I put my kirpan under my pillow and the nurse found it when she was tidying my bed. She grabbed it and called for the sister, saying I was hiding a dagger.

Everyone stared and some people laughed. I was very embarrassed and also angry.'
Sikh man

(see also Chapter 48)

Many of us have grown up with prejudices against different religions, often arising from a history of mutual dislike, misunderstanding and gross misinterpretation. Religious differences continue to be a source of suspicion and conflict, even hatred, murder and war. Members of minority religions, in particular, may feel that their faith is often portrayed only in terms of negative stereotypes and distortions.

'After Rushdie, the Gulf War, and now Bosnia, I have been forced to describe myself in terms of my religion, to proclaim something that was given and understood before. For 20 years I never thought that being a Muslim was a problem. Then it changed. People would say "but you're so educated and reasonable", as if all Muslims are maniacs.'
British Asian academic and consultant (*The Independent* 5 July 1993)

(see also Chapter 44)

Take some time to reflect on your attitudes and feelings about religion and to explore their origins.

- If you are not religious, how do you feel about and react to those who are?
- If you are religious, how do you feel about and react to people who belong to a different faith?
- Are there certain religious groups you find more difficult to accept than others?
- On what do you base your opinions of these groups?
  - personal experience of one or more people who belong to that group?
  - the way the group has been portrayed by the media?
  - other people's views and opinions?
- Would you rely on any of these sources to give a balanced portrayal of your own religion or beliefs?

Difficult issues Health professionals need to demonstrate willingness to learn about each patient's beliefs and needs. Most people are happy to explain provided they are asked in a respectful way and at an appropriate time (see also Chapter 23 *Listening with complete respect*). Sometimes, inevitably, people express beliefs or make decisions for religious reasons that we find difficult to accept. We need temporarily to set aside our own beliefs and values, making a conscious effort to separate our professional responsibilities from our own feelings and views (see also Chapter 8 *Managing negative reactions*).

Practical matters

The value of religious rituals

Religious rituals can have important spiritual, social and emotional significance. They strengthen bonds between members of the group, giving a shared sense of purpose and meaning (Open University 1991). Rituals are very important in most religions: for example, lighting candles, oil lamps or incense; anointing with oil or holy water; the Muslim requirement to wash in a specific way before prayer; the Roman Catholic and Orthodox ritual of making the sign of the cross on entering a church. Religious ceremonies surrounding death often stress forgiveness, preparation for the next world, transcendence and hope.

Religious rituals can be significant even to people whose daily life takes little account of religion. Having a prescribed way of doing things also helps many people deal with the uncertainty and anxiety that accompany new situations, both positive and negative. Rituals around the time of death provide a framework for managing the situation and can give comfort and continuity, reminding people that this has happened to others before them.

> 'If activities and rituals surrounding dying and death appear pointless and unnecessary that is due to our ignorance, not to their emptiness.' (Open University 1991)

Most of the religious rituals that patients and relatives want to perform can easily be accommodated in hospital and other institutions. Many go unnoticed by staff. However, some need special thought and consideration, especially when people are dependent or bed-bound, and a few have implications for health and safety regulations (see below).

Prayer and meditation

Some people pray or meditate at fixed times of the day, others at times to suit themselves. If a religious patient is frail or bed-bound, find out when they want to pray or meditate and if they need help with anything. People may want to:

- wash before praying, usually under running water (eg most Muslims, some Jews, Hindus and Sikhs). Some people may need help with this (see also Chapter 12 *Practical care*);

- cover their heads or put on prayer shawls;
- face in the direction of a holy place (eg Muslims and some Jews);
- adopt certain positions while praying or meditating;
- set up a small shrine;
- light candles, oil lamps or incense.

After a death some relatives also may want to light a candle to symbolise the continuation of the spirit or to light the path for the soul. Lighting lamps, incense or candles often clashes with institutional safety regulations. Most people accept restrictions but occasionally, and especially after a death, people may feel extremely strongly. Their requests should be met with understanding and sympathy, and, wherever possible, accommodated safely (see also Chapter 20).

For more about the requirements of specific religions, see Part Five.

Privacy

However and whenever people pray or meditate, it is important to provide and respect their privacy.

'My husband was in a side ward and one morning a nurse walked in while he was praying. She hastily walked out again. But a few minutes later he noticed several nurses peering at him through the window of his door. They had obviously never seen anyone wearing phylacteries and a prayer shawl before.'
Orthodox Jewish woman

Sometimes a group of visitors will want to gather at a patient's bedside to pray or sing hymns. If available, a side room or day room would give them privacy and peace of mind and reduce disturbance to other people.

'We tried not to sing or pray too loudly but we all felt uncomfortable. It was hard not to be distracted. We could see some staff and patients were angry and we were worried. But we needed to pray with our sister; it was our joy and our duty.'
Jamaican Pentecostalist

Religious items

Religious items such as holy books, holy pictures, statues and beads must be treated with great respect. They should be moved only if it is essential and then only with clean hands. They must never be placed on the floor or near feet, shoes or soiled clothing (see also Chapters 12 *Jewellery and other items* and 20 *The patient's property*).

'The statue of Lord Buddha should always be high up in the room. Nothing should be put above it.'
Thai patient

Religious food restrictions and fasting

For discussion of religious food restrictions and fasting, see Chapter 11 *Fasting patients*.

Holy water

Water from holy places and water that has been blessed may give spiritual comfort and help recovery. It may be sprinkled over the person or used to anoint them. Some Catholics may use water blessed by a priest or from Lourdes to anoint a patient or sprinkle over them; some Muslims may bring water from the holy well Zamzam in Makka for a patient to drink; some Hindus may place a few drops of Ganges water on the lips of a patient at the time of death.

All water is a potential reservoir of pathogens. Pathogens, including *Pseudomonas*, *Enterobacter* and *E coli* have been found in samples of holy water (Daschner 1997, Rees and Allan 1996). Whilst it is necessary to minimise the risks to vulnerable patients, it is also important to respect people's beliefs and practices, especially if the patient's death is inevitable. Although for certain patients there is a risk of acquiring an infection from holy water, the chances of acquiring infections from other sources are probably much greater. Many surfaces and objects in hospitals and other institutions are colonised with similar pathogenic bacteria, making hospital-acquired infection a significant problem. Taps, showers, baths, lavatories, dialysis water, ice and flower water are all possible reservoirs for water-borne infection (Rutala and Weber 1997).

In most cases, the possible risks from holy water are outweighed by the support and comfort it offers. However, for some critically ill people, sprinkling potentially infected water or anointing wounds can pose unacceptable risks. These include patients who are in intensive care, those who are immunosuppressed, those with burns or open wounds, and those with tracheostomies or with venous or arterial lines. Drinking holy water may pose a significant risk to people who are immunosuppressed. Anointing the forehead is unlikely to cause problems.

It is difficult to predict who might use holy water, and how. However, if wound infections worsen after initial response to therapy, or clinical status fluctuates inexplicably, it may be important to ask relatives. This requires great sensitivity. People who believe in the positive power of holy water often find it difficult to accept the idea that it might be dangerous. They may be offended, especially if the suggestion comes from someone who is not of their faith.

'We have been drinking Zamzam water with no ill effects for many years. I can't believe it could harm us.'
Muslim health professional

It is usually easier to talk to patients and relatives about using holy water if it is already clear to them that staff have a positive and supportive attitude to their religion and religious practices. It may be helpful to explain why the patient is particularly vulnerable and the need for stringent precautions to avoid infection from **all** sources, of which holy water is only one. Some patients and relatives may accept an offer to autoclave holy water.

Religious festivals

Just as routine appointments are not given on Christmas Day, it is normally best to avoid making routine appointments for members of minority religions on their major festivals. Many people in hospital or other residential care would also prefer to go home for festivals if possible. Avoid non-urgent tests, operations or investigations if possible and delay routine home visits until the festival is over.

At joyful festivals, patients may receive cards and presents and are likely to be grateful for recognition that this is a special day for them. Visitors may bring in special dishes. Any restrictions should be lifted as far as possible. Some festivals involve fasting (see Chapter 11 *Fasting patients*).

Except in emergencies, try to avoid transferring or discharging people during their major religious festivals, or at least discuss possible difficulties beforehand with the patient and family. Many people have important religious and family obligations at such times and it might be difficult to care properly for a discharged patient while managing everything else. Most Orthodox Jews avoid driving, being driven or carrying anything during Shabbat or other major festivals except when necessary to save life (see Chapter 47 *Shabbat*). Orthodox Jewish relatives may be unable to help with non-emergency moves, discharges and so on at these times. They may also be unable to travel to visit patients.

Knowing the dates One person in each unit could be responsible for finding out the dates of the key religious festivals each year, for circulating this information and for reminding colleagues when an important festival is imminent. Some festivals occur on the same dates every year. The dates of

Hindu, Sikh and Jewish festivals and of certain Christian festivals (including Easter) vary slightly. The dates of Orthodox and Western Christian festivals also differ. The Muslim lunar year is shorter than the Western solar year so the dates of Muslim festivals fall ten or eleven days earlier each year (precise dates for each year are given in the SHAP calendar published annually – see References). It is also helpful to know which festivals are joyful and which solemn so that the festival can be acknowledged appropriately.

Religious leaders and pastoral care

The roles of religious leaders in leading religious rituals and giving pastoral care vary. Most Christian leaders have both a spiritual and a pastoral role. In some other religions, spiritual support is offered mainly or entirely by community members. A person who is employed to lead prayers and care for the place of worship does not necessarily pronounce on religious issues. Practice also changes with changing circumstances. For example, many rabbis and some imams in the UK have taken on pastoral care even though this is not their traditional role.

Visiting chaplains often identify patients to visit from admission lists. Sometimes patients' names are entered automatically on the basis of their answer to the question on religion. But levels of adherence and personal wishes vary. It is important to check with each person whether they would like a religious visitor.

'A nurse came and told me to get into bed and cover my legs properly as I had a knee-length nightie on. Next thing I knew an Orthodox rabbi appeared at my bedside. I don't know who was more embarrassed, him or me. I was angry and humiliated about having been put in such an awkward position.'
Secular Jewish woman

When a person is dying

It is important to support patients and relatives, whatever their religious and spiritual beliefs, and to enable them to carry out important rituals (see also Chapter 18 *Religious ceremonies*).

Good and bad luck

Beliefs about how life should be lived and about what people should and should not do may be linked to ideas of good and bad luck. Western scientific rationalism tends to dismiss these as primitive superstition. In reality, belief in good and bad luck is alive and well in the West, though superstitions are so normal that they often go unnoticed. Few hotels have a room 13; many people are nervous about Friday 13th. People wish each other luck, have lucky charms or mascots, touch wood, avoid walking under ladders and throw spilt salt over their shoulders. Horoscopes abound in magazines and newspapers and have an increasing following. Many people turn to tarot cards and other means of foretelling their future or guiding decisions.

What people believe can have a profound effect on what happens to them. Many health professionals have seen patients with reasonable prognoses give up and die for no apparent clinical reason, while others with very bad prognoses have recovered. In some cultures, belief in good and bad luck is particularly strong. A study among a group of adult Chinese-Americans who were seriously ill, found that those whose year of birth was considered to be ill-fated died significantly earlier than those whose year of birth was considered auspicious. Among the people who were seriously ill, women born in ill-fated years died earlier than men born in the same years. This was thought by the researchers to be due to that fact that the men had had more exposure to Western culture and therefore did not adhere so strongly to traditional Chinese beliefs (Phillips, Todd and Wagner 1993).

Beliefs about good and bad luck and the consequences of 'risky actions' die hard. A modern Italian woman may not believe, as her mother and grand-mother did, that washing her hair when she is ill will make her more vulnerable to infection. But if she washes her hair and then gets worse, she may regret that she did not follow their advice. At vulnerable times such as illness, birth and death, beliefs about bad luck and how to protect oneself may become very important. It is important for health professionals to accept the importance of such beliefs to some people and to respect and accommodate them when possible and appropriate. For example:

- Some English people believe it is unlucky to put red and white flowers together.
- Some people consider certain days, dates or astrological combinations auspicious or inauspicious, and may want to take this into account when elective procedures or surgery is planned. For example, some Jews consider Tuesday particularly auspicious. Some Hindus may prefer to plan elective surgery on auspicious days.
- Some Europeans may be very worried about being in bed, ward or room 13 or about having surgery on Friday 13th. Some Chinese people believe that the number three is lucky; the number four is unlucky because in some dialects it sounds like the word for death.
- Some people believe that anyone particularly precious or beautiful or beloved may be at risk from other people's jealousy or the evil eye. They

may try to protect the people they love by not praising them, or by disguising their beauty by, for example, putting a black mark on the face of a child.

'I was my parent's fourth child. Two boys had died and my sister lived. When I came along they gave me a girl's name to try to fool any evil spirits and protect me.'
Pakistani man

11 Foods and diets

Food, culture and tradition

Food is not simply a matter of nutrition; it often has deep personal significance, symbolising, for example, security, love, moral and religious values
and identity. What we eat also indicates our family's and our community's
history. Different diets reflect climates, seasons and agricultural patterns.
Meals can be important social occasions. In most cultures there are special
dishes for major festivals and family celebrations.

'My children get Western food at school. I cook Nigerian food at home so they
are accustomed to it and like it and won't find it strange when they visit the
family back home.'
Nigerian woman

Almost everywhere women are responsible for preparing food. Most
choose familiar ingredients that they know how to use and familiar cooking methods. They pass their knowledge informally to their children. Food
habits and traditions are a very important part of culture and may be
retained for several generations after a family migrates.

Think about your own attitudes towards food.

- How important were/are meal times in your family?
- What do you like to have for breakfast?
- Which foods do you eat with a knife, fork or spoon, and which
  do you eat with your fingers?
- What sorts of foods do you feel like eating when you are ill or
  sad or vulnerable?
- How do you react when you are given something unfamiliar to
  eat at such times?
- Have you ever been confronted with a menu in a language you
  did not understand? How did you feel? How did you choose,
  and how did you feel when the dish arrived?

Food and well-being

In many cultures, including French and Italian, food is a major topic of interest and pleasure. In others, for example Jewish and African-Caribbean, it is a symbol of health, emotional well-being and security. In many cultures diet is seen as a major influence on health (see below). In English culture, food has not been regarded as particularly important; until recently, interest in food was considered a sign of greed (see Chapter 2 *Not cultural facts but cultural possibilities*).

This disregard for food is still reflected in the lack of attention often paid to assessing and meeting patients' nutritional needs. The nutritional needs of black and minority ethnic patients whose diet is different from the majority are particularly likely to be neglected, especially if they are elderly, incapacitated, have problems with chewing or swallowing or are confused, or if there is a language barrier (ACHC 1997, Barrow 1997).

Manners

Although the concept of good manners related to food is universal, the details vary. In some cultures, great importance is attached to who eats with whom, who serves whom, and the order in which people are served. In some cultures eating noisily indicates that you are enjoying and grateful for your food; in others it is rude. Most Chinese people normally eat with chopsticks and a spoon; most people in the Indian subcontinent eat with their fingers; most Westerners use a knife, fork and spoon. Many people only eat with their right hand (see Chapter 12 *Using the right hand*). In many cultures it is customary always to offer visitors food and drink, and polite for the visitors to accept.

Religious aspects of food

'Food is what binds body and soul together.'
Greek woman

For some people food has a religious significance. Certain foods may be prohibited and there may be religious requirements about the way food is prepared. Jainism, Hinduism, Buddhism and Sikhism all forbid violence against living things and so followers of these faiths may be vegetarian. Some Seventh Day Adventists and Rastafarians may be vegetarian or vegan. Some people of other religions (or none) may be vegetarian or vegan by personal choice. For observant Jews, pork is forbidden and only meat that has been specially slaughtered and prepared is kosher or acceptable. Meat and milk products must be kept strictly separate. Islam also forbids pork and lays down rules for the slaughter and preparation of meat in order to make it halal or acceptable. (For specific religious details, see Part Five.)

Fasting

For discussion of fasting, see *Fasting patients* (below).

Washing before eating

For discussion of washing before eating, see Chapter 12 *Religious requirements*.

Visiting patients at home

Avoid bringing prohibited food into the homes of people who observe dietary restrictions. Before entering the kitchen, find out first if there are any procedures you need to follow: for example, in observant Jewish homes, different worktops, china, utensils and washing-up equipment may be used for milk and for meat (see Chapter 47 *Religious requirements*).

Food and illness

'The importance of food as part of healing is rooted in pre-history, but has been temporarily abandoned in the West in favour of surgery and medicinal treatments.' (Karseras 1991)

Many cultures have strong beliefs about what people should eat or avoid to keep healthy. In traditional Chinese, South Asian and many other cultures, contrasting food types are balanced to achieve maximum health. Certain foods are avoided or increased when someone is ill. For example, in Chinese culture people who have undergone surgery traditionally avoid sour or vinegary foods, which are believed to prevent healing, and eggs, which are thought to inflame wounds. Some patients may also avoid cold drinks which cool the body undesirably and will prefer a thermos of boiled water by their bed (see Chapter 38 *Chinese foods and diets*). In some cultures people who are ill restrict their food intake; in others they are encouraged to eat more.

Giving someone food, especially when they are ill or sad, also symbolises nurturing them and showing them love. Most cultures have special foods for people who are ill. Relatives often take time and trouble to prepare special strengthening food that will tempt patients to eat.

Families for whom food is associated with survival may be particularly concerned that a patient eats and drinks.

> 'My cousin could not bear it that his wife who was dying of cancer had no appetite and had difficulty swallowing. He kept pestering her and forcing her to eat in a way that seemed cruel to me. It was very hard to watch and made me very angry. He could not bear to see that she no longer wanted things that they had both enjoyed together. But if he accepted that she could no longer eat, he would have to accept that she was dying.'
> Jewish woman

Some relatives may feel a religious or cultural requirement to maintain life at all costs, regardless of quality. They may press staff to intervene and, for example, to feed the patient artificially (see also Chapter 18 *Making decisions at the end of life*).

Relatives may become even more distressed if the patient is reluctant to drink or stops completely. Some may insist on offering fluids or ask for fluids to be administered artificially. In some cases it may help to explain that, when someone is dying, enforced drinking is likely to be intrusive and to cause distress.

> 'The … situation is not that the patient is failing to drink and therefore will die, but that the patient is dying and therefore does not wish to drink.' (Lennard-Jones 1999)

In contrast, some relatives may be strongly opposed to artificial feeding or hydration on religious or personal grounds. Many frail older people slowly lose their appetite as well as the capacity to chew or swallow. Some may make a conscious choice to stop eating and drinking (see also Chapter 45 *A holy death*).

Providing food in hospital and other residential care

Familiar food can be especially significant in times of illness and stress.

> 'I got severe flu when I was travelling in the Far East. I couldn't face the local food. All I craved was tinned tomato soup and marmalade sandwiches, which is what my mother used to give me when I was little.'
> English woman

It is important to try to find out for each person what they can and cannot eat and what they would like, and not to make any assumptions.

'When I went into hospital I only got vegetarian food. After a few days I realised other people were getting different meals. When I asked, I discovered that it was because I had given my religion as Muslim. I was brought up a Muslim but I'm not at all religious. I thought you had to give an answer about religion and I didn't know what else to say.'
Iranian woman

Planning and choosing from menus

All patients need food that they find appetising, healthy and acceptable. Anorexia is common in people who are seriously ill, and small quantities of attractive food that the patient likes can be very important in alleviating this (Hockley, Dunlop and Davies 1988). Other family members can often give useful information and ideas, especially if the patient is frail or confused.

Food in hospital and other residential care is often bland and unappetising, due to the undoubted difficulties involved in producing and serving large quantities of safe, nutritious and generally acceptable food three times a day every day of the year on a limited budget. At the same time, menus must offer an increasingly wide range of choices so that everyone can find something that meets their religious and cultural as well as nutritional requirements. Those responsible for catering need to develop, with the help of local people, a range of dishes that are likely to be acceptable to patients of different communities. It is necessary to be specific: a universal 'African', 'South Asian' or 'Indian' diet does not exist any more than a universal 'European' diet. People's customary diet varies according to their religion. For example, depending on their religion, culture and area of family origin, some South Asians are vegetarian. Some do not eat eggs. Some do not eat onions, garlic or root vegetables. Some eat meat but only if it is halal. Others eat all meat, however slaughtered; some refuse beef and pork. Some eat chapatis with their meals, some eat rice, and some eat both. People whose families originated in different areas may use very different ingredients, spices and cooking methods. What suits the members of one community is unlikely to suit others.

'Our local hospital serves different vegetable curries which most of the Indians, Pakistanis and Bangladeshis are happy to eat. Many of the Somalis find them too hot but there isn't anything else really suitable as they are Muslims and most only eat meat if it's halal.'
English community worker

People also have different styles of eating. Those who normally eat with chopsticks, spoons or their fingers need bite-sized food. Those who use only their right hand for eating need to be able to reach their food easily.

People who eat with their fingers need a bowl for washing their hands before and after meals if they cannot get out of bed.

Helping people choose

People who are unfamiliar with English cooking and ingredients may find it difficult to select from menus. If menus do not indicate which dishes are suitable for people who follow specific dietary restrictions, staff may need to find out and offer guidance. It may be necessary to take particular care to ensure that people who are confused or need help with eating are offered food that they like and that is both culturally and religiously acceptable.

'The son of an elderly Hindu vegetarian lady with multi-infarct dementia came to me deeply distressed and agitated because someone had fed her steak and kidney pie. He said that, even though she was unaware of what she was eating and could not be held responsible, she would be unacceptable in the eyes of God because she had eaten meat.'
English staff nurse, medical ward

Religious considerations

When preparing and serving food for people who are vegetarian or vegan or who eat only halal or kosher meat, it is very important to ensure that:

- No prohibited food comes into contact with the food that is being served. A salad from which a slice of ham has simply been removed has already been contaminated and cannot be eaten.
- Separate utensils and dishes are used when preparing and serving food and drink. The same spoon must not be used, for example, to serve meat and potatoes to other people and then potatoes to a Hindu, a Sikh or a Muslim who follows food restrictions. Orthodox Jews may want to use only disposable cups, plates and cutlery when away from home.

Orthodox Jews, some Hindus and some Muslims may refuse any food or drink prepared outside their own home because they cannot be sure that the utensils used at each stage have always been kept separate. They may also avoid all processed and other foods that might contain animal products (eg rennet in cheese, gelatine in jelly, animal fat in cakes, ice creams and soups). Many food additives with E-numbers are unacceptable. E471, for example, is a fatty acid derivative of animal (usually pig) fat, widely used as an emulsifier in bread, cakes and other confectionery. Because it is often very difficult to be absolutely sure that prepared or processed food contains nothing forbidden, many people avoid anything of whose ingredients they are not absolutely sure (London Beth Din 1998) (see also Chapter 14 *Religious dietary restrictions and fasting*).

It may be necessary to keep separate liquidisers for different types of food: for example, vegetarian meals, meals containing halal meat, meals containing kosher meat, and meals for observant Jewish patients containing milk or milk products. Check the contents of proprietary liquid diet supplements to ensure that they contain nothing prohibited on religious grounds (see the chapters on religions in Part Five).

Meal times Islam and Judaism have set prayer times, usually linked to sunrise and sunset. These change with the seasons. If prayer times clash with meal times, arrangements should be made for food to be kept hot until the patient has finished praying.

> 'My mum couldn't feed herself so I went in in the evenings when I could. But sometimes when meal times and prayer times clashed, by the time I'd finished praying the food had been cleared away or was cold. If I fed my mum first, it was often too late to pray afterwards. Eventually I discussed the problem with the nurses and they arranged to keep her meals warm if I was praying.'
> Iraqi man

Fasting patients

Fasting is important in many religions. Some Hindus, a few Sikhs and a few Christians fast or restrict their food intake on certain days. Many Muslims and Jews observe set annual fasts. Most Jewish fasts are also religious festivals during which observant Jews may observe a range of other restrictions. Muslims who fast during Ramadan do not eat or drink between dawn and darkness. People who are ill are usually exempted from stringent fasts if there are genuine medical contra-indications. However, fasts have important spiritual and personal significance for many people and some may be reluctant to miss them. (For specific religious details, see Part Five.)

Find out from fasting patients what they can and cannot eat and drink and how their needs can be accommodated. Patients who are making long fasts – mainly Orthodox Jews and Muslims (see Chapters 47 and 44) – need a good meal before the fast begins and another when it is over. Depending on the time of year, they may miss most set meals and may need food specially served or kept for them (see also Chapter 14 *Religious dietary restrictions and fasting*). Fasting relatives staying with patients may also need special consideration because, depending on the time of year, cafeterias may be closed at the times when they can eat.

Relatives bringing in food

Some families try to solve the problem of food by bringing in meals from home, though this is not always easy. It is also important not to assume that minority patients who are not eating the food provided are being satisfactorily looked after by their families. Torkington (1987) described an incident in which a South Asian women was left for two days without food. Apparently the ward staff knew she was not eating hospital food but presumed that her family were providing something. In fact, her husband was abroad and she had no visitors.

Bringing in food can create its own problems. If food is brought in between meal times, some people feel conspicuous eating it. Although it is possible to draw the curtains round the bed, this is often perceived as unfriendly by other people. It can be difficult to store and heat food for patients and also for relatives who want to stay with a critically ill or dying patient.

Patients who eat food that is spicy or strongly flavoured sometimes receive hostile comments about the smell of their food. Although strong-smelling food can cause problems for patients who are nauseous or anorexic, it is important to remember that all food smells. The only difference is that most of us are usually much less aware of the smell of familiar than of unfamiliar food.

'My grandfather, who came from Austria, was in hospital for some time and was delighted with everything. The only thing he hated was the smell of the food. The smell of things like cabbage and minced beef made him feel really sick. He said even the smell of cigarettes was preferable so he used to go and sit in the day room.'
English woman

Dietary advice

Relatives who bring in food for patients or care for them at home may sometimes need advice on preparing food that is nutritionally suitable or easier to swallow. All advice must be based on a thorough understanding of and respect for the family's existing diet and dietary principles.

'Just because we follow vegetarian or vegan diets, don't assume that we are anaemic or that we don't know how to eat a balanced diet.'
Rastafarian woman

Infection control and food

Since the lifting of Crown immunity from health service premises, local authority officers interpret the relevant health and safety guidelines. Sometimes inflexible interpretations make it difficult to meet people's needs.

'I have been trying in vain to get our local health and safety officers to change their minds and allow us to give soft-boiled eggs to elderly people in long-stay care. Many of them cannot eat protein in any other form. We don't want to have to rely on protein drinks and anyway they like soft-boiled eggs. But the officers insist that all eggs should be hard boiled.'
English consultant physician in public health

Concerns about liability if a patient should acquire a food-borne infection have led some units to forbid relatives from bringing in cooked food altogether. However, these rules are not always applied consistently.

'Our Asian Muslim patients who observe strict dietary laws and cannot eat the food here are not allowed to have cooked food brought in, in case they get an infection. But we don't stop other relatives from bringing in take-away burgers.'
Muslim health professional

Clearly some precautions are necessary. Food should not be stored without careful regulation. Re-heating must be thorough. But rules that prevent patients eating familiar and acceptable food are counter-productive to good care. Unless the institution can guarantee to provide food that is acceptable on cultural, religious and personal grounds for every patient, policies need to allow cooked food to be brought in, stored and heated. Catering managers, dieticians, infection control staff, and health and safety officers need to work together to agree and implement such policies. Although, ideally, relatives could be asked to bring in freshly cooked food at each meal time, this is not realistic, especially for those who live some distance away, for women who have small children or do not travel alone, and for relatives who work full time.

Some units ask relatives who bring in cooked food to sign a disclaimer absolving the institution of any liability if the patient acquires a food-borne infection. If these are considered essential, extreme care must be taken with the tone of the disclaimer and with the way the subject is raised so that there is no implication that the family's food or kitchen is regarded as unhygienic. It is important to get disclaimers from all relatives and not just from black and minority ethnic families.

12 Personal hygiene and grooming

Modesty

'Where I worked in Switzerland there were four-bedded rooms with no curtains between the beds. There was a very small screen that could be put up between a patient's bed and the door when they were using the bedpan or on the commode but otherwise nothing. Elderly patients were examined, treated, washed and put on bedpans in full view of the other three patients in the room and their visitors. I found it really difficult and most inhibiting, especially when I had to examine someone.'
American geriatrician

'[Ethiopian] fathers usually accompany their children to clinic visits. One father with adolescent daughters was appalled when asked if he wished to wait in the waiting room during his daughters' examinations. He said, "I am their father and I should stay here." His daughters emphatically agreed.' (Salzer and Nelson 1983)

Standards of modest behaviour and decency vary enormously. What is perfectly acceptable to some, shocks others deeply.

Take some time to consider your own standards and assumptions.

- When you were growing up, what messages did you receive about modest behaviour and appearance?
- What is important to you in terms of physical modesty? Do you have different standards:
  - at work?
  - in your doctor's surgery?
  - on the beach?
  - at a social event?

- How do you/might you feel if your standards of modesty are violated?
- Have you ever worn a hospital theatre gown? How did you feel? (If you haven't, put one on – without underwear! Try walking, sitting down, climbing onto a bed in it.)

Modesty and health care

Each patient has different standards and different things that matter to them. Respecting a patient's modesty preserves their self-esteem and reduces anxiety and distress.

Some cultures place a particularly high value on personal modesty. Care must be taken to ensure that people always feel decently covered during examinations, treatments and everyday practical care. It is also important to ensure that the patient's environment takes their requirements for modesty into account (see also Chapter 13 *Modesty and physical examination*).

- Many people, especially women of conservative communities, never undress fully except when they are alone. They may be used to uncovering only the relevant part for a medical examination or for treatment.
- Some people never undress completely even to wash. They shower in their clothes, changing into clean dry clothes afterwards.
- For some people it is important that all intimate treatments, examinations and practical care are carried out by someone of the same sex. When there is no health professional of the same sex, some patients may prefer to be washed or helped with washing and using the lavatory by a family member of the same sex if this is possible.
- For some people the idea of being seen in bed or in night-clothes by strangers, and particularly by people of the opposite sex, is very shocking. This is especially likely for people who normally have little contact with people outside their own family. Women and some men of many communities may feel immodest and exposed in their night-clothes and in a public area (see below). Some may want to keep their curtains closed all the time so that they are not exposed to public gaze.

Modesty and mixed-sex environments

Many people in all communities, especially older people and women, dislike or are offended by mixed-sex wards or mixed-sex lavatories and washing facilities. Even where there are single-sex bays and separate washing facilities, mixed-sex wards can cause profound distress to patients and their relatives (Patients' Association 1996).

Wherever possible, both men and women who observe a strict code of modesty and segregation should be cared for in completely single-sex wards. When this is not possible, for example in intensive care units, every effort should be made to preserve each patient's dignity and privacy. Where washing facilities or lavatories are used by both sexes, ensure as much privacy as possible, for example by having doors rather than curtains, and, where there are only curtains, making sure that they close properly. Some women may prefer to wait in a separate area rather than in a mixed-sex waiting room, for example in X-ray departments, especially if they are wearing night-clothes or hospital gowns.

Clothing

Clothes are an important part of identity and comfort. They are strongly influenced by our cultural and religious values, including our ideas of modesty. When the British colonised other countries they rarely adopted the local style of dress. Instead they continued to wear what they were used to and felt comfortable in, sometimes adapted to the local climate.

We tend to judge and categorise other people by the way they dress. Looking a little different may gain approval and admiration; looking very different often attracts criticism and sometimes hostility or anxiety.

'I feel quite threatened by women who wear black from head to foot and cover their faces. I can't make eye contact or see their expressions and I don't know how to relate to them or what they are thinking about me.'
English woman

Modesty and clothing

Many religions and traditional cultures require people to dress more modestly than is customary in the West today. Women in some communities may be expected to dress in certain ways, particularly in the presence of men and in public. Most Orthodox Jewish women and some Muslim and other South Asian women always cover their upper arms and chests, and their legs to below the knee. For some women, uncovering their legs may be as humiliating as for an English woman to walk around in public with her breasts exposed. Some Muslim women cover themselves from head to toe when they leave their homes, to ensure privacy. It is very important to help each patient maintain their normal habits of modesty and comfort.

'When she went into the home Mum was fine all day, but just wouldn't settle at night. She was distressed and restless and nobody could find out why. When I

went in I discovered they had removed her knickers. She always wore a clean pair at night and just didn't feel right without them but felt too embarrassed to ask. Once we put them on for her, she was able to sleep peacefully.'
African-Caribbean nurse

Many people also observe religious requirements in relation to clothing. For example, Orthodox Jewish men cover their heads at all times and may wear a miniature prayer shawl under their shirts. Devout Sikh men and women wear special underpants with religious significance.

Clothing in hospital or other residential care

It is important to advise people who are going into hospital or other residential care to bring clothes in which they will feel comfortable in a public place. Information booklets often assume that everyone wears pyjamas or night-dresses, dressing gowns and slippers. But these are not universal. Most people prefer to wear familiar clothes when they are ill and away from home and should be encouraged to do so. This does not usually cause problems. If, for example, a sari hampers nursing care, ask the patient if she would be willing to wear a shalwar kameez (a loose tunic top and trousers), or a top and a full-length skirt instead (see also Chapter 41 *Clothing*).

Hospital theatre gowns and other institutional clothing, especially garments that tie at the back, are unacceptable to many people. When necessary, hospitals and other residential care institutions should provide clothing that enables people to maintain their self-respect. For women, this means the option of a full-length garment with a high neckline and long sleeves.

Visiting people at home

Professionals visiting conservative families or families with older members need to avoid clothing that may offend or give the wrong impression – for example, for women, tight clothes, short skirts, bare arms or low necklines. Casual clothes may also be seen as unprofessional.

In many cultures people take off their shoes when entering a home. If you see a row of shoes by the door, it is polite to take your own off. If you are unsure, ask.

Personal hygiene

Each of us is used to a routine of washing and keeping clean that keeps us comfortable and feels right.

- When you were a child, what were you taught about:
  - how often you should bath or shower?
  - washing before meals?
  - washing after using the lavatory?
  - washing after touching certain things?
- Do you prefer a bath, a shower or a strip wash? Do you oil your skin after washing?
- Do you bath or shower in the morning, at night, or both? How often do you change your clothes?
- If you go to the doctor's knowing you might be examined, do you wash and put on clean underwear first?
- After using the lavatory, do you clean yourself with paper or with water?
- Do you shave some or all of your body hair?
- What assumptions do you make about the cleanliness and washing habits of people whose skin colour, culture or religion is different from yours?

Practical care

People who feel dirty and possibly polluted may become very distressed if they cannot keep clean as they are used to, especially if they are bed-bound and cannot wash themselves. Being dependent on others for washing, bathing and using the lavatory is humiliating for most people. It is important to protect patients' self-esteem and dignity as far as possible by finding out about and trying to cater for their individual habits and preferences.

Bathing and showering

Different patterns of washing have developed in response to local climates and resources. Most people whose families originated in hot countries place a greater importance on washing than is generally found in traditional English culture (see Chapter 2 *Not cultural facts but cultural possibilities*). Some people feel dirty and uncomfortable if they cannot wash or shower and change their clothes at least twice a day. In most hot countries people do not sit in a bath; they shower or pour water over themselves with a bowl. Some people oil their skin after washing, to keep it soft and supple.

'For me this is very hard. We share one bathroom and one toilet with five other families. There is no shower. The bathroom is locked during the day and is also

very dirty and smelly. I feel dirty all the time here because I cannot wash properly. I feel dirty and uncomfortable, and my children are dirty too.'
Somali refugee in bed-and-breakfast accommodation

Most religions and cultures contain ideas about purity and pollution.
These are explicit in Hinduism, Judaism and Islam and in some forms of
Buddhism. In South Asian culture, all body secretions including saliva,
sweat, urine, faeces, vomit, blood, semen and menstrual fluid are traditionally considered polluting. Running water is believed to be the most
effective cleansing agent. The idea of purity and pollution was also widespread in many Christian denominations: churching ceremonies were held
to remove the pollution of blood loss after childbirth, and menstrual blood
was also regarded as polluting (Cole 1994). Some people feel spiritually
polluted as well as physically dirty if they cannot wash as they are used to
(see also Chapter 13 *History taking*). When patients need help with
bathing and washing, find out what they normally do and try to fit in with
their preferences.

Baths and showers People who believe that only running water gets them
clean may find the idea of sitting in a bath of water in which they have
washed extremely distasteful.

'At first I thought it was very odd if someone objected to sitting in a bath of water.
Then I watched how people scrub up before surgery. They use running water,
being careful to let it run from the fingers and hands down towards their elbows.'
Student nurse

If there are no showers, some people may prefer to have a jug or a large
bowl available in the bathroom so that they can stand or sit in the bath and
pour water over themselves. It is helpful to keep a mop there so that those
who are able to can wipe up any spilt water.

Washing when ill Some cultures limit bathing or showering at certain vulnerable times such as during illness, while menstruating or after childbirth.
Some Chinese people, for example, prefer to wash with a sponge and a
bowl of very hot water when they are ill to avoid the possibility of getting
chilled.

People who are concerned about catching a chill, especially when they are
ill, and those who prefer running water, may prefer a bed bath to a bath of
water. For some this has the additional advantage of enabling them not to
undress completely (see *Modesty and health care*, above).

Religious requirements Many religions have symbolic washing rituals.
Most Muslims wash in a prescribed manner before each of the five daily
prayers. Orthodox Jews wash their hands before eating bread, men may

wash their hands in the morning before getting out of bed. Many Sikhs and Hindus wash before praying. Christians may want to wash their hands before receiving communion. Some dependent patients may need help to wash before praying or eating. Find out from each what is important to them and what they will need (see also below and Part Five).

The importance of being clean to pray or meditate may also mean that some people are more than usually distressed by incontinence and by open or discharging wounds, or if they are unable to wash as prescribed because of plaster casts or lines or because they are receiving radiotherapy.

Oral hygiene

Mouth care is often given a low priority, but it is important both for physical comfort and emotional well-being and to prevent infection (Holmes 1996). People who cannot manage by themselves may want help to maintain their normal method of oral hygiene. Find out what each patient is used to. Some people of South Asian communities, for example, regularly clean their tongues with a U-shaped metal device and may need help with this.

For some people, for example Muslims and some Hindus, cleaning the mouth is an essential part of preparing for prayer (see above). Others, for example Orthodox Jews, do not clean their teeth during fasts in order to prevent the possibility of swallowing water.

Elimination

Many South Asians and Muslims always wash their perineal area with running water after using the lavatory. For many this is both a cultural and a religious requirement. It is also customary to use the left hand for cleaning oneself (see *Using the right hand*, below). At home many people keep jugs with long spouts in the lavatory to pour water over themselves.

> 'I gave an Asian patient a jug to take to the lavatory because I wanted a urine specimen. She seemed unusually delighted and came out with an empty jug. I then realised that I hadn't explained properly what I wanted. She had thought I knew she needed to wash with running water.'
> English health professional

Bidets, taps and jugs Ideally, in hospital and other residential care, there should be a bidet or basin in each lavatory to enable people to wash themselves with running water. Even better, a low-level tap above a small shower tray in the lavatory would enable people to fill their jugs and to wash themselves without wetting the floor (Slater 1993). Such an arrangement would also enable Muslims to perform the ritual wash before prayer in comfort.

Where there is no bidet, basin or tap, invite people who might want to wash after using the lavatory or before praying to bring in their own jug or offer them a jug to use. Water is sometimes spilt when people wash; it is helpful to keep a mop available so that those who are able to can wipe it up.

Dependent patients who normally wash with water after using the lavatory may appreciate having warm water from a jug poured over their perineal area before they are taken off a commode or bedpan. They can then be cleaned and dried with paper before being offered a bowl of water in which to wash their hands. As it is not possible to predict who will want what, it is better to make a gentle tentative offer, which might be refused, than to leave a person feeling uncomfortable and dirty.

Modesty and elimination Many people, for personal, cultural or religious reasons, may be distressed by having to use a bedpan or commode protected only by curtains, or a lavatory that is not completely private. Inhibitions about using lavatories, commodes or bedpans can lead to constipation, which is far better to prevent than to have to treat.

Whenever possible, dependent people for whom privacy is a particular issue should be wheeled to the lavatory either in a chair or on a commode. It is important to ensure that the patient is decently covered. Lavatory doors should normally be closed (see also *Modesty and health care*, above). People who cannot clean themselves after using the lavatory should, if possible, be cared for by someone of the same sex.

It is important to maintain patients' modesty and self-respect as far as possible while they are using a bedpan or commode. They should be decently covered with a blanket and the bed curtains or screens completely closed. Keep catheter bags, which many people find embarrassing or offensive, covered or hidden.

Facilities at home It may be necessary for health professionals to help ensure that ill and frail people who are being cared for at home have access to a lavatory and somewhere to wash.

'It tore me apart to see my mother struggle up the stairs because, due to her religious convictions, she refused to use the commode (as a Muslim you are supposed to wash yourself after using the toilet). I applied to the Social Security for a chair lift and I was told that because she was over 60 she did not qualify for it. They could not understand the importance of her religion.'
Daughter of a woman with cancer (Baxter 1989)

Using the right hand In South Asian and Muslim cultures the left hand is traditionally used for washing after using the lavatory; the right hand is traditionally used for touching clean things and handling food. When handing or receiving anything, some people always use their right hand. It may therefore be necessary to position lockers, food trays and so on within reach of the right hand and, where possible, to insert drips in the left arm. Check with each patient to see if this is important to them.

Skin care

Proper skin and hair care are very important for patients' morale and dignity. It is necessary to maintain each person's normal skin care routines as far as possible and to be aware of people who may be especially vulnerable to skin damage. The skin of older people becomes less resilient and elastic with age. It is also prone to dryness and damage and is slower to heal. **Different skin types may need different care.**

Black or dark skin can be dry and may be particularly affected by such things as hard water, cold, air-conditioning, certain drugs, and by illness and a consequent poor diet. Dry skin is uncomfortable and may also look greyish and 'ashy'. Many people with black or dark skin rub oil or moisturiser into their skin after washing to keep it supple and smooth. People who are not well enough to moisturise their skin may appreciate an offer of help. If they have not brought their own cream, find out what they normally use. Sometimes the combination of skin preparations and the natural shedding of skin leaves marks on bedding, clothing and around baths. This should not be mistaken for dirt (American Academy of Dermatology 1997, Baxter 1992).

It can be more difficult to notice early signs of pressure sores or other skin breakdown, for example around a colostomy site, in black or dark skin. It is important to be aware of this and to be particularly vigilant, avoiding undue pressure, observing pressure areas carefully for any kind of change in feel or colour, however subtle, and for localised heat or coolness, and asking the patient regularly about any soreness. Prompt action is essential even if there are no visible signs (Baxter 1993) (see also Chapter 13 *Recognising clinical signs in skin*).

Hair care

The way we care for and wear our hair is important as part of our personal well-being and self-expression and is also affected by our culture.

Religious considerations Many Muslim and Orthodox Jewish women keep their hair covered. In some cultures long hair is regarded as a symbol of holiness; devout Sikh men and women, particularly those who have taken amrit, never cut or shave any body hair (see Chapter 48 *The five symbols of the Sikh faith*). Rastafarian women and men keep their hair covered, and do not cut it. Orthodox Jewish men may wear side locks and beards and keep their heads covered (for more about specific religious groups, see Part Five). **Never cut or shave any body hair without consent unless there is an immediate threat to life.** If people are concerned about shaving or cutting hair, shave or cut as little as possible.

Dependent patients Caring for a patient's hair in the way they want helps maintain their comfort and self-respect. Ask each patient how they would like their hair to be cared for and arrange for help when necessary.

People who normally keep their head or hair covered, or who oil their hair and scalp, may want help with this. However, some people who regard the head as sacred may be distressed by having their head and hair touched at all. Some may prefer a relative to do their hair for them. Some patients may want to have their hair washed frequently. Others may worry about getting their heads wet when they are ill and it may be important to pay special attention to keeping them warm and avoiding draughts. Some South Asian women, especially older people, may not want their hair washed on certain days of the week, for religious reasons.

Different hair types may require different care. For example, the curly hair of people of African heritage is often very delicate and may require particular care.

- Tightly spiralled hair is fragile and needs combing several times a day to prevent matting. A wide-toothed comb, or a brush with widely spaced bristles, is essential. After washing, the hair must be combed while it is still wet and then oiled with a product designed for black hair, to prevent brittleness. Many people oil their hair and scalp regularly and wash their hair only once a week or fortnight to prevent dryness. In bed, some women cover their heads with a scarf to prevent matting and getting oil on the pillowcase.
- Some people wear their hair in corn rows (braids that lie flat along the scalp) or in plaits. Some women regularly plait their hair before going to bed and may want to have this done when they are ill. Plaiting is a special skill and must be learnt from an expert. Plaits can be left for several days or weeks, and washed and oiled with the braids intact.
- Some people have their hair chemically straightened. Such hair is especially vulnerable and must be treated with great care. The point where straightened and unstraightened hair meet is very delicate and can easily break.

- Most Rastafarians and some other people wear dreadlocks; their hair is not cut or combed. Most people tidy their hair with water. They may apply moisturiser to their hair and scalp after washing (Baxter 1992).

Staff who are unused to grooming black hair should ensure that they learn how from those who are more experienced.

> 'Having lived and grown up with black hair and knowing how to comb it, I can't imagine a white person caring for my hair without having been taught how.'
> Black British health professional

Beards

Ask men with beards whether and how often they would like them brushed and washed. Some devout Sikh men never shave: long beards may be kept rolled and netted (see Chapter 48 *Hair care*). If a beard must be shaved, for example before surgery, explain the need to the patient and obtain his consent. Shave as little as possible if the patient is concerned.

Clean-shaven men may want help with shaving. The choice of method may be important for religious reasons (see Chapter 47 *Washing and cleanliness*) or for more practical reasons. Some men of African heritage whose hair is tightly curled are prone to ingrowing facial hair (razor bumps), which can cause inflammation and infection. It may sometimes help to shave less frequently, to use a safety razor, to wait for the shaving cream or lather to soften the skin first, to shave only in the direction of the hair growth (not against the stubble), and to avoid stretching the skin. If the skin becomes inflamed, do not use a razor. Instead, clip the beard to about 0.6cm long with scissors (American Academy of Dermatology 1997, Baxter 1993).

Jewellery and other items

In most cultures women – and sometimes men – receive special wedding jewellery when they marry. This may be, for example, a ring, bracelets, a necklace or a nose jewel. Most people never remove wedding jewellery and may fear that doing so will bring bad luck. Removing glass bangles almost always breaks them. This may be regarded as a very bad omen.

Religious jewellery may include threads around the body, amulets containing holy texts, pieces of cloth, medals, crucifixes or other sacred items. Many devout Sikhs wear a steel bangle and other religious symbols (see Chapter 48 *The five symbols of the Sikh faith*). Some patients wear religious jewellery especially to protect them against illness and danger, or to help recovery.

'We bought a special piece of cloth which had been blessed by a monk to comfort my aunt. She wore it next to her skin all the time. Somehow it got thrown away in hospital. My aunt was very upset and so were we all.'
Thai man

In most cases there is no need to ask anyone to remove jewellery or other items with religious or cultural significance. If there are genuine medical reasons, find out the significance of the item(s) and, wherever possible, tape them rather than remove them.

13 Clinical care

Patients' personal, cultural and religious beliefs influence their attitudes to the clinical care they are offered and affect the choices they make about investigations, treatments and other interventions (Boston 1993). Taking time to understand what the patient feels and wants both improves care and, in the long run, makes life easier for health professionals.

'The doctor is the expert on history taking, examination, diagnosis and treatment. The patient is the expert on their personal, social, cultural and religious needs and beliefs. We need to be ready to listen, understand and respond appropriately.'
White British specialist in medical ethics

History taking

Different expectations and concerns

Health professionals, especially doctors, have a systematic approach to finding out what is wrong. History taking often consists mainly of closed questions, and examinations usually follow a set pattern. The health professional tends to focus on what they consider significant, and to disregard other factors (see also Chapter 3 *Health beliefs*). Patients may be dismayed or surprised to find that factors that they consider important are of no interest to the health professional, and that their view of the problem and its origins is not shared (Jones 1992). Differences between a health professional's and the patient's analysis of the problem are even more likely when there are cultural and language barriers.

- Some people who are not used to Western medicine may find certain questions and requests bizarre.

'We had a lot of trouble persuading some patients from rural areas of Africa to bring urine samples with them to the clinic. They always smiled but said they had forgotten. Eventually I realised that they could not see the point and what is more they thought we were extremely odd to ask for their urine.

To them it seemed as crazy as we would think a request to bring in our toe-nail clippings. Once we explained, there was no problem.'
Irish registrar in obstetrics and gynaecology

- Certain questions may seem threatening or offensive. For example, asking about family origins, in order to assess the likelihood of genetic disorders such as a haemoglobinopathy, may be perceived as questioning the patient's right to be in the UK or to receive medical care (see also Chapter 23 *Mutual mistrust*). Alternatively, it may be seen as casting aspersions on the patient's family (see *Illness and stigma*, later in this chapter).

- Some people stress physical rather than psychological symptoms, or express psychological distress in terms of physical symptoms. This is especially likely if, for personal, cultural or other reasons:
  - they are used to thinking in terms of physical functioning and well-being rather than feelings;
  - they believe that health professionals are likely to take physical symptoms more seriously than psychological ones;
  - they believe that physical symptoms and physical illness justify their inability to function normally or fulfil their responsibilities, but psychological symptoms do not (Currer 1986);
  - they believe that psychological problems are a sign of weakness and, as such, are stigmatising and debasing (Yung, Lau and Lai 1993).
  Somatisation is also more likely if people also have serious physical symptoms, or if they speak little English and find physical symptoms easier to describe than psychological ones.

- People who believe that their illness is due to witchcraft, the evil eye or a supernatural cause may not tell the professional. They may fear that a Western-trained professional will not understand the significance of these things and will look down on anyone who believes in them.

- People may have different assumptions about normal health. For example, women who are used to being anaemic may take symptoms such as weakness and dizziness for granted; refugees who have lived for some time with inadequate food and in poor sanitary conditions in camps may consider some degree of abdominal cramping normal (Salzer and Nelson 1983).

- People who have been tortured often feel that their health has been irrevocably damaged and never feel completely well. They may be extremely anxious about their health and may consult doctors frequently about minor symptoms, fearing that each is a sign of serious illness or hoping that a physical cause can be found for their chronic feelings of lethargy and discomfort. They may take a lot of medication, both prescription and over-the-counter. It is helpful to try to find out what the patient thinks is wrong and what they are frightened of, and to carry out a full investigation in order to exclude organic disease and to be able to offer meaningful reassurance (see also Chapter 35 *People who have experienced torture or physical abuse*).

Other factors that may affect history taking

Even if professional and patient share the same expectations, other factors may complicate history taking. For example:

Codes of modesty People who observe strict codes of modesty may be reluctant or unwilling to discuss certain symptoms or answer certain questions, especially with someone of the opposite sex (see also Chapter 12 *Modesty*). Women who have undergone genital mutilation, especially those who have been infibulated, may be reluctant to mention it and even more reluctant to be examined, especially by a man (see also Chapter 32 *Physical examination*).

Some people may simply be unable to answer certain questions. For example, a woman who never undresses completely, even to wash, may not be able to say if she has noticed any changes in the appearance of her breasts.

At the same time, it is important not to assume that people of certain communities will not want to talk about potentially embarrassing or distasteful topics on cultural or religious grounds. In India, for example, surgeons and specialist stoma care nurses give full counselling and information to potential ostomists (Bhakta, Probert et al 1992).

Beliefs about pollution People who consider all body secretions to be polluting may sometimes be reluctant to talk about them, and may also be unable to answer certain questions. A person who for cultural or religious reasons never looks at their stools would find it difficult to describe changes in their appearance. Sometimes it helps to explain why you are asking a particular question and why you need to know. It may also be helpful to reduce the pressure to answer by reassuring the patient that it is all right to say if they do not know (see also *Bodily substances and pollution*, below, and Chapter 12 *Bathing and showering*).

Inaccurate or missing information Sometimes important information, such as a patient's age, is inaccurate. Some people do not know their date of birth or have it wrongly entered in their passport (see Chapter 30 *Dates of birth*). People may not always know or remember details of their medical history, especially if they have been cared for in another system or another language or have not been fully informed. Medical records are notoriously difficult to get hold of across national boundaries and do not always contain the necessary information.

'I had a 56-year-old woman with menstrual problems. She turned out to be pregnant and the date of birth in her records was wrong.'
British Asian gynaecologist

Language barriers Language barriers make history taking difficult or impossible, and are extremely frustrating for everyone. If a patient does not speak good English, the best way to obtain an accurate history is to use a professional interpreter or health advocate (see Chapter 27 *Professional interpreters: the benefits*). If there is no interpreter, it may be necessary to carry out a broad range of investigations in order to reach a diagnosis, even though this is likely to increase the patient's distress, lengthen their stay and greatly increase the costs of care.

Even when the patient speaks fluent English, differences in terminology or pronunciation may make it difficult to elicit important information. It can be helpful to have a cultural broker, someone who understands both cultures and their expectations and can help both parties to make the most of the consultation (see also Chapter 23 *Cultural brokers*).

'Two West African patients undergoing rehabilitation following strokes were found to have positive treponemal serology which might indicate syphilis (as a potential cause of their acute neurology) or endemic treponemal disease such as yaws, pinta or bejel. When asked if they had yaws, both said no. Later, an experienced GU physician recognised tribal markings on their legs and asked them if they had had 'yaahs'. They both instantly said they had and were saved from further investigations and from unnecessary and aggressive treatment for syphilis.'
English senior house officer, neurology

Recognising clinical signs in skin

'You only **see** what you have been **taught** to see.' (Zatouroff 1996)

Textbook descriptions of the clinical signs of systemic illness that may be observed in the patient's skin (eg cyanosis, pallor, inflammation and jaundice) are, in the vast majority of publications, based on the assumption that skin is white. This is a graphic demonstration of how 'cultural lenses' operate (see Chapter 1) and results in unintentional discriminatory practice. Not only are descriptions of signs in different colour skins missing, many health professionals seem not to have noticed this omission.

European television engineers installing broadcasting equipment in East Africa were amazed to find that the local people were far more discerning and critical about the different tones of black skin reproduced on the screen than they were. They had to spend a lot of time adjusting the equipment to get the tones just right, though they themselves could not really see the difference.

Both within and between different ethnic groups there is a wide variety of skin tones and colours affecting the way skin looks during illness (Baxter 1993). Failure to observe clinical signs accurately can delay diagnosis and treatment, and may sometimes be life threatening.

Health professionals who are familiar with black skin can usually recognise changes fairly readily.

'I'd recognise skin colour changes at a glance. I've grown up with Chinese, Indians and Malays so I know what the norm is.'
Tamil health professional

However, they may have difficulty in convincing their white colleagues.

'I was working in a very white middle-class area and was the only black person on the staff. During my time there only one black woman was admitted and as soon as I saw the baby I knew something was wrong. The others said the baby was fine. But I just knew his colour wasn't right. Later he was found to have a major heart defect.'
African-Caribbean midwife

Examining or observing people with dark skin, especially very dark or black, requires careful attention and practice. It is not always possible to rely on signs that are more obvious in white skin. However, careful observation may reveal subtle changes. When people are ill, the depth and richness of their normal skin tone may be lost, the skin may lose its sheen and become dull. Nevertheless, unless you know the patient well and have paid attention to the normal colour, tone and quality of their skin, it is easy to miss early changes, even those that are acute and require urgent attention.

Sometimes it is easier to see the first signs of a problem in the patient's general demeanour rather than in colour changes. Observe carefully people who become lethargic, anxious, restless, anorexic or nauseated or who complain of soreness, itching or dyspnoea. Patients or relatives who say that there is something wrong should always be taken seriously. If no problem can be identified after careful evaluation, make sure to keep checking, especially if the symptoms persist or worsen, and to encourage patients and relatives to keep reporting what they notice.

'Recognising skin signs is a matter of experience. It is also important to ask patients and to **listen** to what they say. They will tell you if they have a rash or if an area is sore. Then you can look and learn from them.'
White British GP in East London

In people with dark skins, pay extra attention to those parts of the body with less pigmentation. These vary from person to person: they may be the palms, the tongue, palate and oral mucosa, the conjunctivae, the sclerae and the finger-nail beds.

Nail beds are often an important place for observing skin changes in a person with dark skin. With some women this may be more difficult. Women of several communities, including Somali women, often use henna to stain their finger and toe nails. This takes time to fade. Because it is extremely important to be able to observe the nail beds for cyanosis, dark-skinned women who use henna and are awaiting surgery should be asked to let the henna fade and the reasons explained. Women with dark skins who wear nail varnish can be asked to remove it or let it grow out. Note that asymptomatic pigmentation in the oral mucosa, and dark longitudinal stripes or bands in the nail beds that increase with age, are normal variants in people of African heritage.

Pallor may be due to pigmentation or vasoconstriction as well to a low haemoglobin. In people with dark skins, pallor is usually visible in the conjunctivae, which become pale, and in the oral mucosa, which becomes pale or greyish-white. The skin may look ashen or have a greyish tinge. Depending on the degree of pigmentation, the lips and nail beds may also be ashen. If a patient is in shock, the skin becomes cool and moist.

Cyanosis Depending on the depth of pigmentation, there may be a blue-grey tinge to the skin. Peripheral cyanosis is usually visible in the palms and in the finger-nail beds. In some people the nail beds take on a dark, maroon tinge. However, these changes may not be at all obvious in people with very dark skins or pigmented nail beds. Central cyanosis can be detected in the tongue, gums and palate, which become greyish-white. Depending on the degree of pigmentation, the lips may also become greyish-white or take on a purple tinge.

Jaundice People of Far-Eastern heritage (eg China and Vietnam) who become jaundiced tend to look sun-tanned and/or have a slight orangey tinge to their skin. In dark-skinned people the skin may take on a greenish rather than a yellow tinge. The sclerae are the most sensitive indicator. Observation should be made in good light, preferably daylight, removing any yellow clothing or bed linen first. In the absence of observable skin changes, the first indications of obstructive jaundice can include: itching, especially at night causing insomnia; changes in the colour of the urine and stools; and changes in the distal third of the finger nails, which may become shiny. The sweat of people with severe obstructive jaundice may leave yellowish stains on bed linen.

Rashes In people with very dark skin, raised rashes (such as pustules and vesicles) are more obvious than flat rashes (such as petechiae and macules). However, careful observation may reveal differences between areas with and without the rash. Examine the whole of the patient's skin in a good light, preferably daylight, **and listen carefully to what the patient has observed.**

Inflammation In acute inflammation, swelling may be visible or palpable. The skin may become shiny and smooth looking and hot to the touch. The patient is likely to complain of loss of function and of tenderness. In chronic inflammation, the main symptom is loss of mobility in the affected part; swelling, tenderness and heat may no longer be noticeable. People with dark skins who complain of soreness, for example on pressure areas or around wounds or stoma sites, should be taken seriously even when there are no obvious signs of inflammation (see also Chapter 12 *Skin care*).

Bruising The discoloration that is obvious in white skin may not be easily observed in very dark skin. When bruised, the skin may appear darker or more purple when compared with surrounding skin. It may be necessary in some cases to rely on palpable changes such as hardness or lumpiness and on the patient's own description of tenderness and pain.

(The above is based on descriptions given by health professionals of different ethnicities and on Zatouroff 1996, Archer and Robertson 1995, Baxter 1993, Werner, Thuman and Maxwell 1993and Schull 1987.)

Examination, investigation and treatment

Cultural or religious beliefs and requirements, as well as personal values and experiences, influence patients' attitudes to their illness and to certain investigations and treatments.

Modesty and physical examination People who observe a strict code of modesty (see also Chapter 12 *Modesty and health care*) and are unwilling to undress or be touched, especially by a member of the opposite sex, can make examination very difficult. However, it is important to understand the depth of distress and humiliation that exposure and physical contact can cause and to try to understand the patient's point of view.

It is also necessary to do what you can to minimise causes of distress as far as possible. For example:

- expose only a small part of the body at a time, keeping all other parts, including legs, back and upper arms, covered;
- ensure that doors and windows are closed or screened, and bed curtains completely drawn;
- whenever possible, have a health professional of the same sex carry out the examination. If this is not possible, many people will accept examination by a health professional of the opposite sex provided the medical reasons are fully explained and they are supported throughout by someone of the same sex. Some people may prefer a health professional who does not share their culture or religion, since such a person is less likely to participate in their embarrassment. Some women may cover their faces with a sheet or their sari during intimate examinations to hide their feelings;
- ensure that only essential people are present (if possible, all of the same sex as the patient).

If relatives are present, ask the patient before you begin whether they want the relatives to stay. A relative who is interpreting may feel that they ought to stay and it is tempting to encourage this even if it is completely inappropriate on grounds of modesty and also of patient confidentiality (see Chapters 15 *Maintaining patient confidentiality* and 28 *Using friends and relatives to interpret*).

Vaginal examination can be traumatic for women of all cultures and communities (Schott and Henley 1996). Both men and women may find rectal examinations humiliating and traumatic. Women whose culture or religion requires strict modesty are likely to find intimate examinations particularly traumatic. They may be deeply disturbed about the shame and wrongdoing associated with exposing themselves. Some women are able to accept such examinations but may be very concerned that family members and others do not hear of it.

'We don't tell our mothers that we see male doctors.'
Pathan woman (Currer 1986)

Bodily substances and pollution Certain investigations or treatments may cause additional distress to people who feel polluted or particularly disgusted by bodily substances, especially if they also observe a strict code of physical modesty. For example:

- investigations or treatments that involve rectal, urethral or vaginal examination;

- collection of samples (eg of stools, urine and sputum), especially if they have to carry the specimen to a lab or give it to someone, or of swabs of vaginal or urethral discharges;
- indwelling catheters and drains;
- investigations that involve passing urine when others are present;
- treatments that involve undressing and immersion in a bath or pool (eg baths to help treat open wounds, or hydrotherapy, especially in mixed company;
- pollution and modesty may also be issues for people with a stoma or fistula (see also *Surgery*, below).

It may be possible to help the patient by:

- explaining what is usually done and why, and explaining the potential benefits;
- discussing with the patient what can be done to reduce embarrassment and also to minimise disruption to their usual way of doings things. Urine and stool samples can be left in labelled containers on a shelf in the toilet to be collected by staff, or can be passed to an adjacent laboratory through a hatch from the toilet. It may be helpful to offer special assistance with washing before prayer;
- doing everything possible to preserve the patient's modesty and privacy.

Blood samples and transfusions Some people, for example conservative Chinese people and Muslims who are fasting during Ramadan, may be reluctant to have blood taken in case they become weak. Most Jehovah's Witnesses observe a prohibition against receiving blood transfusions and certain blood products (see Chapter 46 *Blood transfusions*).

Fasting People who are fasting may be unwilling to have any investigations that involve eating or drinking; for example, glucose tolerance tests and barium meals. They may also be unwilling to take medication during fasts (see also Chapter 11 *Fasting patients*).

Radiotherapy People for whom it is important to wash before prayer may be particularly distressed by radiotherapy treatment that prevents them from washing. The same may also apply to people with burns and ulcers (Hammick, Smith et al 1996)

Pregnancy It can be difficult to plan investigations such as X-rays and mammograms well in advance for pre-menopausal women who do not use contraception and may become pregnant.

A pregnant woman with a life-threatening disease may, for religious reasons, refuse treatment that could jeopardise her pregnancy or the health of her baby.

Illness and stigma In all societies, certain diseases and conditions carry a stigma and are therefore particularly feared. The fears of individual patients and their families will depend to some extent on their geographical heritage. Leprosy, for example, carries little stigma these days in European societies where it has largely disappeared, but is greatly feared in many developing countries. Conditions that are particularly likely to carry a stigma include the following.

- Conditions that are disfiguring or which require surgery that will disfigure, whether or not the disfigurement will normally be visible. Fear of stigma may lead some people to refuse a mastectomy, colostomy or other disfiguring surgery.
- Contagious diseases, especially those for which there was or is no certain cure, which are traditionally associated with poverty, and which are perceived to be a threat to the community (eg tuberculosis and leprosy).
- Diseases associated with behaviour that is considered unacceptable, especially in communities with strict codes of conduct (eg sexually transmitted diseases, and alcohol and drug abuse).
- Congenital and hereditary diseases.
- Mental illness.
- Conditions requiring treatment that results in sterility or impotence, especially in societies where everyone is expected to become a parent. Occasionally a patient may refuse treatment even if their illness is life threatening.
- Cancer is almost universally feared. In some cultures it is regarded as unacceptably cruel for health professionals to use the word cancer when talking to patients (Boston 1993) (see also Chapter 15 *Telling patients the truth*). Many people believe that it is always fatal. Some believe that it is contagious; people known to have cancer may become social outcasts.

The consequences of stigma vary in their severity and in whom they affect. Sometimes the personal and social consequences of an illness are worse than the illness itself. Some patients or their families may face rejection and isolation.

'An African woman told us that she could not return to her own country as she would be ostracised by her family and her community because she had had surgery and treatment for breast cancer.'
White British nurse specialist in breast care

'My cousin and her boyfriend were very much in love but then her boyfriend, who was English, broke it off. My aunt suffers from severe depression and alcoholism and the boyfriend said he didn't think it was wise to marry into a family

like that. You couldn't be sure that my cousin wouldn't go the same way. She was heartbroken.'
Scottish woman

Confidentiality is clearly extremely important. It is also essential never to assume that patients have told their families what is wrong with them or what treatment they are receiving (see also Chapter 15 *Maintaining patient confidentiality*).

'An Asian patient who was asked if his family were being supportive following his colostomy, replied that none of them knew that he had a stoma.' (Dawe 1992)

In any situation when a patient declines to give consent to a particular treatment, especially when an illness is life threatening and treatment would be beneficial, it is important to find out their reasons as sensitively as possible and to see whether an alternative way forward can be found. If this is not possible, the patient will continue to require sensitive and sympathetic support from the health professionals caring from them.

Surgery Attitudes to surgery vary enormously between individuals and between cultures. For example, for some traditional Chinese people an operation may be preferable to Western pharmacological treatment. Other people may fear that they will be stigmatised after surgery.

Certain issues may need careful thought and should normally be discussed with the patient well before surgery.

- Black skin has an increased tendency to keloid scarring. If there is a choice, give extra thought to the site of incision in order to prevent scarring that would be visible during daily life and which might restrict flexibility.
- The siting of an arteriovenous fistula for haemodialysis may be important if the patient washes with running water using their left hand after using the lavatory (see also Chapter 12 *Elimination*). Position the fistula so that the risk of splashing with potentially contaminated water is minimised.
- The siting of incisions, and of stomas in particular, may also be critical for people who wear traditional rather than Western dress (eg a sari or shalwar kameez; see Chapter 41 *Clothing*). Position the stoma so that the patient can continue to wear their usual clothes. Muslims who prostrate themselves as part of the five daily prayers need to have the stoma sited to avoid compression and leakage. It is also important to take into account the needs of Muslims to cleanse themselves before each daily prayer and the needs of many people of South Asian origin to keep their

right hand clean (Bhakta, Probert et al 1992, Horsfield-Gardner 1987, Breckman 1981).

For people who, for example, use only their left hand to clean themselves, or who observe the religious requirement to be clean before prayer (in the case of Muslim patients this may be five times a day), it may be preferable to use appliances that can be cleaned out without having to change them completely. This also reduces the risk of damage to the skin around the stoma (Bhakta, Probert et al 1992, Horsfield-Gardner 1987, Breckman 1981).

Prostheses and wigs

Most prostheses are designed on the assumption that the patient has white skin. Every effort should be made to provide people with prostheses of a suitable shade, especially those that will be visible during daily life. The range of health service wigs is often unsuitable for people of minority ethnic groups. In some cases, people have to pay in order to have a wig that is both visually and culturally acceptable (Baxter 1989).

14 Medication, pain and pain relief

This chapter looks first at general issues relating to medication and then at those specific to pain and pain relief.

Patient adherence

Most people comply with medical advice that they understand and that seems sensible to them. Those who do not comply are generally unpopular with health professionals, but research shows that what is interpreted as 'non-adherence' or 'non-compliance' may be due to cultural and linguistic differences. At the most basic level, language and literacy barriers, or poor explanations, may mean that people simply do not understand what they are required to do or why. Sometimes health professionals assume a shared background of knowledge and understanding that does not in fact exist (Buchholz 1990). Sometimes there is an unspoken mistrust or even antagonism between professional and patient (Lowe, Kerridge and Mitchell 1995). One or both people may have stereotyped views and negative expectations of the other. Mutual understanding and co-operation will be achieved only if the professional takes time to try to explore and resolve the issues that are interfering with the relationship (see also Chapter 23 *Mutual mistrust*).

'Patient "irrationality" is often a sign that there are important issues left unstated. Improving communication becomes more important than more rational cognition. Until there is agreement on values, there can be no discussion about logic. Until the physician develops a compassionate understanding of how the patient's decision is made, and the patient's position is openly acknowledged and accepted, the trust necessary to influence patient decisions cannot exist.' (Buchholz 1990)

In prescribing any medication, it is necessary to consider the factors that may affect the patient's willingness or ability to comply. These include the following.

Side effects

Side effects often lead people to stop taking medication. This is more likely if they do not understand why the drug has been prescribed, or have not been warned about possible side effects, or are reluctant to discuss side effects with the doctor. People who are less familiar with Western medication or who speak little or no English may be particularly likely to stop taking medication for these reasons.

There may also be cultural or religious factors. For example:

- People who are used to other medical systems (see Chapter 31) may believe that Western drugs are 'too strong' for them.
- People who observe strict codes of cleanliness and modesty may be especially distressed by side effects such as incontinence secondary to diuresis, diarrhoea or constipation, especially if suppositories or manual evacuation are required.
- People for whom hair has special religious connotations may be particularly upset about hair loss.

Types of medication and their administration

Most people are more comfortable with the types of medication and the methods of administration they are used to. For example, in France and Switzerland many drugs are given by suppository, especially to children; in the UK suppositories are often regarded as strange and most medication is given orally; in many developing countries injections are considered particularly direct and effective. It may sometimes be possible to adjust the method of administration to suit the patient's expectations and preferences.

Some people may also have cultural or religious preferences or requirements. People who dislike eating or drinking anything cold when they are ill may prefer to take tablets with warm water (see Chapter 38 *Chinese foods and diets*). Some Muslims who are fasting may be prepared to take medication by injection (see below).

Possible interactions with other medication or with food

It is important to identify any other medication being prescribed for a patient, as well as any over-the-counter preparations they are taking, and to check for potential adverse reactions. Some patients may also be taking complementary medicines or foods that may affect their medication. Many people are reluctant to disclose that they are taking herbal or other complementary medicines because they know that health professionals may disapprove. In order to find out what a patient may be taking, make it clear that you do not disapprove, that you respect the patient's choices, and that you are genuinely interested and want to work out with the patient what is best for them (see also Chapter 23 *Managing cross-cultural communication well*).

> 'Making teas and soups with various herbal concoctions is a traditional [Chinese] health practice. The team does not discourage [people] from using herbs (in part because experience shows such advice is ignored); instead, the team encourages [people] to tell them what herbs are being used. Such information is vital since many of the herbs contain derivatives similar to compounds found in Western medicines. Armed with this knowledge, the team can watch for side effects, the physicians' prescriptions can be made so as minimise the possibility of overdosage, and drug interactions can be considered.' (Van Steenberg, Ansak and Chin-Hansen 1993)

Possible ethnic differences in response to medication

The effects and effectiveness of different drugs are influenced by many factors, including age, sex, diet, other drugs, diurnal rhythms, menstrual cycle and multiple disease states. Recent pharmacogenetic research has also uncovered significant differences among ethnic groups. Because of genetic differences in metabolism, different ethnic groups may metabolise certain drugs at higher or lower rates; this may alter the clinical effectiveness of the drugs and their side effects. So far, ethnic differences have been identified in responses to certain opioids, cancer chemotherapy, immunosuppressives, antidepressants, anxiolytics, cardiovascular agents, antitubercular drugs, beta-blockers and also alcohol (Levy 1993).

Health professionals need therefore to be alert to atypical drug responses and to unexpected side effects when caring for black and minority ethnic patients. Some people may, for example, require lower or higher doses of a particular drug or may benefit from longer or shorter intervals between doses (O'Hara and Zhan 1994, Kalow 1982). Different brands of the same drug may also be cleared by different metabolic pathways. When, for example, generic drugs are substituted for proprietary drugs, it is important to check that the substitute is as effective and that no dosage adjustments are needed (Levy 1993).

Religious dietary restrictions and fasting

People who restrict their diet for religious reasons (eg some Hindus, Sikhs, Muslims, Jews, some Rastafarians) and people who are vegetarians by personal choice may prefer not to take drugs that contain animal derivatives. These include capsules with gelatine coatings, additives derived from animal fat, and suspensions containing gelatine (see also Chapter 11 *Religious considerations*). Synthetic insulin is likely to be more acceptable than a porcine derivative. If there is no alternative and a drug is considered essential, most people are willing to accept it.

In most religions, people who are ill do not have to fast. However, some may still want to fast as a spiritual and physical sacrifice that may bring them benefit, help their recovery or prepare them for death. Find out how long the patient wants to fast and the details. Then review their medication and explain which drugs they should continue to take during the fast and why. Whenever possible, adjust the timing of doses. For example, if a diabetic Muslim decides to fast during Ramadan, the timing of their medication can be adjusted to fit their altered eating patterns and lifestyle (see Chapter 11 *Fasting patients*). It may also be helpful to review the route of administration. A fasting patient who needs pain control may be willing to receive analgesics by injection, syringe driver or transdermal patch.

Language barriers

Patients who manage their own drugs may need special help to ensure that they understand the timing and dosage of their medication. Those who read little or no English or whose first language is written from right to left (eg Urdu and Arabic) may recognise only the numbers on a label. There is a danger that patients or carers will read them in the wrong order – for example, taking three tablets once a day instead of one tablet three times a day. Wherever possible, labels and other important information regarding medication should be translated for patients and carers who do not read English.

Sometimes pictograms of doses and timing may be more effective than written or verbal information. Werner, Thuman and Maxwell (1993) have suggested using boxes showing simple line drawings of a sun rising, a sun at high noon, a sunset and a crescent moon with the drugs to be taken drawn under the relevant box. If the patient is taking several drugs, the drawings could be matched in colour, size and shape to the actual preparations.

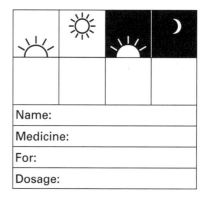

Figure 14.1 A dosage blank (Reproduced, with permission, from *Where There is No Doctor: A village health care handbook* by D Werner, C Thuman and J Maxwell (1993). TALC/Macmillan Education, London)

Pain and pain relief

Culture and expressing pain

The way in which each of us perceives, responds to and expresses pain is highly personal and is influenced by several factors (Melzak and Wall 1996, Brena and Chapman 1991). These include the general norms of our society or community as well as our own childhood experiences: how adults around us responded when we were in pain, and how the adult men and women around us behaved when they were in pain. In some families and cultures, people are brought up not to make a fuss, to be stoical, to show strength and fortitude, or to be a 'good' patient. In other families and cultures, people are brought up to be vocal and demonstrative. It may be normal to display agitation, to moan, cry out, rock, chant, call on God, click fingers or slap oneself. Alternatively, it may be normal to withdraw and remain silent. Our perceptions and expression of pain may also be affected by our religious and spiritual beliefs, as well as by our personality, general physical condition, current emotional state, perceived reasons for the pain, and expectations of whether relief is possible.

Religion and pain

The English word 'pain' is derived from the Latin *poena* which means punishment. Going further back, the Sanskrit root of *poena* is *pu*, meaning sacrifice or purification (Brena and Chapman 1991). This illustrates the deep connection that human beings have long made, and in many cases still make, between pain and spiritual or religious aspects of life. Some people's response to pain may also be influenced by their religious and spiritual beliefs about its meaning and about the kind of response that is appropriate.

None of the major religions proscribes the use of pain-relieving analgesics, including opiates. Most religious people would agree that every effort should be made to control or eliminate pain, although some may be concerned that certain drugs will shorten life. However, some religious people may feel that it is important for them to accept without complaint whatever God sends. Some believe that suffering now will help atone for past misdeeds, will purify them for the life to come, or can be used to help others.

'I offer up my pain to try to help relieve the suffering caused by human wickedness in this world.'
Elderly Roman Catholic man

Language

The language used to describe the intensity and quality of pain varies from culture to culture. Just as Sanskrit has 70 words to describe water, some languages have a richer and more specific pain vocabulary than others (Garro 1990). Cultural and linguistic differences, especially between languages that have very different roots, can make it difficult to translate descriptions of pain in either direction.

'Anyone who has suffered severe pain and tried to describe the experience ... often finds himself at a loss for words.' (Melzack and Katz 1994)

The medical lexicon of English words used to describe pain is vast. However, words that health professionals commonly use to find out about the quality of a patient's pain (such as colicky, dull, crushing, throbbing, griping, burning) are not always readily understood even by English-speaking patients. Such words are even less likely to mean anything to people whose language and culture are very different.

Difficulties in comprehension can work both ways. People may describe pain and other symptoms in ways that do not fit in with the professional's normal range of classifications. For example, some South Asian patients describe their symptoms as 'paining all over' or 'burning all over'. This often baffles health professionals who are used to a more focused description. 'Burning' may indicate generalised feelings of distress or illness rather than a specific pain.

Assessing pain

Understanding ourselves

Our own reactions to other people's pain and the way they express it are also influenced by such factors as our culture and family background. It may be helpful to spend some time thinking about these.

- How do you behave and react when you are in pain?
- How do you prefer people to behave and react towards you when you are in pain?
- If someone underestimates your pain, how do you feel and react?

- How do you feel and react when a patient who shares your culture:
  - is vocal and demonstrative about their pain and distress?
  - is quiet and undemanding about their pain?
- How do you feel and react when a patient who does not share your culture:
  - is vocal and demonstrative about their pain and distress?
  - is quiet and undemanding about their pain?
- Do some ways of expressing or coping with pain make you feel uncomfortable, and others engage more of your sympathy and help? Can you say why?

We inevitably view pain behaviours of other people through our own cultural lenses. The wider the cultural gap, the greater the risk of assumptions and misinterpretation.

Stereotypes and assumptions

Research indicates that health professionals' assessments of and reactions to a patient's pain can be influenced both by the patient's ethnicity and by their own ethnicity. Patients whose culture is different from that of the health professionals caring from them, or whose pain behaviour is unfamiliar or culturally unacceptable, may have their pain inaccurately assessed and receive too little analgesia (see also Chapter 33 *Sickle cell disease*).

- Bond (1980), in a British hospital, noted that patients' stoicism was rewarded with admiration and analgesics. In contrast, patients who were thought to be making too much fuss were met with verbal disapproval, the withholding of analgesics, or even the administration of a placebo!
- Ng, Dimsdale et al (1996) reviewed data from 454 Asian, black, Hispanic and white patients in the USA who had used patient-controlled analgesia for postoperative pain. They found no differences in the amount of narcotic that the patients had administered to themselves, but a significant difference in the amount of narcotic that had been prescribed for patients in the different ethnic groups. The authors concluded that 'ethnicity has a profound influence on the physician's treatment of pain'.

Stereotypes and assumptions about people of different ethnic groups lead to poor care. This is made worse across language barriers.

'I was allocated to a new ward and when I arrived the nurses were casually discussing the fact that an 'Asian' lady had asked for no pain relief following

emergency abdominal surgery the day before. When I saw her I realised she was actually from South America. I asked her in Spanish how she was. She said she had terrible pain and I asked why she had not had anything for it. She said she didn't know how to ask. The nurses had come and said things to her every now and then and to show that she didn't understand she had shrugged her shoulders. Clearly my colleagues had assumed, against all the odds, that this meant, "No, I have no pain". Nobody had bothered to find out where she came from or what language she spoke.'
Black English student nurse

Emotional distress often provides the most significant evidence of pain, though this can be difficult to interpret because of the different ways in which individuals express their emotions. Emotional distress may be conveyed verbally or through non-verbal features such as changes in voice quality, moaning, crying, grimacing, or protective or awkward movements. Fear that pain is about to increase or recur, or that it will not be adequately relieved, also increases people's emotional distress (Craig 1994).

For many people the most difficult and isolating thing about pain is not being believed. People with a lifetime's experience of being ignored or put down because of their ethnicity or religion may respond to scepticism about their pain with anger, increased distress, or silent resignation and withdrawal.

Pain-measurement tools

Experimental work on acute laboratory-induced pain has shown that culture and ethnicity influence people's pain tolerance, though it is not known whether these findings also apply to acute or chronic pain caused by illness (Clark and Clark 1980, Sternbach and Tursky 1965, Hardy, Wolff and Goodell 1952, and Zborowski 1952 cited in Melzak and Wall 1996). However, while cultural variations in pain perception and pain tolerance may be of academic interest, **the practitioner's priority is to relieve each patient's pain regardless of their ethnicity.**

Common methods of measuring pain do not always work. Many people find pain hard to describe even in their mother tongue. There are likely to be additional difficulties across cultural, religious or linguistic barriers.

- Pain assessment charts, such as the McGill Pain Questionnaire, which show the back and front of a naked body may be shocking and unacceptable to people who observe strict codes of modesty or for strict Muslims to whom making images of people is forbidden. Some people may simply find it hard to translate their subjective physical sensations onto a picture that they do not identify with.

- Visual analogue scales work for some people, but others find it hard to relate their subjective sensations to a single point on a horizontal line or on an objective one to ten scale.

  'The doctor asked me to rate my pain one to ten. I was flummoxed. What is ten? Or one? My pain was uncomfortable, not paralysing, so maybe two, but actually very uncomfortable, so maybe six? What would ten be then? I don't see how numbers relate to pain.'

  Elderly English woman

- Some people find it easier to use a practical analogy for the amount of their pain. Salem (1993) suggests using currency. So, for example, if the worst pain imaginable is a pound, how may pennies' worth is the patient experiencing now? After pain relief has been given, has the amount gone down? If so, by how much?
- Although devised for use with children, a Faces Pain Assessment Scale (Bieri, Reeve et al 1990), which consists of a series of faces with expressions indicating no pain through to severe pain, may be useful for some patients who speak little or no English. However the prohibition against depicting people may apply to some conservative Muslim patients.

Objective measurement can help to provide a more consistent and reproducible understanding of a patient's pain experience over time, especially when there are a number of different carers. The important thing is to ask the patient for their own assessment in words that they understand, to listen and take what the patient says seriously, and then to act on it. In practice it is often equally effective to use simpler, non-technical approaches.

'Nowadays when I ask patients about the degree of their pain I simply ask, "Do you have a little pain? Bad pain? Or very bad pain?". And at subsequent assessments I ask, " Is your pain the same? Better? Or worse?" That works just as well as anything else.'
English consultant neurologist, specialising in chronic pain

Treating pain

Although culture, religion and ethnicity may all influence people's perceptions, reactions and expression of pain, it is never possible to predict on the basis of their 'group' what pain relief an individual patient will want or what concerns they will have. Because pain is by definition subjective, **understanding the patient's own perception of their pain and what it means to them** is the only logical starting point for trying to relieve it. It is helpful when talking to the patient to be aware of the many factors that may influence them, but important not to make assumptions.

People who do not want pain relief

Some people may not ask for or may refuse pain relief. This may be for the religious or cultural reasons mentioned above. It may also be because:

- they may fear that the side effects will be more distressing than the pain. Many older people witnessed the terminal illness of their parents at a time when it was customary to give high does of opiates which resulted in unconsciousness;
- they may worry about being drowsy and out of control;
- they may want to be aware and in control, especially when approaching death (Baxter 1989);
- they may have low expectations of pain relief;
- they may be concerned about becoming addicted to or tolerant of opiates;
- they may fear that opiates or other medication will shorten their life – the double effect;
- they may prefer to try alternative approaches to pain relief (eg prayer, meditation or chanting).

Try to find out the patient's reasons. Sometimes explanation or discussion of alternatives may lead the patient to change their mind. If patients then continue to refuse pain relief, find out what other forms of support they would like (see also Chapter 18 *A 'good death'*).

15 Consent, telling the truth and confidentiality

Attitudes towards issues such as informed consent, confidentiality and whether it is right to tell patients their diagnosis and prognosis are very much influenced by culture. In the UK in recent years, the relationship between patients and health professionals has changed radically, reflecting a growing emphasis in society on individual freedom and rights and on consumerism (Kohner 1996). The traditional paternalistic and protective relationship of professionals towards their patients is gradually being replaced by a more balanced relationship based on patient autonomy and their right to ask questions and make informed choices. Patients are generally expected to make their own decisions about their care and should be given the information they need in order to do so. Relatives are expected to be supportive but not to take over or to make decisions for patients. Nevertheless, among professionals, patients and families, individual attitudes and expectations still vary a good deal.

Other cultures do not necessarily place the same value on autonomy and independence. In many societies each person is traditionally regarded more as part of a mutually dependent, mutually supportive family group than as an autonomous individual. Those with authority, generally older people and often men, may expect to take responsibility for, or at least to be closely involved in, all important decisions affecting other family members. They may find current UK practice and expectations hard to understand.

Informed consent

In Britain, competent adults have a right to full information about their condition and about their treatment and care options. They also have the right to refuse examination, diagnostic procedures and treatment. Attending for diagnosis and care does not constitute implicit consent for physical examination or for a particular treatment (GMC 1998a, UKCC 1996, BMA and RCN 1995).

The limits of truly informed consent are difficult to define. How much patients want to know about their condition and the degree of autonomy they want to exercise also vary (see also *Telling patients the truth*, below). Some people want detailed information about their options and to partici-pate fully in all decisions, others strongly prefer to follow advice or to have some or all decisions made for them by people they trust. As they try to provide appropriate information for informed consent, health profession-als run the risk of imposing their own cultural values, both in the choice of how much autonomy a patient 'should' exercise and in the information presented.

Possible cultural issues

- Older and more conservative people who have lived mainly within their own community may not be familiar with the concept of informed con-sent. Some may feel obliged to accept whatever is suggested to them. They may not be aware that they have a right to ask questions and to refuse treatment. Do not assume that a patient who does not ask ques-tions does not want information (Davey 1993).
- In some cultures, independent decision making is highly valued and patients may want to make all decisions about their care by themselves. They may also wish to ensure control over their future by making an advance directive (see below).
- In some cultures, major decisions are normally taken by senior family members or by the whole family. Patients who are used to this may find it hard to take decisions on their own behalf or may not want to. They may delegate authority and decisions, explicitly or implicitly, to other people. They may not expect to deal with distressing information or dif-ficult choices and may be ill-equipped to do so. Respecting the patient's wishes and autonomy includes respecting the wish to delegate that autonomy (Pellegrino 1992). At the same time it is important never to assume, purely on the basis of culture, religion, sex or age, that individ-ual patients will not want to make their own decisions.
- Obtaining informed consent and assessing a patient's capacity to give consent are clearly far more difficult across a language barrier. Patients who are dependent on others to interpret for them may also find it dif-ficult to assert their rights, especially if the interpreter is not a professional (see Chapter 27).

When a patient cannot give consent

When a patient is too ill to consent to treatment and care, health professionals have a duty to act in their best interests, based, whenever possible, on what they know about the patient's previous wishes and preferences. The patient may have discussed these wishes earlier with relatives or health professionals, or may have written them in an advance directive (see below). Although it is often both helpful and prudent to involve relatives in decisions about the care of a patient who is too ill to consent, under UK law no person can give consent to treatment on behalf of another adult. The professional's duty of care is always to the patient (BMA and RCN 1995).

Advance directives

Advance directives, or living wills, state what medical treatment a patient accepts or refuses if they become too ill to make their wishes known. The use of advance directives is likely to grow as the technical ability to prolong life increases. It may also grow among people who observe specific religious requirements in relation to medical care. For example, Jehovah's Witnesses are now encouraged by medical liaison committees to state in an advance directive their objection to blood transfusion (see Chapter 46 *Blood transfusions*). Some Orthodox Jews who observe the requirement to preserve life at all costs may use living wills to request that everything possible is done to extend life (see Chapter 47 *Attitudes to life and illness*). In contrast, people who believe that any discussion of negative events or death may cause them to happen are likely to find the subject of advance directives unacceptable (see also *Telling patients the truth*, below).

An advance directive usually sets limits on life-prolonging treatments, in particular, antibiotics, tube feeding, prolonged life support and resuscitation. It is not possible to refuse basic hygiene measures in an advance directive, nor the offer of oral feeding, nor to ask for any treatment that is unavailable at the time when the directive is written (Patients Association 1996). Advance directives that apply to the patient's current condition and that refuse treatments or interventions should be respected and complied with in the same way as refusal by a competent patient.

Advance directives that request every possible life-prolonging treatment are more problematic. The treatment requested may be clinically inappropriate or useless; there may also be resource implications (BMA 1993). It has been suggested that, although there is a requirement to respect requests for life-prolonging treatment, health professionals are not obliged to provide treatment that would be futile (NCHSPCS 1993).

Understanding our own values in relation to informed consent

Respecting a patient's autonomy and right to choose means accepting their right to refuse treatment or care (Kohner 1996). It also means respecting their right to seek a second opinion with the hope of receiving further treatment, even when there is no realistic hope of benefit. It can be hard to continue to offer good care when a patient has made choices that conflict with our own beliefs. Understanding our own views and feelings is an important step towards understanding and respecting other people's different choices.

How do/would you feel and react:

- When, before consenting, a patient wants to know about their choices in great detail?
- When a patient wants you or their relative to make the decision for them?
- When a patient refuses a life-saving intervention?
- When a patient or family insists on treatment even when there is no hope of benefit?
- When a patient or relative presents you with an advance directive?

If you were to write an advance directive, what interventions or treatments would you refuse and what would you ask for?

Telling patients the truth

Nowadays health professionals are routinely faced with decisions about what and how much to tell patients. It is no longer normal to shield patients from difficult truths or from the knowledge that they are going to die. For many health professionals and patients this is a huge relief.

'When I was a student in the 1960s we were never allowed to say. I shall never forget one man who, during his frequent sleepless nights, regularly asked me, "Am I going to die? ... I'm dying, aren't I? What will happen to me? What will it be like?" It was awful not to be able to listen to his fears and to talk honestly with him. I shall always remember the fear in his eyes, his growing mistrust of all of us and his increasing isolation.'
English ex-nurse

However, the trend towards openness in the USA and UK is not necessarily shared by other countries that practise Western medicine. In Italy and Japan, for example, 'honest' styles of disclosure are generally regarded as cruel (Del Vecchio Good, Good et al 1990). Even in the UK, despite a radical shift in cultural attitudes towards telling the truth, there are still enormous variations both in professional practice and in public expectations. The old idea that it is courageous for dying people not to talk about death has largely gone. Now it is generally considered courageous, even morally superior, to talk about death (Walter 1994). But this view is as limiting as the other.

> 'We've talked for years now about the patient's right to know and in doing so have lost sight of the patient's right not to know.'
> English woman

Individual patients differ a great deal in how much they want to know, and in the pace at which they can or want to take in painful information. Many want to be told everything from the beginning. Some need time and a gradual build-up of information. However, some people do not want at any time to be told their prognosis or that they are dying (see also Chapter 18 *Emotional and spiritual care*). This choice may be based on the patient's sound understanding of themselves and of what they can manage. It is not uncommon for patients who, in medical opinion, have months or years to live, to give up and die soon after learning their diagnosis. Some people suffer more anguish from knowing the prognosis than from the illness itself (Charlton 1994).

Possible cultural and religious factors

Whether people want or expect to be told their diagnosis and prognosis is also influenced by cultural and religious beliefs.

> 'In our culture we never talk about death, we try to block it. And if someone is very ill and asks, we reassure them, we comfort them, we don't say yes. But I know that when I am interpreting, if a patient mentions death, the Western way is for the professional to pounce on it, to talk about it openly. But usually, in our culture, that isn't what the patient expects or wants. They mention death in order to be given reassurance, to be comforted.'
> Iraqi interpreter

For people of many cultures telling the truth can seem vindictive and irresponsible rather than principled and honest. Some people find it difficult to believe that health professionals can predict death. Some feel that predicting death is wicked or negligent. People who have experienced racism and discrimination may also be suspicious of health professionals' motives and commitment.

> 'I had to tell the family that their father was going to die. They were angry. "Who are you to tell us that? Only God can know when someone will die. Everything comes from God." They begged me to ask the doctors to try to save him. They were angry and hurt that I was so negative; they felt I didn't care. "How can any human being know that someone will die until it happens?" To them, saying he was going to die was exactly the same as saying that the doctors weren't going to try to cure him, that they had decided to let him die although they could cure him if they wanted to. The family was absolutely sure that Western medicine could cure anything. Some family members thought that we were giving up on the patient because he was a refugee and a Muslim, because he was black.'
> Eritrean nurse

In some cultures, talking or thinking about negative things may be seen as inviting or causing bad things to happen. Any discussion that implies that a patient is going to die, including, for example, discussion about cardiopulmonary resuscitation (see Chapter 18) or making a will, may be seen as inviting a self-fulfilling prophecy.

Many people whose illness is terminal know that they are dying even if they have not been told. They interpret the signs and notice changed behaviour and visiting patterns in those close to them. But not all cultures place the same value on words and on spelling things out clearly. Knowing things doesn't always mean that they have to be brought out into the open or discussed (see also Chapter 18 *Coming to terms with dying*).

> 'I was visiting a Turkish family where the daughter-in-law was dying of cancer. I felt unsure that the patient really knew and I started to talk to the woman's brother-in-law who spoke good English. I wanted him to interpret. He stopped me. He said, "You can't talk about that. We all know it but we don't discuss it."'
> Swiss palliative care nurse

Relatives' wishes and fears

Relatives who know or suspect that a patient is terminally ill may try to prevent professionals from telling the patient. Many people in all cultures feel that it is wrong and cruel to take away the hope of recovery from a patient.

> 'I tell the truth if they want to know it but I never try to take away hope, the hope that there may somehow be a miracle. Hope is useful and helpful, it helps people take a holiday from their illness sometimes and step outside it.'
> English palliative care nurse

Sometimes, however, relatives' requests have more to do with their own fears about whether they can cope with the patient knowing than with the patient's wishes or best interests (see also *Maintaining patient confidentiality*, below). What people decide is appropriate for others is not always what they would choose for themselves. In a UK study of 100 relatives of patients with Alzheimer's disease, 83 said they did not want the patient to be told their diagnosis. However, 71 also said that if they had Alzheimer's disease they would want to be told their diagnosis. Most felt that it was their right to be told (Maguire, Kirby et al 1996).

For some people, maintaining hope is a religious requirement. Judaism, for example, teaches that nothing, including the removal of hope, should be done that might hasten death. Balancing the cultural or religious imperative to maintain hope of recovery with the patient's wishes can cause ethical problems for health professionals.

> 'A Jewish patient was dying of cancer and his wife and son were adamant that he should not be told. His wife was quite obsessed with the idea that he must never know and kept saying, "It would kill him if you told him". This was hard as it is contrary to our usual approach. I found it particularly awful because he kept asking me, "Am I dying? I am dying, aren't I?" and I felt I had to jolly him along, especially as the doctor hadn't told him.'
> Jewish nurse

Maintaining hope of other things

Many people assume that 'hope' when someone is dying can only mean hope of recovery. However, Scanlon (1989) suggests that often 'hope is not based on false optimism, but is built instead on the belief that better days or moments can come in spite of the prognosis'. Blanket assumptions about the meaning of 'maintaining hope' and fear of the effects of exploring further can prevent professionals from finding out people's real needs and wishes. Patients who know that their prognosis is poor may still hope for many other things. Giving them an opportunity to talk about these may make it possible to help some of them come true. A patient may, for example, have an ambition to swim with dolphins, to live until their daughter's wedding or the birth of a grandchild, to take a holiday with their family or to make a pilgrimage. Most people faced with serious illness hope that they will not be a burden or lose their autonomy and dignity. Dying people may hope to die at home, to have their pain controlled and to have a peaceful death.

Identifying our own views

Our own beliefs and assumptions about what is helpful and good for people profoundly affect our approach to telling patients the truth. They also influence our reactions to people with different beliefs and wishes from our own.

Patients should always know the truth	Patients should never be told the truth even if this means lying to them

- Where do you stand on this spectrum of truth telling? Should patients always be told their diagnosis and prognosis? Or should they always be shielded from the truth?
- On what is your own practice based?
- If your practice is always the same, why is this? Whose needs are you meeting?
- If you had a terminal illness, what would you like to be told?

Telling the truth: the principles

Despite the current emphasis on the patient's right to know and on patient autonomy, professional practices and attitudes vary and sometimes conflict. Doctors bear the main responsibility for informing patients but some find this too difficult. Because nurses and other professionals are often more available and approachable, patients who want to know more or who want clarification often turn to them. Although nurses and other professionals have their own ethical guidelines, they are often compelled to follow the doctor's lead. The UKCC (1996) states that, if there is conflict, nurses must stress that under their professional guidelines they are first and foremost accountable to the patient.

For all professionals, deciding what to say to patients and relatives who are facing very painful and difficult situations can be very hard, especially across cultural barriers. It is important that all the professionals involved, including social workers, counsellors and interpreters:

- share a basic commitment to the duty to care, to patient autonomy, confidentiality and informed consent, and to responding honestly to patients (see also *Giving bad news*, below);
- understand the importance of respecting different cultural and religious values as part of their duty of care to the patient;

- are well informed about the needs and wishes of each patient and of their relatives;
- are kept informed about how much each patient and their relatives know about the diagnosis and prognosis, and their wishes and fears;
- are able to explain their reasons and actions to the relatives;
- give other support to relatives whose wishes conflict with the professional's understanding of what the patient wants.

'To preserve both autonomy and beneficence, physicians must get to know their patients well enough to discern when, and if, those patients wish to contravene the mores of prevailing medical culture. This requires a degree of familiarity and sensitivity increasingly difficult to come by, but morally inescapable for every physician who practices in today's morally and culturally diverse world society.' (Pellegrino 1992)

Giving bad news

Buckman (1984) defines bad news as 'any news that drastically and negatively alters the patient's view of her or his future'. The impact of any news on an individual depends on their personality, lifestyle and aspirations, as well as on their cultural, spiritual and religious values. For example, although it is not life-threatening, being told that they are medically unfit to drive is devastating to someone whose lifestyle or job relies on driving. In communities where marriage is the only acceptable state for a woman, disfiguring treatment or surgery that might make her unmarriageable may be a particular catastrophe. In contrast, for a very old person in failing health who has strong religious or spiritual beliefs, death may be a friend rather than an enemy.

The effects of receiving bad news

Bad news is hard to give and harder still to receive. The way it is given can have a profound and lasting effect on people's lives; it is important to do it well.

'In Eritrea you don't use words, just words just like that. You break bad news through your own emotion. You go to see them and you cry, everybody cries, so the person who has to receive the bad news knows. And usually this is done by older people. You don't offer tea or coffee until after they have cried and wailed and released their feelings. Then you offer tea or coffee. Here you offer it first. It's different.'
Eritrean nurse

Think back to a time when you received some bad news. It might have been expected – or unexpected. Perhaps it was some disappointing exam results, or the break-up of an important relationship. Perhaps it was the illness or death of someone you loved.

Now jot down words to describe how you felt, and how you reacted, both at the time and in the following hours and days.

Look at the words you have written. Ask yourself, when you feel like this:

- can you listen and remember?
- can you understand what is being said to you?
- can you think clearly and objectively?
- can you make sound decisions?

Good practice in giving bad news

'... disclosure needs to be considered as part of a complex and on-going process, not a single event that does or does not occur.' (Del Vecchio Good, Good et al 1990)

Good practice includes:

- Offering privacy, time and attentive listening, sitting down at the same level (see also Chapter 23 *Listening with complete respect*).
- Finding out who, if anybody, the patient would like to have with them (see *Maintaining patient confidentiality*, below).
- Finding out how the patient views their situation and what they have already been told, trying to assess how much information they want.
- Letting the patient set the pace, tailoring the rate and depth of information to the patient's needs, not necessarily saying everything or saying everything now.
- Using open questions, matching language to individual needs, avoiding euphemisms, especially if there is a language barrier (see below).
- Accepting and adapting to the way the patient reacts, conveying empathy in a way that is appropriate to the patient's personality and culture.
- Not assuming that everybody wants to talk about their feelings, especially to people outside their family, or feels better for doing so (see Chapter 9 *Different families*), allowing time for silence and time for questions.
- Remembering that most people only take in and remember a small proportion of what they are told, especially when they are frightened or upset.

- Arranging a time to talk again later, and ensuring that the patient knows whom to contact and talk to in the meantime if they want to.
- Ensuring that the relevant staff know what the patient has been told and recording the discussion in the patient's notes.

Both the patient and the relatives (if they are present) may have practical and emotional concerns that they do not want to raise in front of each other to avoid distressing them. Offer each opportunities to talk to a key health professional in private.

Language barriers

Many people find it hard to discuss death and dying openly, especially when it relates to themselves or those they love. Traditionally, many use euphemisms such as 'go', 'pass away' or 'pass on'. The current move in English culture towards greater directness is probably helpful but hurts and shocks some people (see Chapter 2 Not cultural facts but cultural possibilities). Health professionals have to draw a fine line between respecting individual sensibilities and ensuring that what they say is clearly understood. Such a line is even more difficult to draw with someone whose English is patchy. Anxiety, shock and distress affect people's ability to understand what is said to them or to express themselves, even more so in a foreign language. If you are not confident that the person you are speaking to really understands what you are saying, a professional interpreter or a health advocate is essential.

When you have to give bad news through an interpreter or health advocate, try to talk to them before the interview. Explain what you intend to say and find out if there are any cultural or religious factors that would make the person unwilling to translate bad news to the patient or would affect the way they do it. Try to ensure that the same interpreter will be present next time you see the patient (see Chapter 27 Working well with a professional interpreter).

If the patient brings an English-speaking relative whom you might use to interpret, you need first to find out from the patient through a professional interpreter whether this is acceptable (see Maintaining patient confidentiality, below). Whenever a family member or friend interprets, the patient's confidentiality and autonomy are automatically breached. Many patients bring someone to interpret because they have been told to do so. This does not mean that they are happy for the person they have brought to be given personal, confidential information about them (see also Chapter 28 Using friends and relatives to interpret). Bear in mind, too, that, even if the patient is willing for a relative to interpret, the 'interpreter' may be unable to do so properly in distressing and difficult situations.

It is never acceptable to use a child to interpret anything that may be confidential, distressing, personal or sensitive, or that they would not normally know about or be party to (see Chapter 28 *Children*).

Training and support for health professionals

'A patient can be given bad news in many different ways – none can make it good!' (Goldie 1982)

However well it is done, giving bad news is always hard, very time consuming and stressful. Nobody wants to cause pain and anguish; most of us find it hard to witness people's shock, disbelief, grief and anger. We may also worry that we might be blamed, or that we simply do not know how to give bad news well (Buckman 1996). All health professionals should be offered training on giving bad news, including across cultural and language barriers. All health professionals should also have access to professional support and help whenever they need it.

Maintaining patient confidentiality

All patients have a right to expect confidentiality (UKCC 1996, BMA and RCN 1995). However, maintaining confidentiality has become increasingly complex with the proliferation of bureaucracy in health and social services. Guidance issued by the General Medical Council (GMC 1998b) clarifies the duty of doctors in relation to confidentiality. It states, among other things, that:

- In all normal circumstances the patient's agreement should be obtained before information is given to the patient's partner or family.
- Relevant information should be shared with other health professionals involved in caring for the patient, unless the patient objects. Only information that is relevant may be disclosed.
- Consent is not required when a doctor has a statutory obligation to disclose information; for example, when notifying a communicable disease or when required to disclose information by a judge, a coroner or a procurator fiscal.
- Consent is not required when disclosure of information would prevent serious harm to a third party (see, for example, Chapter 20 *Infection control issues*).

The views and needs of relatives

The illness and impending death of a family member or loved one is a major life crisis that may have serious practical and financial implications for relatives, as well as long-term emotional and personal consequences. Understandably, most relatives want to know the likely course and length of the patient's illness so that they can give the patient the support they need and can try to plan and to pace themselves both practically and emotionally. This is especially important if they are to be involved in some or all of the patient's practical care. However, sometimes patients do not want to know their own diagnosis and prognosis, or are unwilling to give consent to relatives being informed about their condition. Sometimes relatives are adamant that it would be culturally or religiously unacceptable to tell the patient the truth. These situations raise major problems related to patient confidentiality.

As a general principle, it is wrong to give relatives information about a patient's condition or prognosis without telling the patient, or without the patient's consent. This does however, happen, particularly when the patient is old and frail (BMA, personal communication 1998). If a decision is made to withhold information from a patient but to give it to the relatives, it is always necessary both to be absolutely clear about the reasons and to be sure that the decision is genuinely in the patient's own best interests. The decision should never be made purely because the patient is old, or belongs to a certain ethnic or religious group, or because of relatives' anxieties about their own ability to cope with the patient knowing the truth (see also *Telling patients the truth*, earlier).

Possible cultural and religious factors

Managing confidentiality can be particularly complex when caring for patients whose families have a hierarchy of authority, or where decisions are made by the family rather than by the individual. Senior family members may feel that they have a right to information as part of taking responsibility for the care and protection of the patient. They may find the idea of patient confidentiality strange or misguided.

'An elderly Asian woman was due to see me following a hysterectomy. I planned to discuss management options with her as the histology confirmed an aggressive malignancy. I was surprised when her husband and sons appeared instead. They said they had come for the results and that the patient was at home. I had to explain gently but firmly that I could not discuss any medical details or treatment options with them and that I needed to see the patient herself.'
British Asian consultant gynaecologist

As in this case, it may sometimes be necessary to explain that your duty of care and confidentiality is to the patient and that their consent is needed before you can talk to anyone else.

Some patients or families ask their religious leader for advice or to act as advocates for them. Occasionally a religious leader may ask professionals for information about the patient's condition or treatment options in order to clarify their own understanding. Consent should first be obtained from the patient or, if the patient is not competent, from the next of kin.

16 The place of care

When there is a choice to be made about the place of care, those responsible need to ensure that both the patient and the relatives are well informed about the different options. This may be particularly important for black and minority ethnic families who may know less about different possibilities and what they involve.

Care at home

Many patients want to stay at home if they can, maintaining familiar routines with people they are used to, and retaining as much privacy and independence as possible. They may see a hospital, and almost certainly a hospice, as a place where people only go to die. For some people the idea of leaving home for such a place is terrifying.

> 'I think they should not build all these old people's homes. Give the people a home that all the family can live together and die together. How nice it is for an old person in her bed with her grandchildren around her, and she die in peace with her grandchildren around her.'
> Elderly Jamaican woman (Age Exchange 1994)

From a practical point of view, however, care at home is often impossible, especially when the patient's condition becomes more serious. Many older people in all communities live alone and have no one to look after them. Others live with an equally old and often frail spouse for whom the practical tasks of caring may be too much. In many households all adults of working age are out all day; there is no one to look after a seriously ill or dependent person. Poorer families may simply be unable to afford the costs of a family member at home who needs extra laundry, extra heating, a special diet, repeat prescriptions and so on. People who live in overcrowded accommodation may have insufficient privacy or space for someone who is seriously ill. They may lack adequate washing, cooking, storage and other facilities.

For black and minority ethnic families, there may sometimes be additional considerations.

- In many cultures it is traditional for people to grow old and die at home and for the adult women of the family to provide all the necessary care. Older people and those who are very ill may expect to die at home surrounded by the people who love them.
- Patients may fear that their cultural and religious needs will not be fully understood or met away from home. They worry that they will encounter prejudice, insensitivity and racism from staff and other patients when they are already most vulnerable. Their families may share their fears.

> 'My mother was in an old people's home where the staff were kind and did their best but there were two old ladies who were very rude to her. They called her "Black cow" and much worse things. The manager said it was to be expected because they were old and they probably didn't mean to hurt. I found it strange; why should people be allowed to be racist and unpleasant and make other people unhappy just because they're old? It didn't get any better and she was miserable so in the end she came home.'
> Indian woman

- Some family members who cannot care for a relative at home may feel guilty at what they may see as an extreme failure of duty. They may also be judged harshly by other members of their community. Some older people who have to go into hospital or other residential care may feel ashamed and humiliated at their family's failure to carry out their moral and/or religious obligations towards them.
- For older refugees, even those who have lived in Britain for many years and who seem perfectly at home, the losses associated with ageing and illness – physical losses, illness and dependency – as well as separation from familiar people and places, may trigger intense and profoundly disturbing feelings. A study of ageing survivors of Nazi concentration camps found that it was very difficult for people to accept illness. In the camps, illness meant an automatic death sentence, whilst health meant possible survival. The prospect of leaving home and going into hospital or other residential care may also terrify some people (Hirschfeld 1977).
- In communities where death traditionally carries a stigma, for example in some Chinese communities, some families may very much want a seriously ill or dying person to be cared for in hospital so that the bad luck associated with death does not affect their home (see Chapter 38 *Attitudes towards death and dying*).

Support for relatives caring at home

'Sometimes I visit a home and the patient is lying in bed, the focus of attention, grapes, flowers, everyone running around meeting his needs. And at the foot of the bed is his wife, anxious and weepy, hasn't slept through the night in months, can't go out of the house, has a bad back, isn't eating properly, shaking with exhaustion, and no one is looking after her. I ask you, who is the patient here?'
Community palliative care nurse

Many carers in all communities are lonely, socially isolated, anxious and exhausted. Black and minority ethnic carers may experience additional problems due to isolation from wider society, language barriers, unfamiliarity with sources of available support or support that is inappropriate (eg unsuitable meals-on-wheels or day care provision). Research confirms that many black and minority ethnic carers find it difficult to get access to the services available; many also know little about the services or financial help they or the patient are entitled to (Yee 1995). It is important to help make sure both that patients and carers receive the support they need and are entitled to, and that this support meets their personal, religious and cultural needs.

'Carer' is a relatively new bureaucratic term for relatives or friends who care for people at home, coined to meet the needs of statutory services. Although it is gaining acceptance outside professional circles, many people find it awkward and unfamiliar and do not identify themselves as carers. Black and minority ethnic relatives may be unfamiliar with the word 'carer' as applied to themselves and may not understand how, for example, carers' associations, carers' support schemes or carers' forums could be of help to them (Yee 1995).

'Community' support? The use of the term 'communities' in relation to black and minority ethnic groups can seem to imply that families within these groups are embedded in a close and supportive network. This is no more likely to be true than among the white 'communities'. People who share a language, a culture and possibly a religion **may** form a mutually supportive group but this cannot be assumed. All 'communities', minority or majority, are in fact made up of disparate individuals and families with different backgrounds, areas of origin, concerns, values and interests. Economic pressures and social mobility can lead to the weakening of social and religious bonds. People who simply look similar to outsiders may have little or nothing in common and are unlikely to feel a sense of mutual responsibility simply because of their skin colour. Many black and minority ethnic families also live in areas where there are few or no other families of their 'community'.

Even where there is a clear local minority community, this does not guarantee mutual support or involvement. Most families in all communities are busy with their own responsibilities and duties and have no time or energy to reach out to others. Degrees of neighbourliness and mutual support vary a good deal everywhere; long-term practical support across family boundaries is generally rare. Members of black and minority ethnic groups may find less support in Britain than in their country of origin.

'We were much closer back home. The children were in and out of each other's houses. When there was trouble in a family, everybody knew and people would stop by and offer to help. They would maybe cook a pot of food and send it round with one of the children. Here it's different. Everybody is so busy and there is no time for people or for dropping in. It can be very lonely here.'

Jamaican woman

Do not assume that black and minority ethnic carers have more access to wider community support than white majority carers. Because they often feel marginalised and excluded by the white 'community', they may have less.

Hospital and residential care

When a patient is seriously ill or dying, many people feel that a hospital or hospice will give the best care. For black and minority ethnic patients and families there may be particular considerations.

- If people are to be able to choose the place of care, they need detailed information about the extent to which the different options will cater for their cultural and religious needs (see Chapters 9 to 12). If the patient speaks little or no English, it is also important to find out whether an appropriate interpreter will be available.

'These people came over to Britain to work and have contributed a great deal to society. They have adapted and fitted in [to British culture] all

through their adult lives and now that they have retired it is time they were able to be themselves.'
Manager, residential care home (Mangan 1988)

- People who have experienced extreme loss and separation in their lives (eg asylum seekers and refugees) may find further isolation terrifying and unbearable. Wherever possible, flexible arrangements should be made for family members to stay with patients or to visit as often as they can (Hirschfeld 1977).
- Moving from a familiar to an unfamiliar environment is a common cause of confusion for older people, even more so for people who are already confused.

   '... environmental factors may play a considerable part in the process of dementia; ... the elderly person can be very sensitive to environmental influences; if these are negative they may accelerate normal cerebral ageing to a considerable degree.' (Bram 1983)

Hospital wards, for example, can be disorientating even for patients of the majority culture. For many black and minority ethnic patients, everything may be less familiar and more confusing. It may be necessary to pay special attention to ways of reducing the stress caused by unfamiliarity and to try to ensure that as much as possible in the daily routine is familiar to the patient. This may include food, washing arrangements, religious observances, clothing, and cultural and religious symbols. It helps, too, if there are people who understand and even share their values, experiences and interests.

Familiar language also helps. A research study of people with dementia found that language that was more complex than they could understand significantly increased restlessness and agitation (Hart and Wells 1997). This has particular implications for people with dementia who speak little or no English. People with dementia may also become even more distressed and confused if they are cut off from all communication.

'Sometimes people think that the distress shown by someone who cannot speak English is due to their dementia, when in fact it is related to their absolute isolation and the fact that they have been deprived of human interaction.' (Kratiuk-Wall, Shanley and Russell 1997)

- When people are moved out of their home, discharged from hospital or moved from one facility to another, it is important to ensure that their care continues smoothly and to a high standard. The professional who takes responsibility for initiating, co-ordinating, planning and organising the discharge process needs a complete picture of the whole patient and their situation (Nazarko 1997). All this is even more significant when there are particular cultural or religious needs to take into account, and when these may be unfamiliar to the receiving health professionals and may require special consideration or provision.

Hospice and other palliative care

Research indicates that black and minority ethnic patients are currently under-represented in hospices and other specialist services for people who are dying. This is true even when allowance is made for age and class differences and some different patterns of disease. Various reasons have been suggested for the failure, up to now, of most hospice and similar services to reach those black and minority ethnic people who need them (Haroon-Iqbal, Field et al 1995, Hill and Penso 1995, O'Neill 1994). These include:

- Different patterns of referral, possibly because of assumptions by GPs and other health professionals that black and minority ethnic patients and families will find hospices and similar services alien and unfamiliar, that hospices will not cater for minority cultural and religious requirements, or that black and minority ethnic families prefer to care for patients at home.
- Patients and families may also worry that practical provision for patients will not meet their cultural needs.
- Many hospices have had an overtly religious, usually Christian, image and atmosphere, which may make people of other religions or of no religion feel unwelcome and ill at ease. Even if the religious orientation of the hospice is not overt or if insiders are not aware of it, it may seem intrusive and oppressive to people of other faiths (O'Neill 1994).
- Only a few hospices or other similar services currently provide interpreters in minority languages.
- Information about hospice and other palliative care services is often spread by word of mouth, which may mean that it does not reach minority communities. Publicity material is generally in English and may give a very 'English' image of the care available. There is very little information in minority languages or through channels that may be more accessible to black and minority ethnic people.

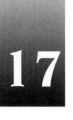

17 The needs of relatives of people in hospital and other residential care

'Admission to hospital has a profound effect on all family members, even though only one person is being treated.' (Altschuler 1997)

Until recently, admission to hospital or residential care and the resulting focus on the patient often meant the marginalisation of the family. However, whenever an individual becomes ill or dependent, other family members are affected, often severely and permanently. The needs and problems of patient and family members are usually bound up with each other. Caring for a dependent, ill or dying patient may, therefore, also involve supporting and looking after the family. (Here and in the rest of this book the words 'family' or 'relatives' are used to mean all the people who are close to the patient.)

Whereas health professionals often have fairly short-term contact with a patient, relatives have known that person all their lives. How family members see and respond to their responsibilities reflects years of shared history, the details of which are not known to health professionals, and can sometimes result in behaviour that is difficult, baffling and even destructive. Nevertheless, relatives are a crucial part of the picture. They usually understand the patient's personal, cultural and religious needs, and generally continue to feel a strong responsibility for the patient. Relatives in all communities who feel informed, listened to and valued are more likely to be able to support and care for the patient in their turn. Many patients are also very anxious about the effects of their illness on their relatives. Knowing that health professionals are aware of their relatives' needs and are supporting them can give great comfort.

Relatives as 'visitors'

In an institution there is usually little physical space for close family members and friends. They are often labelled 'visitors', a term that in no way indicates their importance or their closeness to the patient. In most places, visitors have to follow explicit and implicit rules about what they can and cannot do, and how they should behave. Visitors are also expected to be self-policing. Breaking the rules is usually assumed to be a conscious and ill-mannered act.

However, 'correct' visitors' behaviour varies a good deal. In many parts of the world, families are responsible for much of the practical day-to-day care that, in the UK, is given by professional staff and care assistants. Hospitals are open and family members may be expected or even required to stay 24 hours a day. There are no visiting times or restrictions on numbers.

> 'I was in a bad car crash in Italy and spent five months in hospital, most of the time unable to move. I discovered that the family was supposed to feed the patient. I would literally have starved if my kind friends hadn't organised a rota of people to come and feed me every day.'
> English woman

People from countries where health care is private or paid for through private insurance schemes may, in contrast, expect a high level of hotel-type services.

What are your assumptions about how visitors should behave?

- What is the normal number of visitors? How long should they stay and what should they do or not do? When should they not be there?
- Under what circumstances might visitors stay overnight? How many? What can they reasonably ask for?
- Should visitors care for the patients' physical needs? What should they do or not do?
- Should visitors bring in food? When? What kinds? What practical help can they reasonably ask for?
- What can visitors reasonably expect you to do? What requests or demands do you consider unacceptable?

How do you feel when visitors do things outside the bounds of what you consider acceptable? How do you respond?

Most people work out what is expected by watching, listening and asking other patients and relatives. This is far more difficult across language and cultural barriers. A survey of minority ethnic parents with children in hospital found that half the parents had not been told about doctors' rounds, mealtimes or the availability of a hospital social worker (Slater 1993). Staff may need to help patients and relatives who are unfamiliar with their situation by offering sensitive explanations and giving them opportunities to ask questions. Try not to assume that seemingly 'inappropriate' behaviour is intentional.

'We had a lot of Bengali women on our ward and most of them kept their curtains shut all the time. When their husbands came in they would walk up the ward opening all the curtains. We were furious. If they were so worried about modesty, how could they be so insensitive? Why didn't the cultural rules on modesty apply to them? Then an interpreter pointed out that it wasn't a cultural thing. They were just looking for their wives. Now we have the names outside the curtains and everyone is happy again.'
English health professional

Working together

In many cases, health professionals and relatives work well together in caring for a patient. However, there is often an inherent tension between them over responsibility for care, information and 'ownership' of the patient, especially in a long-term relationship (Relatives Association 1997). Many relatives feel that they no longer have the same rights with regard to the patient: they cannot care for or relate to the patient in the same way, and physical contact is often difficult, especially under public scrutiny. Many feel awkward and inhibited. When there are cultural differences between family and staff, there is even more potential for mutual misunderstanding, distress and hostility. The following can usually help to minimise possible problems.

- Create an atmosphere in which relatives feel welcomed and validated. This is especially important for black and minority ethnic relatives, who may feel under particular scrutiny from other patients, families and staff.
- Value and use the knowledge that relatives have about the patient and his or her normal habits and wishes, especially if the patient has different cultural or religious needs and/or there is a language barrier. Most relatives are grateful for respectful and sensitive requests for information and advice.

'The staff were great. They asked us all about my father's preferences and what was important to him, and then they really tried to make everything

right. I can't tell you how much better I felt. I was feeling so guilty but they did a very good job to make things familiar for him and make him feel comfortable so that he felt all right there. That took a load off my mind.'
Sri Lankan woman

- Make sure that relatives know who is who and who does what. Because of traditional hierarchies, male health professionals may be assumed to have more authority than their female counterparts. Older people, in particular, may assume that women doctors are nurses, or are subordinate to junior male colleagues. Doctors may be seen as having knowledge and authority on all matters. The role of the nurse may not be understood. Problems are likely to be exacerbated if people do not understand the meanings of the different titles used in the health service, cannot read name badges, or if proper introductions have not been made.

  'On a ward round, a patient questioned my decisions about her management, saying that the doctor (indicating the pre-registration house officer) had decided to do something quite different. The patient assumed that, because the house officer was male and I was female, he must be the one in charge.'
  British Asian consultant gynaecologist

- Make sure that relatives know whom they can talk to if they have worries or problems. If they speak little or no English, it may be necessary to communicate through an interpreter (see also Chapter 28 *Working well with a professional interpreter*).
- Find out whether relatives who have been caring for the patient at home would like to continue with certain aspects of practical care, and help make this possible. On the other hand, recognise that they may be extremely grateful to be able to hand over practical care to other people.
- Try not to see family members' concern about the patient's care or treatment as criticism, but listen and accept their concern positively (Relatives Association 1997). Although most family members have no medical expertise, they are the experts on their own relative. They usually have more time than busy health professionals and may be better observers of subtle changes in the patient's condition (see, for example, Chapter 13 *Recognising clinical signs in skin*). Wherever possible, take advantage of the relatives' attention and contribution, making time to listen to them and regarding them as partners in care.

Visiting restrictions

If the patient is part of a large close-knit family or community, there may be large numbers of visitors. They may also feel an obligation to visit outside normal visiting hours (see Chapter 9 *Different families*). People who work shifts or long hours, for example in the catering or retail trades, may need to visit in the mornings. The continual presence of visitors can cause problems on a public ward or in a shared room, and staff may have to make very difficult decisions, trying to understand and balance the needs and obligations of everyone involved (Murphy and Macleod Clark 1993).

- The patient may be very grateful for the company and support of family members, especially if they speak little or no English or feel culturally or socially isolated. They may be afraid to be left alone. On the other hand, they may also need rest and peace and quiet. Wherever possible, it should be the patient's needs and wishes that determine the visiting arrangements.
- The relatives may want to be there all the time to look after the patient, and may worry about leaving the patient alone. They may feel under a moral or religious obligation to be there 24 hours a day. In some communities it is very important that the family is present when a patient dies. There may also be religious rites to be carried out (see Chapter 18 *Religious ceremonies*).
- However, the constant presence of large numbers of people can cause problems for the patient and their immediate relatives, who may want time alone together in private.

> 'When my mum was very ill it was really difficult for my brother, me or my dad to be alone with her or have any private time with her. There were so many people around all the time and we wanted to say things we couldn't say with them there. But we couldn't ask the rest of the family to stay away. They would have been hurt and scandalised. Finally I asked one of the nurses if she could have a word and say that my mum needed fewer visitors for a bit. She did it very tactfully and we were able to have some time in peace with my mum before she died.'
> South Asian woman

- Large numbers of visitors can also cause problems for other people who may find it difficult to sleep or rest, may feel their privacy intruded upon, or may find the situation unfair. They may also cause problems for staff and disturb routines. It may sometimes be possible to move the patient into a side room, or to ask visitors to visit a little less while still meeting the patient's needs. When explaining any restrictions, make it clear that you understand the difficulty and distress these may cause, and try to find creative solutions together.

Many wards and units have signs outside restricting numbers and times of visitors. If some patients and their visitors regularly observe these restrictions and others do not, this can cause understandable and lasting resentment and bad feeling. In general, it is wise to avoid setting up restrictions that people of different communities are almost bound to break. It may be better to have a more general sign inviting people to ask about visiting arrangements, or stating a general policy on visiting and inviting visitors to discuss their particular needs with staff.

Visitors from far away

Black and minority ethnic patients may be more likely to have visitors who fly in from overseas. If a patient is seriously ill and deteriorating, or near death, it is clearly very important that the visitor is allowed to see the patient as soon as possible, even at unusual hours. In extended families, people outside the nuclear family grouping may be considered very close relatives.

> 'My uncle had a heart attack and my aunt phoned me. I set off at once but it was a long journey and then I had to wait for a place on a flight. On the night when I finally got to the hospital it was midnight and he was still alive but they would not let me see him because I was not his son, only the son of his second cousin. In the morning he was dead and I never said goodbye.'
> Bangladeshi man

Sometimes immigration officials may require information from doctors before granting a visa to a visitor from abroad wishing to visit a seriously ill or dying relative. In some cases visas have been refused; in others, administrative delay has meant that they were issued too late.

Giving information to relatives

Informing relatives about the progress and condition of different patients can be a major strain for busy staff. If a large number of people are concerned about the same patient it can be particularly difficult. There may also be issues of confidentiality when professionals do not know all the people they are talking to or are not sure about their relationship with the patient (see also Chapter 15 *Maintaining patient confidentiality*). It is often best to identify a single family member to act as the focal point for communication. Such a person can pass on information about the patient's condition to other family members, and can pass on questions and concerns from the family to the health professionals caring for the patient. If the family chooses an older person who speaks little English, on grounds of seniority, a second family member may be needed to interpret. It may also be helpful to arrange an occasional family meeting if patient care issues become complex and if many people are likely to have concerns and questions.

Expressing emotion

Cultural and religious differences may lead relatives to express their grief and concern in ways that health professionals may not understand or find difficult to accept. Some may express their feelings loudly, cry openly or shout, and seem, to many white English eyes at least, alarmingly out of control and threatening (see also Chapter 21 *Culture and the expression of grief*). Others may show little or nothing and seem strangely unconcerned. Across cultural and language barriers it can be very hard to know whether relatives need help. If professionals are seriously worried, it may be helpful to consult, in complete confidence, a professional interpreter or a cultural broker (see Chapter 23 *Cultural brokers*).

Facilities for visitors

Many relatives visiting patients suffer from lack of privacy, lack of food and lack of overnight facilities (Townsend, Frank et al 1990). These problems may be more acute for black and ethnic minority families. If the patient speaks little or no English or feels anxious about being in an unfamiliar environment, relatives often feel that it is particularly important for someone to stay with them all the time, including overnight. Even if food is available for relatives, it is not always suitable in cultural and religious terms (see also Chapter 11). There may be nowhere suitable to pray or to wash before praying (see also Chapters 10 *Prayer and meditation* and 12 *Bathing and showering*). All hospitals and residential care institutions need to review their provision for relatives of all communities who visit or want to stay overnight, and make sure that their basic needs are met.

Wherever possible, there should be a quiet room where relatives can go to be alone, to rest or to make themselves something to drink. Ideally, such rooms should be large enough to accommodate larger families, with enough seating for men and women to sit separately. Disposable cups should be available so that people who do not use cutlery or crockery that may have been in contact with prohibited food (eg observant Jews) can make themselves a hot or cold drink (see Chapter 47 *Religious requirements*).

18 Care for people who are dying

•••

'We have to take a good hard look at our own attitude to death and dying before we can sit quietly and without anxiety next to a terminally ill patient.' (Kübler-Ross 1970)

Caring for people in the final stages of their lives requires special skills and sensitivity. Identifying and meeting individual cultural or religious needs and wishes is an important part of that care.

'However many dying people I've known, this person is dying for the first time and I don't know what they need: everyone has different needs. You must hold your previous experience of dying patterns very lightly, so that if they prove incorrect for this person then you can shift very quickly.'
Hospice project administrator (Walter 1994)

Cultural and professional attitudes towards death

'There are many ways in which human beings can approach their own and others' mortality, but no one chooses their approach independently of others. True, we each die alone. But we also die as we live, as social beings.' (Walter 1996)

Beliefs and attitudes towards death and dying are very personal. However, Western societies seem, at present, to find it easier to accept death as 'entertainment' rather than as the inevitable and natural conclusion to life. Most children have seen many thousands of violent deaths on screen before they reach adulthood. At the same time, increasing longevity means that many people have little or no real contact with dying people or with death until they are well into middle age. In addition, death is now largely dealt with away from everyday life. It has become institutionalised and the province of professionals (see also Chapter 21 *Mourning rituals*).

'In the nineteenth century it had been the physician's role to minister over or administer a peaceful death; his modern successor seemed to promise to overcome death. Rendered a mark of failure, death became a taboo, something to be deferred.' (Porter 1997)

Expectations of medical science have risen enormously. Some people appear to feel that, with the right doctor and the right treatment, death can and should be postponed almost indefinitely. It is possible that a decline in religious belief in the West has also made it more difficult for people to accept death. Death is less often seen as a transition to a better life than as an enemy to be fought until the bitter end. Dying can be seen as losing the battle.

> 'I feel so ashamed; I feel I'm letting my children and my husband down. I should be able to beat this, and if I can't I am failing them.'
> English woman with cancer

Health professionals share aspects of the culture in which they live. It seems that many health professionals also find death particularly hard to accept.

> 'Much has been written about patients denying a lethal prognosis, but little about physicians doing so.' (Higgs 1999)

It is possible that people who choose a profession that enables them to care and to save lives may be more likely to experience death as a failure and an insult, and dying patients as people 'for whom nothing can be done' (Buckman 1996).

> 'Most of us are not very good at dealing with death. We want to make things better and everything to be OK. I didn't get a lot of preparation as a student. We had training days on death and saw a few videos, but it doesn't really prepare you properly, especially when you are young and haven't had much life experience.'
> British Jewish staff nurse

Religious beliefs

All major religions teach that physical death is not the end. However, the precise form that continued existence takes varies between different religions and sometimes between different denominations (see also Part Five). Major themes include:

- belief in the cycle of birth, death and rebirth (reincarnation);
- being united with God;
- being re-united with loved ones who have died earlier;
- being judged and rewarded or punished for past deeds and thoughts, possibly in hell or in heaven, in purgatory, or in the next life;
- going to heaven or hell;
- sleeping or resting until spiritually or physically resurrected by God.

Strong religious faith brings great comfort to some patients and their relatives.

> 'We have some African-Caribbean Christian patients who have a really strong faith. When they are terminally ill, they almost welcome the prospect of death, as they will be united with God. It is quite humbling to see such radiant faith.'
> Irish Macmillan nurse

However, not everyone with strong religious beliefs faces the finality of death calmly. Even strong faith can waver. Many people are daunted by the prospect of being judged and rewarded or punished for the lives they have led. For many, the idea of leaving everyone and everything they know is terrible. Each person has their own fears and anxieties.

> 'My mother-in-law said she was frightened of death. I asked if she meant the process of dying or being dead. She assured me she meant being dead. I asked why, since I know she doesn't believe in an afterlife. She replied "I can't bear to think of it all going on down here and I won't know about it."'
> English woman

Individuals of any religion or denomination (or of none) vary in what they want to talk about. Some people feel better for talking about their feelings and fears, especially to a respectful and sensitive listener. Some feel that religious and spiritual matters are personal; others prefer to keep quiet with people who do not share their faith for fear of being misunderstood. Some find that they cannot believe what their religion teaches and feel frightened or guilty. The only way to find out about a person's beliefs or fears and whether you can help in any way is to listen respectfully to what they choose to tell you.

A 'good death'

> 'Approaching one's own death or the death of a loved one is among the greatest times of stress we face as human beings.' (O'Rawe Amenta 1997)

In recent years health professionals, especially those working in palliative care, have focused on the idea of a good death. Definitions tend to emphasise physical and psychological rather than religious or social perspectives. They often include good symptom control, maintaining autonomy and control, emotional support and comfort, family involvement, accepting death, setting practical affairs in order and resolving unfinished business (Payne, Langley-Evans and Hillier 1996, Payne, Hillier et al 1996, BMA 1993, Pickett 1993). However, patients' ideas about a good death may differ.

In one study, Payne, Langley-Evans and Hillier (1996) found that patients placed less importance on awareness and conscious involvement. They were more likely to value a sudden death, dying in one's sleep, dying quietly and in dignity, and being free of pain.

Personal beliefs, values and experiences, as well as cultural and religious norms, all influence people's priorities and needs, and their ideas about a good death. Indeed, for some people there is no such thing as a good death. It is important to avoid assumptions about what will be right or wrong for any individual and to try to find out from them. For example:

- Some people may want – for personal, cultural or religious reasons – to avoid pharmacological symptom control and pain relief (see also Chapter 14 *Pain and pain relief*).
- Dignity, privacy and cleanliness are important to most people. However, particular aspects may be very important to people who observe strict codes of modesty and personal hygiene (see Chapter 12 *Modesty* and *Personal hygiene*).
- Patients who see themselves as part of an interdependent family group may be unused to making decisions by themselves. Those for whom serious illness or old age involves withdrawing from responsibility may not want to make decisions. Some people may prefer to let others decide on their behalf (see Chapter 9 *Different families*).
- Most people prefer to die in a place where they feel that they belong and are accepted and loved, and where things are familiar and cherished. Some black and minority ethnic patients may very much want to go to their own or their family's country of origin to die.
- If a patient is unaware of or does not want to know their prognosis (see Chapter 15 *Telling patients the truth*), it can be difficult or impossible to help them come to terms with their approaching death, set their practical affairs in order, or deal with unfinished business. However, they will still have many practical and emotional needs that can be met with respect and understanding.
- Some people have a religious requirement to ask forgiveness of others and to make peace before they die. Some may be more concerned about getting practical and business matters settled.
- In some religions a good death involves opportunities for reflection, meditation or repentance, with the aim of reaching spiritual peace and acceptance. A sudden or unexpected death may be viewed by some people as disastrous and as having very bad consequences for the soul of the person who has died (see Chapter 19 *Sudden death*).
- For many patients and relatives it is very important to ensure a good death and, sometimes, to help the progress of the soul by performing

religious ceremonies and rituals immediately before and/or immediately after the death.

Making decisions at the end of life

Advances in medical science and technology have made it possible in some cases to prolong life even when there is little or no hope of recovery. Discussing the withdrawal or withholding of active treatment confronts people with the reality of impending death. Some patients and some relatives find this very hard to accept. They may want to continue active and sometimes aggressive treatment. In some cases their wishes are based on deeply rooted cultural norms or religious requirements.

- People who feel a duty to preserve life at all costs, to maintain hope and never give up, may be particularly anxious to continue aggressive treatment even when they are told that there is no hope of benefit (see also Chapter 47 *Attitudes to life and illness*). Some may seek second and third opinions or complementary treatments. Some may want the patient to receive intravenous or subcutaneous fluids, and others may ask for the patient to be tube fed (NCHSPCS 1997).
- Relatives who believe that the patient should be protected from the knowledge that they are dying, or who have a duty to maintain hope, may be very distressed by proposals to stop active treatment and may not want the patient to be included in decisions about, for example, cardiopulmonary resuscitation.

Discussing cardiopulmonary resuscitation (CPR)

Decisions about CPR must be taken on an individual basis, normally after discussion with the patient themselves. Some people prefer a peaceful death with dignity rather than to be resuscitated. Others, even those who know they are dying, will want CPR. In a study comparing relatives' and patients' views, Mead and Turnbull (1995) noted that, although 86 per cent of older patients were willing to be consulted about their own CPR status, their relatives were much less enthusiastic about them being asked. Mead and Turnbull concluded that mentally competent, older patients should be asked for their views.

However, discussing resuscitation with patients is a difficult and sensitive task. Some relatives, especially those who feel – for cultural, religious or personal reasons – that people who are dying should be protected, may object particularly strongly. Whenever possible, discussions about CPR should be held as part of wider conversation with the patient about how they see their situation and what is important to them. Ideally, such discussions should take place at a time when the patient is relatively well and the question is less likely to cause alarm, but this is not always possible. It is also important to remember that people may change their minds when their circumstances change.

Symptom control

Most people of all cultures and religions are willing to accept whatever will relieve their symptoms. However, some may be concerned about accepting pain relief, particularly opiates and sedatives because of the double effect (see Chapter 14 *Treating pain*). In some cases giving the patient more information, allaying specific fears, or adjusting the medication or the method of administration may help. In other cases, people may make decisions that you find difficult to accept. It is important to support the patient's preferred coping strategies even if they are unfamiliar.

Emotional and spiritual care

Although Western medicine divides up the physical, social, emotional and spiritual aspects of the self and usually pays most attention to the physical, in fact, all these aspects interrelate and affect each other (Baines 1990). Psychological pain, for example, can exacerbate or exceed physical pain. Everyone, therefore, needs holistic care: to be treated not just in terms of their illness but as an individual with their own beliefs and values and their own unique needs for emotional as well as physical care. Emotional and spiritual needs cannot be categorised or anticipated; it is important not to assume on the basis of ethnicity, social situation or religion what they are (NHS Confederation 1996).

'An elderly Jewish lady, originally from Vienna, flatly refused an offer to see any of our chaplains. However, she went downhill very quickly and asked to see a priest. Because she was Jewish the nurse assumed she meant a rabbi and asked one to see her. The old lady was deeply offended and insisted that she wanted to see a priest. It turned out that she had been protected by a Catholic priest as a child and wanted to say thank you before she died.'
Hospice manager

Coming to terms with dying

The range of feelings experienced by people who are approaching death have been described by Kübler-Ross (1970) as a grief process. She observed that people often experience five stages: denial, anger, bargaining, depression and, finally, acceptance. These insights revolutionised people's understanding of the emotional process of dying and have enabled health professionals and others to provide more understanding and supportive emotional and spiritual care.

Kübler-Ross makes it clear that these stages are not a blueprint, and that not every dying person experiences every stage. However, as with many valuable insights, her findings are sometimes simplified and reduced, giving the impression that it is normal and desirable for everyone who is dying to move step by step through a simple process of stages towards acceptance. In reality, patients and their feelings vary a good deal, influenced by factors such as their personality, the nature of their condition, their age and life experience, their culture and their religion. Although many people who know that they are dying do experience denial, anger, bargaining, depression and acceptance, it is unhelpful to expect and encourage all patients to go through them, or to assume that there is a problem if they do not. In addition, people may sometimes be angry or depressed about things that need urgent practical action by health professionals, for example poor communication, failures of care, or insensitive or inappropriate care.

Denial, sometimes considered a harmful or bizarre reaction, can in fact be a protective mechanism that enables people to face their situation at their own pace. Denial can give people the hope and courage to endure suffering by alleviating the external reality of illness (Davidhizar and Newman Giger 1998). People often take in only as much information as they can cope with at a particular time, and may later ask for information that they have already been given. They may move in and out of denial, depending on how much painful reality they can deal with and giving themselves time, consciously or unconsciously, to get used to the facts. Some people remain hopeful of recovery to the end.

'My mother, who was a psychotherapist, knew that she had cancer secondaries and that she was very ill. But she was talking cheerfully about coming home to turn her PhD thesis into a book only a couple of days before she died. I'm glad we didn't confront her with the fact that she was bound to die soon. She was happy and optimistic right to the end.'
English woman

In some cultures and for some individuals, denial is accepted as a normal, long-term protective mechanism and may be considered the best or only way of maintaining hope and courage. People who believe that it is essential to preserve hope at all costs may simply decline to face the reality of their situation. Relatives may also see it as their duty to protect the patient from such awareness (see also Chapter 15 *Telling patients the truth*). People who believe that it is unlucky to contemplate anything negative may also refuse to consider anything but full recovery.

It is important for health professionals to attune themselves to the patient at any particular time and to offer whatever information or response they believe will be most helpful. Maguire and Faulkner (1993) suggest that **'denial should not be challenged unless it is creating serious problems for the patient or relatives' and that, if it must be challenged, this must be done gently and with sensitivity.**

Anger and bargaining Many people, especially those whose death is untimely, feel great anger at their approaching death and at the loss they are facing. This anger may be turned inwards or may be directed outwards, sometimes at family members, employers or at health professionals. However, not everyone feels anger.

- People who feel that they have had a good life and are ready to die may see no cause for anger or bargaining (Walter 1994). Religious people who feel a great trust in God's plan for them may also accept their death without anger or bargaining. However, some religious people who feel that they should trust in God's will and cannot, or who feel that anger is wrong, may feel guilty and ashamed. They may welcome an opportunity to talk to someone who will not judge them (see also *Religious beliefs*, earlier).
- Anger often arises from the sense that an injustice has been committed against oneself. In some cultures, injustice is more often attributed to one's own lack of vigilance or failure to prevent the problem early enough. Some people may therefore see no reason for anger when they are approaching death.

  'Encouraging such an individual to express an anger he does not feel, but the caregiver feels he should have, may result in his feeling even more insecure within his environment.' (Kagawa-Singer 1987)

- In some cultures the expression of anger is traditionally not acceptable (see, for example, Chapter 38 *Gaining consent*).

Depression It can be hard to assess depression in patients who are terminally ill (Hanratty and Higginson 1994). Depression in black and minority ethnic patients is even more likely to be missed, for a variety of reasons.

- Many Westerners wrongly assume that people from other cultures do not experience depression as a psychological condition (CRE 1993).
- Language differences may mean that some people do not identify their subjective experience of distress with words such as 'depression' or 'depressed'. In many languages there is no single word for depression; different words or expressions may be used. The word 'depression' has been used in its current medical sense in English only since the early twentieth century (OUP 1996). A study of Asian women found that they described symptoms that, if they had been reported by fluent English speakers, would have been diagnosed as depression (CRE 1993, Rack 1991) (see also Chapter 27 *What an interpreter does*).
- The idea that some black and minority ethnic communities are particularly cohesive and supportive can lead to the assumption that patients of these communities are less likely to feel isolated and depressed or to need professional support (see Chapter 16 *'Community' support?*). In reality, their experience of racial discrimination and exclusion may lead them to feel more isolated and distressed.
- Some people may be more likely to present psychological distress in terms of physical symptoms (see Chapter 13 *Different expectations and concerns*).
- Some people may see depression as a spiritual issue and may prefer to turn to spiritual sources of help rather than discuss their feelings with health professionals.

There is also wide variation, partly due to culture, in the way people express or discuss their feelings. Overt or vocal expression of grief does not necessarily mean that the person is out of control or that they are overwhelmed by their feelings. Equally, lack of expression does not necessarily mean that they do not have strong feelings (see also Chapter 21 *The experience and expression of grief*).

Understanding ourselves

Our own reactions to other people's expression of emotion (or to their lack of expression) are influenced by our own culture, experience and personality. Understanding how we react is an important step in enabling us to extend the range of emotions we can accept and support.

> How do you/might you feel and react when a patient:
> - is unwilling to face the fact that they are dying?
> - is unwilling to talk or express their feelings?

- is vocal, demonstrative and highly emotional?
- sees their situation as God's will, which must be accepted without protest?
- is obviously frightened?

- Which of these do/might you find easier to deal with?
  Which (might) engage your empathy and support?

- Which do/might you find difficult?
  Which make you/might make you tend to avoid the patient?

Meeting spiritual needs

Spiritual care is difficult to define, precisely because it encompasses the immeasurable and often unspoken aspects of our humanity. Spiritual needs are not necessarily the same as religious needs. Many people with no religious affiliation lead deeply spiritual lives. People who would not define themselves as religious or spiritual may still have spiritual needs.

Health professionals often assume that spiritual care is the province of religious leaders or the patient's religious community, and that religious practices and rituals will meet patients' spiritual needs. Although this is true for some, it does not help people with no religious affiliation or belief, or those whose religious faith is unorthodox. People with a formal religion may also find that their religion does not always help. Some people may worry that their fear of death implies a lack of faith (Grey 1994). Some may be relieved to talk to health professionals about feelings that they cannot reveal to relatives or religious leaders. Spiritual care is therefore everyone's responsibility.

'We are all different, but what we have in common is our mortality, our vulnerability, our need for kindness and understanding.' (Lister 1997)

Weaving spiritual care into all other aspects of care

The quality of every verbal and physical interaction has the potential to enhance or diminish spiritual comfort. Ways of enhancing spiritual comfort include:

- identifying and accommodating the patient's personal, cultural and religious needs, for example in relation to privacy, modesty, personal grooming and diet (see the earlier chapters in this Part);
- listening (see also Chapter 23 *Listening with complete respect*);
- respecting their choices;

- meeting their physical needs with gentleness and respect;
- paying attention to detail and to the patient's personal preferences;
- preserving their chosen level of autonomy for as long as possible.

Talking and listening

Most people have a need to make sense of their life. Talking often helps people to sort out their feelings and thoughts and to become reconciled with past events. Many people think more clearly when someone is listening to them than they do alone. Having someone really listen and try to understand without criticism or judgement can validate people and strengthen them.

However, it is unhelpful to assume that talking is always a good thing, and intrusive to expect it of everyone. For some people, the last thing they want to do, or are able to do, is to talk about their feelings. For example, people who have been through terrible experiences in their lives may have managed to survive precisely because they have cut themselves off from their feelings and have not allowed themselves to think about what happened (Chodoff 1970).

Other ways of enhancing spiritual comfort

Some patients are uplifted by music, art, poetry or by photographs of favourite places and of the people they are close to. However, some may find secular music or depictions of people unacceptable for religious reasons. Other patients find comfort through physical contact, for example a massage or having their hand held. Stanworth (1997) describes giving a middle-aged builder a hand massage, during which he began to reciprocate. When asked which he preferred, he said that both giving and receiving were for him the essence of spirituality. However, touch by a relative stranger, especially someone of the opposite sex, may sometimes be unacceptable or an intrusion on the privacy of people who are normally physically reserved or who observe strict modesty codes.

Some patients gain comfort from revisiting a place that holds special meaning for them. This might be, for example, going home for a short time, going to their usual place of worship, or even returning to their country of origin. Some patients choose to focus their attention on the needs and feelings of people who will survive them, especially their children and grandchildren. Some people may spend time creating a memory store for future generations by writing letters and memoirs or recording their life stories onto tape or video (Rosenbluth 1997). It may be particularly important to some people of some minority cultures, especially those who came to Britain from other parts of the world, to record their family history and their personal story for posterity (but see *Talking and listening, above*).

Care when death is imminent

Approaching death

Near-death experiences have been reported by people of many different cultures, by those with strong religious beliefs and those with none, and by people who had never heard of a near-death experience before their own. The experiences vary a good deal but typically include some of the following: leaving the physical body and watching with detachment what is going on; travelling through a tunnel towards a bright light; the presence of a bright white light or a being who, depending on the person's beliefs, might be an angel, a religious figure or a prophet; meeting loved ones who have died; experiencing a rapid, detailed life review; and returning with reluctance (Brinkley 1995, Kübler-Ross 1995, Moody 1975).

A common feature, regardless of religious belief, is that for most people a near-death experience lessens their fear of death. Some, however, find the experience terrifying. Many people fear that if they talk about their experience, others will not believe them or will think they are mad. People may feel even more isolated if their experiences do not correspond with their religious faith, if the fact that they are dying is not openly acknowledged, or if they feel that what they say will be dismissed as superstitious or 'primitive'.

The origins of near-death experiences have been interpreted in several ways. Many people dismiss them as hallucinations or imagination, or the product of an anoxic brain. Some believe them to be the work of evil spirits. Others regard them as a sign that there is life after death. For individual patients, the 'scientific' cause is far less important than the emotional, social and spiritual impact of their experience.

Some health professionals see near-death experiences as the province of religious leaders, who in their turn may regard them as medical phenomena and outside their scope, or even as evil. The patient may be unwilling to talk about their experience with their family or with a religious leader, or may have no religious affiliation. It is therefore essential to listen without judgement (see also Chapter 23 *Listening with complete respect*).

Sometimes people who are approaching death become agitated and worried. Calanan and Kelley (1992), two experienced hospice nurses, describe behaviour they have observed in people who are very near death. They note that many people talk about journeys and seem uncertain how to get to their destination. They may worry about catching a train, finding tickets or a map. They may speak to someone nobody else can see, often someone they have known who is now dead. People are rarely able to explain these experiences; usually they go unnoticed or are dismissed as due to confusion, 'culture' or communication problems. However, theories about the origin or meaning of these experiences are less important than listening and responding respectfully.

> 'The day before my father-in-law died he was clearly agitated. He said that he couldn't find his way, didn't know how to get there. We were embarrassed and thought he'd lost his mind, we tried to hush him up. Now I know a bit more, I think I would respond better. He needed sympathy and reassurance that he would find his way and that it would be all right.'
> English woman

Practical care

The physical needs of patients and their relatives when death is very near are broadly similar, regardless of culture or religion. Privacy, dignity, a peaceful atmosphere, basic hygiene and good symptom control are always important. There may be some additional cultural or religious considerations.

- For some people it may be particularly important to hear the last words a dying relative says. These words may, for example, contain an important message or may indicate the spiritual state in which the person died.
- Some people, for example some Orthodox Jews, may follow the religious requirement to preserve a peaceful and undisturbed environment for a person who is dying. Some may also want the patient touched or moved as little as possible (see Chapter 47 *The last few days*).
- In some communities it is traditional to die on the floor rather than on the bed. Very rarely, a patient may get out of bed and lie on the floor, or the relatives may place them there. Just as midwives have learnt to be flexible about where and in what position women give birth, health professionals need to adapt their care to meet the needs of patients who want to die on the floor.

Religious ceremonies

Religious ceremonies around the time of death vary. In some religions they are carried out by religious leaders, in others by the family and members of the religious community. In most cases it is very important for the relatives to be present.

For some people it is very important to die with their attention focused on God. There may be special prayers or texts to be recited by or for the patient. Some Muslims want to whisper the call to prayer into the ear of a dying person. Some Christians may want a minister to give the last rites, hear the patient's confession and anoint them. Some Hindus may place a drop of holy water on the lips of the dying person. In Judaism it is traditional for the eldest son to close the patient's eyes immediately after death. If possible, ask relatives in advance what they might want when death is imminent, whether the family or a religious leader should be called, and what staff can do to help.

Many families will appreciate privacy during these ceremonies. However, some, especially those who have never seen anyone die, may be reassured by the quiet presence of a health professional.

The needs of relatives

Many relatives want to be present when a loved one dies. For some this has a strong cultural or religious imperative. Being absent at the moment of death can cause lasting distress and resentment. In such cases, sending exhausted relatives home to rest, although well meant, may not be helpful.

Sometimes a large number of people may want to be at the patient's bedside. Every effort should be made to accommodate them. If one is available, a side room can be used so that the family has privacy and so that the disruption to other patients is kept to a minimum (see also Chapter 17 *Visiting restrictions*).

It is important to keep relatives informed about the patient's condition and to prepare them for the physical changes they may see in the patient as death approaches. Information should be clear and unambiguous, avoiding euphemisms and medical jargon. These can be misunderstood by people who speak English fluently and are especially misleading when the relatives speak little or no English (see also Chapter 15 *Language barriers*).

19 Organ donation, euthanasia, suicide and sudden death

Organ donation and transplantation

Definitions of death

For some people the acceptability of organ donation hinges on the definition of death. Death has traditionally been defined as the irreversible cessation of breathing and circulation. The idea of brain stem death, that is the irreversible cessation of brain stem function, is relatively new (Department of Health 1983).

For most lay people a person is dead when they stop breathing and their heart stops working. Many are unfamiliar with the idea of brain stem death and find it difficult to understand. It can be especially hard for relatives to accept, because the patient looks the same as they did before they were pronounced dead, and because care and treatment continue. Sometimes, relatives' concerns about whether the patient is really dead may be allayed if they are invited to be present when brain stem function is tested, so that they can see for themselves that the patient does not respond or breathe unaided. It may also be helpful to emphasise that the continued care and treatment are to maintain the organs and cannot benefit the patient in any way.

Some relatives may have religious or spiritual concerns about the moment of death.

'A Christian woman asked me when the soul would leave her husband's body, as she was anxious that we did not take any organs before this had happened.'
Transplant co-ordinator

Religious and cultural beliefs

Organ donation and transplantation are not forbidden in principle by any of the major religions in the UK. However, there are certain variations in the details of what is and is not acceptable within each religion (see Part Five). There are also wide variations in how individuals of different faiths and communities view the issues involved, and the importance they attach to particular religious practices and traditions. People in more isolated communities, or those who are cut off from general discussion of these issues by language barriers, may know little about transplants or their benefits.

Respect for the body

Throughout the world, cultures and religions stress the importance of treating the dead with complete respect and of protecting their bodies from disturbance or harm. This is part of the basis for the requirement in many cultures and religions to hold the funeral as soon as possible. There is an almost universal taboo against any mutilation. Throughout history, desecration of the dead and of burial sites has been used as a weapon to humiliate and devastate oppressed groups and defeated armies.

Many people feel strongly that bodies should be complete and whole for burial or cremation. Lord Nelson, who lost his right arm eight years before he was killed at the Battle of Trafalgar, asked that it be buried with him when he died. Some people have a deeply felt personal need to preserve the body of someone they love from any interference. Others have religious beliefs about physical resurrection or about the importance of the body being complete in order to enter the next world.

> 'Some years ago I was supporting an elderly lady who had nursed her son through a long and distressing illness. A few weeks after his death she received a letter from the hospital to say thank you for her son's corneas. As was common at that time in that hospital, the corneas had been taken without her knowledge or consent. She was distraught because "He won't be able to see in heaven".'
> Bereavement counsellor

However, treating the sick and preserving life are also universal values. For many people the possibility of saving another life may override concerns about urgent burial or keeping the body intact. Relatives of all religions and cultures may gain comfort from the realisation that, out of their personal tragedy, the lives of others could be saved or improved. Sometimes, people who believe that the body should be complete and whole at burial are willing to compromise. They may, for example, agree to the donation of one kidney, since in life a person can remain healthy with only one.

Demand and supply of organs for transplantation

There is a shortage of organs for transplantation, and it is also commonly assumed that the problem would be completely solved if more people agreed to donate. In reality, the number of people awaiting transplantation will probably always exceed the number of available organs. Nearly all donated vital organs are taken from people who are brain stem dead due to intracranial haemorrhage or head injury. Brain stem death accounts for only one per cent of all deaths; sometimes the organs of people who are brain stem dead cannot be used for clinical reasons such as major trauma to other parts of the body, infection or malignancy.

There is a particular need for suitably matched organs for patients of black and minority ethnic groups, mainly because the tissue types of these patients differ from those of the majority population (UKTSSA 1996). The incidence of disease predisposing to life-threatening organ damage is also higher among certain minority groups in the UK. For example, there is higher incidence of hypertension and diabetes with consequent renal failure in the South Asian and African-Caribbean communities. However, these populations are small; nine out of ten people diagnosed as brain stem dead are white. The number of potential donors whose blood group and tissue type are a suitable match for black and minority ethnic patients is consequently very small (UKTCA 1995).

One reason often cited for the shortage of donors is relatives' refusal. In fact, 70 per cent of all relatives who are approached for donation agree. Although there is a higher refusal rate among black and minority ethnic groups, research shows that relatives in these groups are also less likely to be approached (UKTCA 1995). In addition, some health professionals do not ask any relatives about donation because they themselves object to transplantation for personal, ethical or religious reasons. In relation to black and minority ethnic groups, the assumption that the shortage of organs is due to their unwillingness to donate can lead to the victims being blamed. This compounds the pain and distress of potential organ recipients and alienates the black and minority ethnic communities.

Approaching the relatives

Although there is no legal requirement to 'establish lack of objection' from relatives if the patient has recorded their wishes about organ donation or has signed a donor card, it is good practice to consider their views and feelings (Department of Health 1983). The decision to agree to the donation of a loved one's organs is very personal; it can raise complex feelings and issues at a time of crisis and distress. What is technically possible and logical to many people, as it may save another life, must be balanced with ethical issues and cultural and religious traditions.

It is therefore important to listen to and respect individual sensitivities and the values of the people directly involved. If an interpreter is required, ensure that the interpreter accepts the principle of organ donation and transplantation and will not be constrained by his or her own religious or cultural beliefs from discussing the issue with the relatives (see also Chapter 27 *What an interpreter does*).

It is not uncommon for different family members to have differing views. In some communities and families, decisions are often taken by older people, who may be more conservative.

> 'When my daughter came home with a donor card and wanted to register her name, my wife and I were horrified that she wanted to do such a strange thing. Now that I have kidney failure I realise that she was right, she was doing the right thing.'
> Elderly Sikh man

Individuals may have a variety of other concerns, which need to be addressed to help them make a decision about organ donation.

- Some people want to be present at the moment of death. This is complicated when medical and lay definitions of death differ, and when the physical functioning of the body will be maintained for some time in order to preserve the organs. It may be helpful to explain that death will be certified on completion of the second set of brain stem tests, after which the relatives can spend time with the body and say their goodbyes. A few people may want to stay until the body is taken to the operating theatre.
- Rarely, a relative might want to come into the operating theatre at the moment the ventilator is switched off. It is important to prepare them for what will happen, to explain that there will be a long wait, and that the ventilator will be turned off only when the organs have been removed.
- Some relatives may worry that they will be unable to carry out religious ceremonies after the surgery is completed and after the ventilator is removed, especially those that involve touching the body or placing items on the body (see Part Five). They may worry about the correct timing of prayer and other rituals.
- Relatives may be concerned about what the body will look like afterwards and whether they can see and touch it. This is particularly important for families who want to wash and prepare the body for the funeral themselves (see Chapter 20 *Possible cultural and religious wishes*). In such cases it is helpful to explain when and where the relatives will be able to see and touch the body, that although the body will

look very different it will be carefully stitched and restored (and to ensure that this happens), and that the usual ceremonies can be performed before the funeral.

- Some relatives may have doubts about how the donated organs will be used, or whether they will be used at all. This may be a significant issue for people who have had negative experiences of health services in the past, or may simply be the consequence of poor communication.

Professionals' attitudes and feelings

Approaching distressed relatives about organ donation is very hard. It can be more daunting when there are cultural and religious differences or language barriers. Some health professionals assume that people of certain cultures or religions will not consent and therefore do not raise the issue with them (UKTCA 1995).

'A four-year-old Bangladeshi girl was certified brain dead and nobody thought to ask about organ donation. Her father rushed in and asked about donating her organs. We were only just in time to retrieve them. We later discovered that the father was on renal dialysis awaiting a donor and was only too aware that his daughter's organs could change the lives of other people in his situation.'
Transplant co-ordinator

Some health professionals are particularly reluctant to approach families who are expressing grief openly and loudly, for fear of increasing their distress. However, ways of expressing grief are cultural as well as personal (see Chapter 21 *Culture and the expression of grief*). Overt expressions of grief do not necessarily mean that relatives will be any more distressed by the suggestion of organ donation than those whose culture conditions them to grieve in more restrained and private ways.

Although some relatives will not agree, it is important not to assume refusal in advance. In addition, automatically avoiding the issue with relatives of certain groups is discriminatory. Even if people refuse, raising the issue increases people's awareness of the value of transplants and the shortage of minority group donors, and may in the long run change attitudes.

Xenotransplantation

Although there are prohibitions in Judaism and Islam against the consumption of pork and pork products, in both faiths the requirement to preserve life overrides other considerations. Transplanting pig organs is likely to be acceptable to most people if there is no alternative.

Euthanasia

'Often ... it is not death itself that people dread, but the manner, time and even the place of death.' (BMA 1993)

Euthanasia – in Greek literally a good death – has come to mean hastening death. The term 'voluntary euthanasia' means that the decision is taken by the patient; 'involuntary euthanasia' means that it is taken by someone else without the patient's consent (Voluntary Euthanasia Society 1998). Many people hold strong personal views about euthanasia. Whether it is legal or illegal, it is likely to remain a controversial issue. In the media, health professionals frequently assure the public that nobody needs to die in pain, indignity and distress. However, many people are well aware that, for whatever reason, such deaths do occur. Some become advocates of euthanasia precisely because they have seen the suffering of a loved one.

Euthanasia, both voluntary and involuntary, is forbidden by all major religions. However, individuals vary in their views and may sometimes change them if faced with a distressing terminal illness.

Suicide

'One of the saddest things about suicide is that it may be the only thing that is remembered about the victim, and remembered with fear.' (Murray Parkes 1975)

There are between 4,000 and 5,000 suicides every year in England and Wales. The official figures are thought by many to be an underestimate of the actual rate, because, if there is no clear-cut evidence, a possible suicide may be classified as misadventure, open verdict or accidental death. Suicide trends in minority ethnic groups tend to reflect national trends. However, there is a higher incidence of suicide among young people in some minority ethnic groups, notably young African-Caribbeans and young women of South Asian origin (Soni Raleigh 1996).

All major religions forbid suicide. In former times, most religions and societies inflicted severe punishments. In Britain, for example, people who committed suicide were refused a religious funeral and in some cases burial in sacred ground. Their bodies were desecrated and their families suffered extreme disgrace and sometimes lost their home and all their possessions. People who attempted suicide but lived were severely punished (Wertheimer 1991). Nowadays, most societies and religions regard people who attempt or commit suicide less severely. Rather than sinful or wicked, they are often considered to be mentally ill or suffering from extreme stress. Nevertheless, the anguish and pain experienced by relatives of people who kill themselves is still considerable. In many cases this is compounded by social stigma and fears about the spiritual consequences for the person who has died.

People who attempt suicide are sometimes treated with less compassion and respect than other patients. When a black or minority ethnic person attempts or commits suicide there is also a tendency to assume that the cause must be 'their culture' that is in some way particularly unreasonable, difficult or oppressive. Social pressures and stresses are likely to be strong contributory factors for people of any culture, including those who belong to the majority. Judgemental assumptions about 'cultural' causes and negative stereotypical images of their 'community' do not help patients or their families.

Sudden death

'Sudden death is well recognised as one of the most traumatic crisis events that can be experienced.' (Wright 1996)

Shock, numbness and disbelief are common reactions to an expected death. They are greatly magnified when death occurs suddenly and unexpectedly; relatives are likely to have much greater difficulty coming to terms with what has happened. The way they are treated during the time surrounding the death is therefore of the utmost importance. There may be particular considerations for relatives who are unfamiliar with the British system of health care and for those who have experienced insensitive services, discrimination or racism in the past. Relatives often go over and over events during the following months or sometimes years, trying to make sense of what happened and to regain some sense of order and control (Wright 1996). Everything that is done or not done now, everything that is said or left unsaid, may be indelibly etched into their memories.

Communication The increased shock and trauma of sudden and unexpected death also make it even harder for relatives to listen, hear and remember what is being said to them. People need time to assimilate what has happened and time to formulate as well as to ask questions. Shock, anxiety and fear all seriously affect people's language ability. A professional interpreter is essential for people whose English is not completely fluent (see Chapter 27 *Professional interpreters: the benefits*). Written information of what relatives have to do after a sudden death is needed in all the main languages spoken in the area (see also Chapters 20 *Written information* and 29 *Materials in other languages*).

Religious implications

For some people a sudden death may have particular religious significance. Sudden, unexpected death may be believed to cause additional suffering to the dead person's soul in a future life; the fact that the person had no time to pray or prepare their soul may be regarded as particularly tragic; if the death has already occurred, the family may be very upset that they were not there to hear any last words or to pray or carry out religious rituals. If the family was not present, it may be very important that a health professional describes to them exactly what happened and any words the patient said before they died.

Resuscitation: the presence of relatives

There has been much debate about allowing relatives to witness resuscitation attempts. The evidence so far indicates that the advantages to relatives who want to be present outweigh any disadvantages, and that relatives should normally be offered the opportunity, accompanied by a chaperone who can give emotional support and provide technical information on the resuscitation. Most relatives who have witnessed resuscitation attempts appreciate seeing what happened rather than relying on their imagination and on what others tell them. Many feel that their presence was a support to the patient. Some have found it helpful to speak to the patient during the last few minutes. Staff also benefit because the time spent with the family during resuscitation creates a rapport with the family and places the patient in context within the family. The staff are then more able to care for the family as a whole (Robinson, Mackenzie-Ross et al 1998, Wright 1996, RCN and BAAEM 1995).

Sometimes there are additional cultural, religious or personal issues:

- In some communities it is extremely important that family members remain with a dying person until the death and that they hear any last words (see Chapter 18 *Care when death is imminent*).
- For some people the future of the soul depends on certain prayers and rituals being performed around the time of death. For some it is important to be there to help the dying person focus on God.
- Families who observe strict codes of modesty may feel that it is inappropriate for a member of the opposite sex to be present during resuscitation, especially if the patient is a woman, because it is inevitable that at least the chest will be exposed.
- Being present may also be important for black and minority ethnic relatives who fear racial discrimination and that their relative will not receive the same care and attention as other patients.

Wherever possible, relatives should be offered the opportunity to be present when the patient is resuscitated; they can then make up their own minds.

There is evidence that relatives who chose not to be present during resuscitation, or who arrived after the death, find it helpful to talk later to a member of staff who was present. Some people are anxious to know exactly what happened and whether the patient said anything. It may also help to see the person's body in the room where they died (Wright 1996).

Seeing the body

Seeing the body after death often helps people to realise what has happened, both at an emotional and at an intellectual level. This can be an important step towards grieving. Seeing the body is especially important to people who have a religious obligation to perform certain rituals. Relatives, including children who want to, should always be offered an opportunity to see the body as soon as possible after the death.

In many accident and emergency departments it is common for a body to be cleaned and tidied and even wrapped first in order to avoid adding to the relatives' distress (RCN and BAAEM 1995) (and see below). If the head or face is disfigured or mutilated, the relatives should be told in advance so that they can decide whether they want to see the body. If they prefer, the injuries can be covered so that they can at least hold their loved one's hand. Some people, however, may want to perform religious rituals that may involve, for example, touching the face, body or feet.

If the room must be cleared urgently, the body should be moved to another, designated, room where relatives can stay as long as they want without feeling rushed. Relatives who are religious may appreciate having religious items and holy books available (see Chapter 20 *The chapel of rest*). It is most important that relatives have as much time as they want to be with the body now, as it is very likely that a sudden death will be referred to the coroner. Viewing facilities at public mortuaries are designed for identification rather than for the emotional task of saying farewell to a loved one.

Some families may be particularly distressed at the prospect of referral to the coroner, because this is likely to delay the funeral and to involve a post mortem. They may need extra time, support and explanation (see Chapter 20 *Referral to the coroner*).

Last offices, clothing and photographs

Relatives should always be consulted before the body is washed or prepared for removal and asked if they have any particular requirements, especially in relation to touching and positioning the body and religious items. They should also be asked if they want to help wash and prepare the body (see Chapter 20 *Possible cultural and religious wishes*).

- For some Orthodox Jews, it is crucial that all body parts and fragments, however small, are buried with the body (see Chapter 47 *Preparation for the funeral*). Check first before discarding any tissue of an Orthodox Jew who has died.
- It is essential to check with the relatives before discarding any clothing, even if heavily torn or soiled, because some people want to have it for personal or for religious reasons (see Chapter 47 *Preparation for the funeral*).
- In some accident and emergency units, photographs are taken of the dead person and are either offered to the relatives or kept on file. This may be unacceptable to certain people for cultural and religious reasons. Some Muslims regard taking photographs as unacceptable, because representations of the human form are traditionally forbidden in Islam (Gatrad 1994). Some Chinese families may also regard taking photographs of a dead person as completely unacceptable. Even if taking photographs is routine, it is prudent to explain why and seek permission first. If the family refuses, find out whether there is a religious reason, in which case the photograph should not be taken.

Going home

Before relatives leave, check that they have no more questions for the time being and that they know whom to contact if they want to ask questions later. They also need to know what they have to do and what will happen to the body (see also Chapter 20 *Paperwork and certificates*). This is particularly important if they are unfamiliar with British systems or speak little or no English.

Many relatives find it hard to leave. They may need permission to go, or help with travel arrangements and finding someone to accompany them. Women from certain communities who usually lead a secluded life and who are unused to going out alone will be in special need of help.

In many cultures, men traditionally protect women from trauma and distress, in others there is a cultural or religious prohibition against the overt expression of grief. Sometimes people who hope to alleviate the distress of those relatives most closely affected by the death may ask for sedatives to be prescribed for them. Such requests are made with the best of intentions. However, it is important for health professionals, wherever possible, to weigh their knowledge of the bereaved person and what is likely to be best for them against the possibility that the request for sedation may be more to protect others from the pain of witnessing the distress of bereavement. Tactful discussion rather than a prescription may be required.

20 After a death: procedures and paperwork

When a patient has died, there is pressure to deal with the body, the property and the paperwork as quickly as possible. Although these are important tasks, the focus throughout must be on the relatives. Their needs must be reflected in the way the body and the property are handled and the paperwork is done. Inappropriate care after a death is a frequent cause of complaints.

Some families may have cultural or religious requirements that are not met by standard procedures. It may be helpful to explain what usually happens after a death before asking if relatives have any special wishes (see also Chapter 8 *Asking effective questions*).

Some families, for example Orthodox Jews and Muslims and some Sikhs and Hindus, may need everything completed very quickly so that the funeral can take place within 24 or 48 hours of the death. Others need plenty of time. It is important that people do not feel rushed into hasty decisions and actions that they might later regret (see also *Post mortems*, later in this chapter). If this is the first time they have dealt with a death, they may want to consult other family members or religious leaders before deciding.

If the relatives speak little or no English, an interpreter is needed. Even people who are normally fluent in English may find that shock and grief impair their ability to communicate or to understand what is said to them (see also Chapter 26 *Stress and language*).

Care of the body

All communities throughout history have created rituals and procedures for handling the bodies of people who have died, and for meeting the practical and emotional needs of bereaved people. These rituals and procedures have developed in response to local conditions, history, and religious and cultural beliefs, and may vary a good deal.

The relatives' involvement

In Britain and most other industrialised countries, the management of death has become professionalised and institutionalised. Dying people are usually cared for by professionals in hospitals or other residential care. After death, the body is usually handled and housed by people who did not know the living person. If relatives see the body, they normally do so only after the body has been carefully washed, prepared and dressed. The family becomes more involved at the funeral but most practical matters are dealt with by funeral directors, religious leaders and cemetery or crematorium staff. As a result, few English people know much about or have anything to do with the care and disposal of bodies after death. For many, these are areas of uncertainty and fear (see also Chapter 2 *Not cultural facts but cultural possibilities*).

In contrast, in some religious and cultural groups it is traditional for relatives or other members of the community to keep watch over the body until the funeral, as a sign of respect and to ensure that the body comes to no harm. They may also wash and prepare the body for the funeral themselves. In the period following the death, they may carry out ceremonies and rituals to benefit the spirit of the person who has died. Relatives who are unable to perform these essential duties may feel lasting distress and guilt. A small but growing number of people of all communities manage funerals themselves, collecting and preparing the body and organising everything. Relatives should be given the facilities and support to carry out whatever duties they want in caring for the body.

Immediately after the death and last offices

The way the body is treated after death is of vital importance. Everything must be done with respect and dignity. The way the body is washed, dressed and groomed is not only a conclusion of care for the patient but also a continuation of care for the relatives. Many people will also want to spend time with the body before the last offices are carried out. Excellent care during life can be permanently negated in the eyes of the relatives if the treatment of the body is inadequate, hurried or culturally offensive.

'We used to take pride in doing last offices. It was the last thing we could do for the patient. A sort of respectful farewell and something that might in some small way comfort the relatives, especially those whom we knew well.'
Retired Welsh ward sister

Procedures for last offices vary but, unless there are religious or cultural reasons for doing things differently (see below), good practice normally includes the following. Close the eyes, replace dentures, close the mouth and support the jaw, taking care to avoid creating pressure marks on the skin. Raise the head above chest level to prevent blood pooling and discolouring the face. Straighten the body and limbs and place the hands on the abdomen to prevent discoloration of the fingers.

Unless the death is to be referred to the coroner (see below), pack the orifices if leakage is anticipated, remove lines, tubes and drains, and seal wounds (Mallet and Bailey 1996). Releasing a body with lines and tubes in situ or with unsealed wounds exposes people who prepare the body for the funeral to unnecessary hazards and additional distress (see *Infection control issues*, later). It is important, therefore, to find out in advance whether the death will be reported to the coroner. With the family's consent, the body should then be washed, dressed and wrapped before removal to the mortuary. List and pack the property (see *The patient's property*, below).

Possible cultural and religious wishes

Customs immediately after death vary enormously and are to some extent a matter of personal choice. Ask relatives if they have any special wishes.

- **Immediately after the death** it may be important for a close relative to close the eyes. Traditionally the mouth is also closed and the jaw supported. Apart from aesthetic reasons, this was traditionally done because of the belief that the soul rests in the eyes and departs through the mouth with the last breath (Gaster 1955). (See also Part Five.)
- Some people follow certain rituals or traditions to allow the release of the soul and/or to keep out negative influences and evil spirits. For example, they may open a window and then close it. They may want to close curtains and blinds and to cover mirrors. A few people may want any water in jugs or vases to be discarded. Some may want to cover the dead person's face.
- The position of the body and the limbs may be important. Some families may want the bed turned so that the dead person's feet face the door. A

few may want to place the body on the floor. Muslims traditionally turn the head towards the right shoulder and position the body so that the head is facing the Ka'ba in Makka (see Chapter 44 *When someone is ill or dying*). Some people may want the arms placed along the sides. Do not place the hands and fingers under the body, because this may cause discolouring (see above). Some people will want health professionals to wear gloves when touching the body.

- In some communities it is traditional for large numbers of people to gather at the bedside of a person who has died. This can cause difficulties for other patients and families and for staff, but it is important to understand that people have a social obligation to come; not to come would cause enormous and lasting offence. Every effort should be made to accommodate people who arrive after the death, if possible in a side room or in a dedicated room in the mortuary.

> 'A Ghanaian man died in the care home. The family were all gathered round and wanted to stay with the body. But there was an Orthodox Jewish man and a Chinese man in the same room and we were concerned that they might find it unacceptable to be near a dead body for any length of time. So we explained to the family that we would move the body to a another room so that they could spend as much time as they wanted with the body in privacy without having to worry about other people's reactions.'
> Care assistant

- **Last offices** in some communities, it is customary for family or community members to wash and prepare the body for the funeral themselves, either immediately or just before the funeral. There may be a prescribed ritual for washing; some people use water from holy places. Families who wash and prepare the body themselves may want health professionals to do as little as possible. This can upset nurses, for whom last offices are part of completing their care for the patient and relatives as well as a source of personal and professional satisfaction and closure (Katz 1996). They may also see last offices as an unsuitable task for relatives and lay people. Nevertheless, it is necessary to recognise the responsibilities and needs of relatives and to accept their wishes. It is generally acceptable to clean up anything (eg vomit) that is likely to distress relatives and leave a lasting bad memory. Ask the relatives whether they would also like you to remove lines and tubes, and to seal wounds. Most families prefer this as it reduces soiling and the risk of infection, and causes less distress to those who prepare the body. Body bags should not be used unless absolutely essential (see *Infection control issues*, later).
- Some people who do not want to carry out the whole procedure themselves may want to be present while the nurse does it, or may want to

help. It may be necessary to support and guide them sensitively, especially if they have never done this before.

- Many people prefer the body of the dead person to be dressed in their own clothing or wrapped in a plain sheet. This may be on religious grounds or for aesthetic reasons.

  'My father would have looked like a ridiculously overgrown choir boy in a hospital shroud with a frilly neck. So we asked the nurses to dress him in his pyjamas.'
  English woman

- Most people will want religious or wedding jewellery left in place. Some religious and cultural groups place certain additional items on the body or in the coffin prior to the funeral. Some people will not want flowers placed on or near the body.

The patient's property

When packing a patient's property, bear in mind that distressed relatives will unpack it.

'As a nurse I had often packed patient's property, mostly without much thought. But when my aunt died and I was on the receiving end I got a quite different view. It was the hardest thing in the world to empty that plastic bag. I felt like a voyeur. Seeing the night things and knickers she had worn was upsetting, especially the ones that needed washing which were all mixed up with the clean ones. And there was a half-eaten apple in there, too'.
English nurse

What relatives want varies enormously. Some want everything, including items of food and half-used toiletries; others only want valuables. Whenever possible, ask before packing the property. If this is not possible, separate perishable or used items, and soiled clothing, into different labelled packages so that relatives can choose whether to open or discard them. Religious items and holy books should be treated with great care, wrapped and kept separate.

Some people may consider it essential to have all clothing returned even if it has been cut or torn, or is heavily blood-stained. In some cases there is a religious duty to bury blood-stained clothing with the body (see Chapter 47 *Preparation for the funeral*). If possible, check with relatives as to whether they want all the clothing, pack it separately and mark it, and warn them that it is soiled when they collect the property.

Property bags should be discreet and durable and should have handles.

'In one hospital where I worked, all the property was just dumped together in bin liners. People had to go home, sometimes on public transport, with black rubbish bags tied with bits of string. It was as if all that was left of their loved one was just rubbish. In another hospital the bags had 'Patients Property' blazoned in huge letters. Imagine walking through the streets with that. I'd worry people would think I'd stolen it or that everyone would know that I was newly bereaved.'
Health professional

Transfer to the mortuary

'When somebody died on our ward we first had to go round closing all the curtains, without saying why. Then we called the porter and he came with the mortuary trolley. It was called a concealment trolley because you closed it and put a pillow and blanket over it so that it looked like an empty trolley and no one knew there was a body inside. Then the porter would lift the body in and close the lid which was often quite a noisy performance. He would wheel the trolley out – the wheels always squeaked – and we would tidy up the bed. And then we went round opening everybody's curtains again. The other patients could all see that the bed was empty but usually nothing was said. Some were obviously terrified but I don't think they dared say anything because we clearly didn't want to talk.'
Retired English nurse

Bodies must be removed, and be seen to be removed, with dignity and respect. Procedures must take into account the needs and feelings of the patient's relatives. They should also take into account the feelings of other patients who may be facing their own deaths and who need to know their bodies will be treated with respect and not smuggled shamefully away. Hurried or insensitive handling, or attempts to conceal what is happening, can cause lasting distress and anxiety. The needs and feelings of staff should also be considered. This includes porters, who are usually summoned at short notice to perform a stressful task, often with no preparation or support.

'I hate it. We always send the new porters because it's such a horrible job.'
Hospital porter

The nursing staff need to inform the mortuary staff of any special cultural or religious requirements in relation to the care and handling of the body.

Post mortems

In many hospitals it is routine to ask for a post mortem. However, many relatives find post mortems abhorrent; to some they are unacceptable on religious grounds. According to Jewish law the body must be complete and whole when buried; a post mortem is considered a desecration. Many Muslims also refuse post mortems on religious grounds. For people whose religion requires burial as soon as possible, a post mortem may cause unacceptable delay. However, for some people in all communities, the need to understand exactly why the person has died overrides religious and other considerations. (See also *Referral to the coroner*, later).

After a post mortem, all organs should be replaced and the body carefully stitched and restored. This is especially important if the relatives are going to prepare the body for the funeral themselves. The pathologist should be informed of this in advance, and the relatives warned that there will be stitch lines. If a full repair is not possible the family should be sensitively told before they see the body.

Cremation

If the body is to be cremated, relatives should be informed that implants, such as pacemakers and radioactive material, must be removed beforehand. This may be important for those who object to the body being touched or disturbed in any way.

Spending time with the body

Spending time with the body of a loved one may help people accept the reality of the death. It is also often important for cultural or religious reasons. Everything should be done to enable relatives to express their grief and pay their respects in the way they wish, and to perform customary ceremonies and rituals.

Some people will want to see the body several times before the funeral. They may appreciate time to sit with the body before the body is moved from the bed, in familiar surroundings and supported by staff they know. This is especially important if the death is to be referred to the coroner, because viewing facilities at most coroner's courts are suitable only for identification, and it may be some time before the body is released to the funeral director again (see *Referral to the coroner*, later).

Relatives may also want to see the body in the mortuary. Many hospitals and other residential care institutions have a room set aside for this purpose (see below) and relatives are usually offered the opportunity to 'view' the body. The term 'viewing' implies taking an objective look from a distance. This may shape staff's assumptions about what relatives should or should not do, and may also inhibit relatives. This is unhelpful. It is important that the environment and the support the relatives receive enable them to grieve in their own way. Some may want to touch the dead person's face, hands or feet. Others may want to embrace and hold them. Some may want to pray or meditate, silently or out loud. Some may want to sing or to wail.

However, not everyone will want to see or spend time with the body. Some people may prefer to remember the person as they were in life. Others may avoid contact with the dead for religious or cultural reasons.

Some families may want to keep the body at home or to take the body home before the funeral. In some communities it is traditional to keep the coffin open until and during the funeral service.

The chapel of rest

The room where relatives can spend time with the person who has died should be quiet and private, and relatives should have complete access to the body. Routine separation by glass screens is unnecessary and causes great distress. Wash-hand basins should be available for relatives and friends to use before leaving if they want (see *Routine hygiene precautions*, below).

It is important that the room is visibly non-denominational. The person responsible for the chapel of rest needs to consult leaders from all the religious groups in the area about appropriate religious symbols, books and other items. All religious symbols should be removable and stored out of sight when not in use. It is also helpful to have religious items available such as skull caps, prayer mats, compasses and shawls as well as suitable scripture and prayer books. The latter could include, for example, copies of the Bible, the Qur'an, the Gita, the Pentateuch and the Psalms (see Part Five). Purchase all such items with a member of the relevant religious group to ensure that they are appropriate. Discuss acceptable storage arrangements.

The term 'chapel' has strong Christian connotations. Some people of other religions may not understand the term, and a few may find it off-putting and inappropriate. It may be helpful to try to find a different name in discussion with leaders of local religious groups.

Paperwork and certificates

The patients' affairs officer

After a death, the next of kin have to deal with a large number of unfamiliar tasks at a time when they are often unable to think clearly. Patients' affairs (or relatives') officers play a crucial role, helping relatives to find their way through complex processes. This is especially necessary when relatives are unfamiliar with the systems for registering death and arranging funerals, when they have special cultural or religious needs, or when they speak little or no English. For some people speed is essential; some may be worried about post mortems; some may want frequent or continuous access to the body (see above). Family members abroad may have to submit a copy of the death certificate to British immigration authorities before they are granted a visa to attend a funeral in the UK; relatives in the UK may need help to organise this.

Some patients' affairs officers provide information about local funeral directors. Because prices vary widely, and because not all funeral directors offer services that meet the needs of cultural and religious minorities, it is essential that patients' affairs officers are independent and give absolutely unbiased information. The practice of contracting out the work of a patients' affairs officer to a funeral company is therefore questionable.

Written information

Relatives need clear, practical, written information to back up the verbal information they receive from the patients' affairs officer. This includes maps and directions to the register office and other key places, and information about transport and parking facilities as well as office opening hours. Someone who does not know the area should try out all the maps and directions and check them for accuracy before the leaflets are printed. There should also be information about completing formalities out of hours. Leaflets must be available in the languages needed by the local communities (see Chapter 29 *Materials in other languages*).

Communication with the patients' affairs officer

It is particularly important that the people who have been caring for a patient and their family tell the patients' affairs officer when relatives have specific personal, cultural or religious needs, and if there are language barriers.

Because most patients' affairs officers are available only during normal working hours, nurses must also be equipped to give advice and guidance to bereaved relatives. They need to know:

- who can register a death, where and when;
- what information and documentation the person registering the death must take;
- what facilities are available locally for out-of-hours registration (see below);
- what to do after registering the death.

They also need copies of any written information to give to relatives.

Registering a death out of hours

Office opening times and the availability of the registrar are decided by the local authority. There is no legal obligation on them to provide an out-of-hours service, though some do. However, where there is no out-of-hours service, families who need to hold the funeral within 24 or 48 hours (see above) face major problems, because they must register the death before they can hold the funeral.

If current services are not meeting the needs of minority groups, it is necessary for those responsible and those affected to work together to find a solution. Discussions should involve the relevant community representatives and religious leaders, in particular Muslim and Jewish representatives, the patients' affairs officer, mortuary staff, the registrar and the local authority officer responsible for register office hours.

Collecting the body from the mortuary

In most cases, the funeral director collects the body from the mortuary. Occasionally, family or community members want to collect the body. It must be possible for them to do this, including out of hours.

Before releasing the body, most institutions ask to see the disposal certificate (green form) signed by the registrar. Although this is not legally necessary, it enables staff to be sure that the correct procedures have been followed and that the body will not be required by the coroner. Problems occur if the relatives have been unable to register the death, for example because the register office is closed (see above), and so cannot present the green form.

Hospitals and other residential institutions with no mortuary or with limited storage space sometimes have a contract to use the premises of a local funeral director. Here again it is essential to ensure that relatives can have

24-hour access, and that those who want to can sit with the body, wash the body themselves and perform religious rituals. Relatives should feel under no obligation to use the services of the contract funeral director for the funeral. It should be made clear to them that they are free to choose another funeral director or to organise the funeral themselves.

Infection control issues

In recent years, infection control issues have come to the fore and many procedures have changed accordingly. However, some procedures unnecessarily prevent relatives from having full access to the body and from performing the customary religious and cultural rituals. When reviewing and developing procedures to ensure effective infection control, it is important to bear in mind that, in most cases, living patients with diseases present a far greater hazard to the healthy than dead patients (Healing, Hoffman and Young 1995), and that, nowadays, most deaths in the UK are due to non-infectious causes.

- In the vast majority of cases a body poses a **low infection risk** to relatives who want to sit with or wash the body and to the people who prepare the body for burial or cremation, provided routine hygiene precautions are observed (see below).
- A body poses a **medium infection risk** if the patient had hepatitis B, C, non-A or non-B, or had HIV/AIDS. People with AIDS are also highly likely to have had other concurrent infections. Embalming is contraindicated, but relatives can sit with and wash and dress the body for the funeral, provided they observe routine hygiene precautions (Healing, Hoffman and Young 1995).
- A body poses a **high infection risk** only if the patient had any of the following diseases: anthrax, plague, rabies, smallpox, viral haemorrhagic fever, yellow fever, transmissible spongiform encephalopathies such as Creutzfeldt–Jakob disease, or invasive group A streptococcal infection (Healing, Hoffman and Young 1995). In these cases a body bag is recommended. Spending time with the body, preparing the body for burial or cremation, and embalming are all contraindicated.

If the patient was cared for in an open ward or at home, relatives naturally find it hard to accept that after death the risk of infection prevents them from touching the body, or from seeing the body except through glass (Young and Healing 1995). In contrast, most relatives of patients who had a highly infectious disease are already used to stringent barrier precautions and are likely to find it easier to accept restrictions.

Routine hygiene precautions

In all cases, people who touch the body should be advised to wash their hands afterwards, and facilities should be made available for this. Community and family members who prepare the body for burial or cremation should be sensitively advised about routine hygiene precautions. This means:

- ensuring that any cuts or abrasions on their hands are covered with waterproof plaster;
- wearing gloves and an apron;
- washing their hands carefully afterwards and especially before eating, drinking or smoking (Health Services Advisory Committee 1991).

Embalming

Embalming (sometimes called hygienic preparation) involves removing the blood from the body and replacing it with a mixture of formalin and other substances. It is carried out by specialist embalmers who work with funeral directors. It is commonly practised in the UK because it delays deterioration, thus enabling relatives to see the body several days after the death and to have the coffin open at the funeral. Embalming is unacceptable to some people on religious grounds. If the body is to be buried in a green or woodland site, embalming may be prohibited in case the chemicals damage the environment (Albery, Elliot and Elliot 1997). However, embalming is always required when a body is to be repatriated (see later).

Informing people about infection risks: the issues

Employers (in this case hospital trusts and other institutions releasing bodies) **have a legal duty to protect their own workers, and also to ensure that their working practices do not expose people who are not employed by them to risk** (HSE 1994, Health and Safety at Work Act 1974). Although funeral directors, embalmers and some relatives need to know for their own safety if a body carries a medium or high risk of infection, there are at present no standard procedures for informing them. Funeral directors do not see the Cause of Death Certificate, which anyway may not be explicit about any infection. Relatives, who may see it, may not understand the significance of the information it contains. As a result, professionals and members of the public who prepare bodies for funerals are placed at risk.

The requirement to keep patient information confidential, which persists beyond death, is often given as a reason for not informing funeral directors or other key people about cases of infection risk. However, the General

Medical Council (1998b) states that consent to disclose information is not required when the disclosure would prevent serious harm to a third party. In the interests of public health, people who collect and prepare the body for the funeral need to know so that they can take precautions to protect themselves and others. A degree of confidentiality can be maintained by giving information only about the level of risk (low, medium or high) rather than naming a specific infection or cause.

Universal infection control precautions Some hospitals justify their failure to tell funeral directors and others about infection risks on the grounds that everyone ought to be using universal infection control precautions. However, these involve very severe restrictions, which are unnecessary in most cases (see above) and are very distressing to most relatives. For example, under universal infection control precautions, relatives cannot see or touch the body; the body cannot be washed or dressed for the funeral; coffins cannot not be kept open during religious rituals or up to or during the funeral. In addition, the body cannot be embalmed, so, if there is not enough refrigeration space, the family may have to hold the funeral urgently and relatives who live far away may be unable to attend. Because universal precautions cause such distress and difficulty, and are in most cases unnecessary, most family members and most funeral directors disregard them unless they are convinced that there is a real risk.

Body bags Hospitals and other residential care institutions that follow universal infection control precautions routinely place bodies in body bags. However, this practice causes more problems than it solves. Formerly, the use of a body bag indicated a 'high-infection risk' and served as a warning in itself. Universal use removes this significance: funeral directors have to decide for themselves whether to open a bag to allow relatives to see the body, and whether it is safe to wash, prepare and embalm the body.

The routine use of body bags also has other disadvantages:

- distress to staff placing the body in the bag and to those having to open it;
- distress to relatives if the bag is insufficiently hidden when they see it;
- increased speed of decomposition because of condensation and heat retention;
- deterioration of samples that may be required for histopathology;
- increased costs to the health service;
- poor-quality body bags split easily;
- body bags made of polyvinyl chloride should not be cremated because they release dioxin when burned (Young and Healing 1995).

Funeral directors' practice

Because there are no standard procedures for indicating the level of risk, current practice varies. Some funeral directors try to find out if there is a genuine risk of infection, though this is not easy.

> 'We want to serve families and help them to do what they want to do. But we have to go round the back door to find out if there is a risk of infection. Sometimes the mortuary staff will drop a hint. Sometimes we ring the GP or the hospital doctor, but that depends on our having a good relationship with them. We are the ones facing distraught relatives, and we do not actually have the right to stop them seeing, touching or preparing their relative for the funeral.'
> English funeral director

Some treat all bodies in body bags as high risk. This unnecessarily prevents families from paying the usual respect to the body or holding a normal funeral. Some funeral directors treat all bodies as low risk unless they have information to the contrary. If body bags are used routinely irrespective of risk, some funeral directors simply remove them, as do most families and community groups who take charge of the body themselves.

Devising rational infection control policies and procedures

Fear of the spread of infection can sometimes obliterate professionals' sensitivity to the feelings and needs of the people for whom their services exist. In most cases it is safe for relatives to see and touch the body, and there are no risks to those who prepare the body for the funeral.

Policies and procedures must differentiate between different levels of risk. They should both protect those who come into contact with the body and enable families to carry out their wishes in relation to the handling of the body **unless there are clear clinical contraindications**. Restrictions should not be imposed unless they are essential. If the patient had a medium- or high-risk infection, the family and the funeral director should be clearly informed. Body bags should be reserved for high-risk infections.

There is a clear need for a standard method of informing the people who take charge of a body about its infection status. Marking the body in any way is likely to distress all relatives and could be highly offensive to some. If the body is in a body bag, the bag would have to be opened to see the mark, which would be counter-productive if there were a high risk of infection ('high infection risk').

One possibility is to produce a certificate that defines the degree of infection risk (low, medium or high) and also gives the appropriate infection control advice. This could be issued by the doctor who signs the Cause of Death Certificate and taped to the shroud (or, when a body bag is essential, to the outside of the bag). The new certificate should be different from the Cause of Death Certificate, which does not accompany the body.

Consultation Representatives of everyone involved at any stage between the death and the funeral should be included in discussions **before** policies are drafted and implemented. This includes people working on the ground such as infection control staff, medical and nursing staff, porters and mortuary attendants, as well as funeral directors, embalmers and representatives of local religious and community groups, especially of those who may want to prepare bodies themselves or to keep the coffin open before or during the funeral.

Referral to the coroner

Referral to the coroner is usually an additional source of stress for relatives. Explain why the referral is necessary and what is likely to happen, and identify and acknowledge relatives' concerns. If it is probable that the death will have to be referred, it is helpful for staff to warn relatives about this in advance. The likely delay may be particularly upsetting for people who may already be preparing to hold the funeral as soon as possible. However, many coroner's court staff are aware of the urgency of the funeral for some religious groups and do everything they can to speed the process.

Seeing the body

If the identity of the dead person is uncertain, the next of kin may be asked to attend the coroner's court to identify the body. Relatives can also visit simply to see the body. However, in many coroners' offices this is possible only through a glass screen. It is therefore very important that, whenever possible, relatives are able to spend time with the body before removal to the coroner's court. Otherwise, they have to wait until the body has been released again. In some cases the whole process can be completed and the body released within 24 hours. However, it often takes longer, for example while a pathologist is found to perform the post mortem, or if a crime is suspected (see below).

Coroner's post mortems

In most cases referred to the coroner, a post mortem is required by law in order to establish the cause of death. Some people, for religious, cultural or personal reasons, object strongly to post mortems (see above). They may be asked to put their objections in writing for the coroner. If the coroner still decides that a post mortem is essential, the relatives can appeal to the Divisional Court. However, this will involve further delay.

Relatives who want to see the body after the post mortem, or to prepare the body for the funeral themselves, should be told in advance what to expect. Sometimes a family member tries to shield others from the distressing knowledge that a post mortem has taken place; they need to know that the stitches will be obvious to anyone who washes and dresses the body or arranges the hair. Normally, all the organs are replaced, though sometimes body fluid samples are retained for analysis. On rare occasions an organ may be retained in order to establish the cause of death. The pathologist should be informed if the relatives are likely to want to wash or prepare the body for the funeral themselves, so that special care can be taken with repair (see also *Post mortems*, earlier).

Coroners' inquests

An inquest must be held in cases of sudden unexplained deaths, deaths under suspicious circumstances, deaths during surgery or under anaesthetic, deaths in police custody, and deaths that could be due to industrial injury, violence or neglect (Home Office 1996).

If murder or manslaughter is suspected, the defence has a right to a second post mortem. This can result in further delay. To prevent this, it is possible to arrange for an independent pathologist to be present at the coroner's post mortem, or to arrange a second post mortem as soon as possible. This is customary in Northern Ireland and in Scotland. However, in England and Wales the body may not be released until after the case comes to trial, which can be many months. Relatives who are already traumatised by loss and by the circumstances in which the person died often experience additional anguish because of long delays before they can hold the funeral.

Repatriating the body

'As I've grown older and when my children left school, there was a terrible longing to go back to Ireland. But as they grew older and got married, the grandchildren came, so you were more or less hooked. But I've given them strict instructions that I'm to be buried in Ireland, come what may. I've saved enough to take my remains back to Ireland. They may have to pay their own fare.'
Irish woman (Schweitzer 1989)

Some families may send the body to their country of origin for burial or cremation. The bodies of foreign nationals who die while living in or visiting the UK are also repatriated. Repatriation is a complex, bureaucratic process and relatives need extra support and guidance. It is usually arranged by funeral directors with specialist knowledge of the regulations and an understanding of and respect for different cultural and religious requirements.

Regulations and requirements

Before repatriation can take place, the regulations of the country where the death occurred, of the airline and of the receiving country have to be met. For example, in England and Wales the following documents must be obtained:

1 The Death Certificate or 'Certified Copy of an Entry' issued by the registrar of births, marriages and deaths.
2 An Out of England order (OOE), issued by the coroner.
3 A Freedom From Infection certificate (FFI), issued either by the doctor who certified the death or by the pathologist who performed the post mortem.
4 An Embalming Certificate, which is an overseas state or government requirement but can also be required by the airline. This is issued by the embalmer (see *Embalming*, earlier).
5 A Funeral Director's Declaration.

Different receiving countries have different requirements and regulations. Some require all documents to be legalised by their consulate or embassy in the UK, and require the coffin to be officially sealed. Some require additional documents, for example from the Home Office. Some countries' requirements for special documentation cause delays.

Airlines require the body to be embalmed and placed in a hermetically sealed coffin. Nowadays, most coffins of this type can be reopened so that relatives can pay their last respects at the funeral in the receiving country, though this also depends on local regulations.

If the death occurred under suspicious circumstances or could be due to unnatural causes, the body cannot be repatriated until the coroner's inquest has been adjourned (see above).

Transporting ashes

There is wide variation in national regulations. All countries require a Cremation Certificate and a Death Certificate before ashes can be imported. Some require the papers to be legalised and the urn to be sealed by their embassy in the UK before transportation.

21 After a death: bereavement and mourning

The experience and expression of grief

Grief is a normal reaction to loss, the price we pay for commitment and love. The experiences of bereaved people are both universal and highly individual. Grief can generate a wide range of feelings and physical symptoms (Scrutton 1995, Wortman and Silver 1989). Its length and depth may be influenced by many factors, including the intensity and significance of the relationship with the person who has died, the age at which they died, and the personality and life experiences of the bereaved. People who have devoted all their time and attention to the person who has died may have to make more adaptations than those whose daily lives have not been so fundamentally disrupted. The emotional response to a sudden and unexpected death is likely to differ from the response to a death after a long and difficult illness (Wright 1996). Death as a result of suicide or violence is likely to generate intense distress (see Chapter 19 *Suicide* and *Sudden death*).

Previous experience of loss can also influence people's reactions. Those who have had many bereavements may be completely overwhelmed by yet another death. Refugees and asylum seekers who have already suffered repeated losses may be especially vulnerable. They are also less likely to have emotional and social support networks (Eisenbruch 1984).

Current ideas about grief

Much has been written about the feelings and reactions of people who have been bereaved. Grief has been described as a series of stages or phases through which people move to varying degrees at varying rates over a period of time. These stages offer a useful foundation for thinking about grief and for understanding how bereaved people might feel and react.

However, there is a danger that some people may ignore the variability of grief responses that have been described, imposing a framework of 'normal grieving' on bereaved people and expecting them to progress through a series of prescribed stages rather than listening to them and responding to their real needs (Davies 1990, Wortman and Silver 1989, Murray Parkes 1985) (see also Chapter 18 *Emotional and spiritual care*).

'Grief simply does not follow any kind of ordered, linear progression. If anything, the experiences of grief are better characterised in terms of wave after wave of violently contradictory emotional impulses. Paradoxically, the stage/phase presentation may only ever make sense to people who have not had the experience, ie in all probability, most young to middle-aged health professionals.' (Littlewood 1992)

Other common assumptions include:

- A belief that people must experience painful feelings in order to come to terms with their loss. However, there is little evidence to substantiate this. Some people who are grieving never show intense distress; others are distressed for much longer than is believed to be normal (Walter 1994, Davies 1990, Wortman and Silver 1989). The former may be labelled 'in denial', the latter 'pathological'.
- A conviction that after a period of time the mourner should reach 'resolution', letting go of the person who has died and moving on to other relationships. This belief is not shared in all cultures. Whatever their culture, many people benefit more from reassurance that they can keep the person who has died somewhere in their mind or heart rather than relinquishing them completely. Imposing culture-based requirements as part of 'healthy grieving' can be damaging (Worden 1996, Walter 1994).

Culture and the experience of grief

Research indicates that grief is experienced in similar ways across all cultures, and that within each culture there is also a huge range of individual responses (Murray Parkes 1975). Cowles (1996), in focus-group interviews with people of six different cultural heritages, found no differences in people's ideas about and experiences of grief. The participants in all the cultural groups generally agreed that grief has the potential to affect every area of a person's existence – physical, psychological, emotional, spiritual, social and behavioural – and that it is dynamic. It changes with time, but not along a rigid, linear progression. The course of grief was likened to the healing of a physical wound; the wound can be re-opened many times. However, all the groups stressed the highly individual nature of grief and the variety of ways in which people deal with it.

'Don't fit me into your stages of grief. Listen to me, understand my beliefs and
the way I view things.'
Chinese woman

Culture and religion do, however, influence the way that people explain
the causes of their loss to themselves and how the loss fits into their system
of values. Every culture and religion teaches different ways of trying to reconcile the pain of loss. For each culture and religion there are also,
therefore, some losses that are more distressing or challenging to people's
values, both to lay people and to health professionals (Eisenbruch 1984).

Culture and the expression of grief

'All individuals ... can expect to experience some forms of loss. The response
to this experience ... is not universal, and may be as varied as the different individuals and their cultures.' (Eisenbruch 1984)

Although the experience of grief is similar across different cultures, there
are many factors that may influence the way people express their grief.
Children learn how to mourn by observing mourning behaviour in adults.
Cultural conditioning and social norms are a strong determinant of the way
grief is or is not expressed. Mourning behaviour is, therefore, not simply a
matter of conscious choice, but is influenced by 'mental programming' (see
Chapter 1).

'How a person mourns is determined to some extent by the way he is expected to mourn.' (Murray Parkes 1985)

In the UK, bereavement has traditionally been regarded as private and
personal. English culture valued reserve and stoicism rather than open
expression. Mourners were expected to demonstrate outward control
and to show their distress in subtle ways, for example with downcast eyes
and subdued voices. People familiar with the cultural norms knew how to
interpret these. Public weeping and grieving caused embarrassment, and
people who had temporarily 'lost control' often felt bound to apologise.
Loud crying and wailing were disapproved of unless feelings were clearly
so unbearably strong that they could not be contained. Men were brought
up to keep a stiff upper lip and to take charge; as a result, they tended to
have different coping strategies from women (Cline 1995, Murray Parkes
1985). (See also Chapter 2 *Not cultural facts but cultural possibilities*.)

In recent years it has become more acceptable for people in the UK to show
their grief and even for men to cry. At the same time, ritual is increasingly
seen as meaningless and empty. Individual expression is valued and is often
thought to be more sincere. People who display control and reserve may

now be regarded as unhealthily inhibited rather than admirably stoical (Walter 1994).

> 'When my wife died, I just about managed to avoid breaking down. We had been inseparable for forty years. I found that younger people, I suppose they thought they were being helpful, kept urging me to cry, especially at the funeral. I didn't want to, it would have made things even worse. It may be all right for people nowadays but it's not the right thing for me.'
> Elderly English man

> 'For me personally it's much better to let it out than bottle it up. It's brilliant to be able to cry and not to care who hears you. I think it's much healthier in the long run.'
> African-Caribbean nurse

In many cultures, people expect and are expected to grieve openly, both physically and loudly. They may, for example, moan, rock, sob, shout, walk up and down, wring their hands or throw themselves on the floor. In some communities wailing is seen as the normal expression of grief. In some societies official wailers may be hired for funerals (a contrast with British funeral directors' silent pallbearers).

> 'Wailing is what some people have been brought up to do. Sometimes staff think people put it on, especially when they see someone switch from being calm to sudden wailing. But that's what grief is like. It comes in waves and if that's how you've been brought up to show it, or if it is what is expected of you by friends and family, that is what you will do. It's still real grief.'
> Patients' affairs officer

In some communities, people who do not express their grief loudly and openly may be thought peculiar or unhealthy. They may also be thought to have had a poor relationship with the person who has died.

> 'In this country most people don't express their feelings in public. They might express them in private I suppose, when they are at home or alone, but for us grief is a public thing, you show and share your feelings. It is important to let people be themselves when they are so sad and shocked, to hug, cry, shout, weep. It is important not to make them feel ashamed.'
> Iraqi interpreter

Religious and cultural customs

Religious and cultural customs and beliefs also influence the expression of grief. Observant Jews may suspend outward mourning on the Sabbath. Devout Muslims and some Christians who believe that everything must be accepted as the will of God may subdue their grief. However, individual reactions do not always coincide with religious teaching. Some people may still be overwhelmed by the need to express their anguish openly.

'Outwardly I was calm and accepting. But I was screaming and furious inside.' Muslim woman

The different ways in which bereaved people are expected to behave in public, the restrictions that they are expected to observe and the clothes they are expected to wear, how funerals are organised, and many other external expressions of grief are largely determined by culture and history. **They do not necessarily indicate what individuals are experiencing or what they need.**

'To assume that a [person] is experiencing grief in a certain manner, or to attribute his or her behaviour or expressions of need solely to ethnic or cultural heritage, precludes any attempt to understand the very individual, intrapersonal aspects of grief.' (Cowles 1996)

Grief and older people

Ageist assumptions may influence the way health professionals and others respond to older people at times of serious illness and loss (see Chapter 4 *Ageism*). Some may assume that older people have less strength and ability to cope, whereas others believe that they should expect illness and loss and should accept them without fuss. Whatever their age, people who are facing serious illness, death or bereavement need to be listened to and responded to as individuals.

Grief and children

In any family or close-knit community, children are deeply affected by the death of someone they love. The most profound loss for a child is usually the death of a parent. However, depending on patterns of child care, a child may be equally devastated by the death of another person, perhaps a grandmother, who has been their prime carer.

The involvement of children after a death depends to some extent on cultural norms and expectations. Some people actively include babies and children after a death; children witness the grief of adults, attend wakes and listen to stories about the person who has died. They may see the body and attend the funeral. Others try to shield children from death and extreme grief. Some people encourage children to make their own choices about matters such as seeing the body, helping to plan the funeral and attending it, and visiting the grave.

Like adults, children have to accept the reality of their loss, to cope with their feelings and to adjust to life without the person who has died. They also need to find a new place in their emotional life for that person. Research indicates that they can be helped to do this by having a choice about their level of involvement (Worden 1996). However, cultural or religious norms both define the options available to the family and to the child, and sometimes override the child's wishes. Children are generally helped by having the consistent support of an adult who is close to them and who is able to listen and respond to them.

Witnessing grief and offering support

'The loss of a loved one is ... not only painful to experience, but also painful to witness, if only because we are so impotent to help.' (Bowlby 1980)

Worden (1991) has listed four factors that make it hard for health professionals to witness the grief of others:

- We are likely to experience feelings of helplessness.
- We have been conditioned by the culture of health care, which demands detachment and also focuses on **doing** things to or for people rather than just **being** with them.
- We may feel that it is our role to remove pain and distress. When people are grieving we cannot do this.
- We may also be reminded of the losses we ourselves have experienced and of the losses we fear. Our own mortality may be brought into sharp focus.

As a result, it can be tempting to erect barriers between ourselves and people who are distressed in order to protect ourselves.

Understanding ourselves

Our cultural conditioning and social norms are derived from our upbringing and our own experience of loss, as well as from our professional training. These influence the judgements we make about the ways in which people express grief, and our ability to offer support. It may be helpful to take some time to think about our reactions to different behaviour and what lies behind them.

Arrange some time and privacy for this reflection. You may find it helpful to write down your thoughts and feelings on your own. Alternatively, you may prefer to work with a friend or colleague, taking turns to talk and to listen (see also Chapter 8 *Finding a good listener*). Even if we have not been bereaved, each of us has experienced the feelings associated with loss. These can be triggered by any change that we experienced as negative; for example, changing schools, the loss of a friend who moved away, the separation or divorce of parents, the end of a romance, moving countries. Reflecting on our own experiences can be sad and difficult, but it can help us deal better with painful memories that may be triggered unexpectedly when we are trying to care for others.

- What losses have you experienced?
- How did you feel and react?
- What helped you to cope?
- What did you find unhelpful?

The right kind of support

When we do feel able to offer support, we tend to offer what we ourselves would want, but this is not necessarily appropriate. The kind of support people need varies from individual to individual and from culture to culture. Think about your own answers to the following questions. Then ask friends and colleagues, both men and women, of different age groups and different heritages what their preferences would be.

When you are upset what do you need?

- Do you like a matter-of-fact business-like approach?
- Do you prefer to be alone or to have someone supportive with you?
- Do you want to be touched? If so, how? By whom?
- Do you want to talk or to be quiet?
- Do you welcome encouragement to express your feelings?
- Do you want reassurance, advice or information?
- Do you appreciate reassurances or explanations based on religious beliefs?

Our own feelings and needs and the way we handle grief also affect our reactions to others. If you have been brought up to be reserved, you may be relieved if relatives seem to 'be taking it well' and anxious when they are expressive. If you prefer to express your feelings openly, and believe that doing so is important and cathartic, you may find it hard to accept that some people cope just as well by being very quiet.

Think about how you would feel and react if you were caring for the bereaved people in the following list. Notice your thoughts and assumptions:

- a woman who is crying
- a man who is crying
- a person who is sobbing and wailing
- a person who throws themselves on the floor
- a person who is unexpressive and matter of fact.

Everyone needs to be able to handle and express their grief in their own way and at their own pace. Culture and religious or spiritual beliefs are important, but they do not define how any individual will react or what they will need. It is essential not to make assumptions about how to help but to watch and listen. When you are unsure, ask what they would prefer.

- Most people need time in a place where they feel able to do what feels right for them. For some this means complete privacy, for others being alone in a room is lonely and frightening.
- Many people appreciate the presence or availability of someone who is supportive and understanding. Offering your time and full attention, and demonstrating a willingness to listen and respond, is the best you can do.
- Be aware that physical ways of offering comfort are not universal. For some people physical contact or eye contact with a stranger, particularly someone of the opposite sex, is unacceptable. Try to be alert to the other person's body language.
- Comfort based on religious beliefs and values is a very sensitive issue. Some people may welcome words of spiritual comfort, even across religious barriers. Others may find them distressing and inappropriate. Try to pick up the person's cues before saying anything.

Mourning rituals

Rituals, whether secular or religious, can help people manage life crises with a sense of meaning and continuity (see also Chapter 10 *The value of religious rituals*). In English culture, mourning rituals have been increasingly reduced. In most cases, funerals are small and muted, involving only close relatives; other people may feel they should not intrude. Public mourning ends after the funeral. Bereaved relatives are no longer expected to wear black, even to the funeral. The bereaved household is not marked out in any formal way. This trend towards playing down the public recognition of death seems to have begun during the First World War. Until then, most English people wore elaborate mourning dress and funeral processions were public events. However, the huge numbers of deaths of young men at the battle front affected virtually every family; it was considered too depressing and demoralising for the nation for so many families to be in formal mourning all at the same time (Gorer 1965).

With the loss of much of traditional ritual and ceremony, many people simply do not know what to do. They have to create their own individual rituals and ceremonies in order to give meaning and resonance to what has happened. This can be hard. Saying the right things to bereaved people has also become a task for each individual; the old formulae are often considered meaningless and empty. Many people find this very difficult and avoid the grieving person altogether, even at a formal event such as a funeral (Walter 1994).

'When someone in your family dies, people are frightened to talk to you. They don't know what to say and are frightened of upsetting you. I find it much more upsetting to be ignored and treated as though nothing has happened.'
African-Caribbean nurse

In some communities, formal grieving is regarded as very important. All the members of the family, friends, neighbours and sometimes the whole community may be involved. Large numbers of people may visit the family home to pay their respects to the person who has died and to offer support. There may be a set period during which close relatives remain quietly at home, followed by a gradual return to normal life, sometimes marked by religious ceremonies. There may be formal arrangements for giving the family emotional and practical support.

'You don't get invited when somebody dies back home, you just go, everybody goes, the whole community. And you make the family cry, you make them laugh. You cry with them, you laugh with them, you eat with them. People bring food for themselves and the family and they sit with them for days. And often there is someone who is very good at making people laugh and they help the family. They make them laugh as well as crying.'
Eritrean nurse

In some communities, bereaved relatives wear special clothes.

'My mother and aunts wore black for a year when any close relative died. I hardly remember my mother ever out of black. But it meant that everyone knew and I think people were more supportive.'
Austrian woman

Many people derive support and comfort from these traditions and customs. However, they may not meet everyone's needs. It is important, for example, not to assume that a person will not need support from you because their own culture traditionally offers a structure for grieving.

Funerals

Ceremonies and services

The move towards secularism and individualism in English culture has also affected funerals. Although many English people find religious and formal funerals comforting and meaningful, many do not. Increasingly, especially for people with no formal religious or spiritual beliefs, the purpose of a funeral is to benefit the survivors rather than the soul of the person who has died. There is a small but growing trend for families and friends to arrange and officiate at funerals themselves.

In contrast, for many religious groups the main purpose of the funeral rites is to benefit the soul of the person who has died. Many people also find great meaning and comfort in traditional ways of doing things, perhaps especially if they are part of a cultural minority. In many minority communities, funerals are more formal and more traditional. It may be customary to have the body at home before the funeral, often in the open coffin. Large numbers of people may visit the home to pay their last respects, and there may be prayers and ceremonies. In some communities it is customary to take photographs of the dead person and to photograph or video the funeral.

'I was talking to a West African family about their grandfather's funeral. They showed me a photograph album with pictures of everybody who came to the funeral and of him lying in the open coffin. They asked if I would like to see the video of the funeral. I asked about the coffin being open and they were astounded and shocked to learn that coffins are usually closed in the UK. They asked, "If the coffin is closed, how can you believe deep down in your heart that the person has died? And how can you remember the funeral or grieve properly later if you don't have photos or a video?"'
English woman

In some communities only men attend funerals; it is considered that women should be protected from witnessing the harsh reality of seeing a burial or cremation. While many women accept this, some very much want to be present.

'Sometimes women ask me to be their advocate and explain to their family that it can be very helpful to be at the burial.'
Muslim health professional

Although in the UK it is traditional to send flowers unless specifically asked not to, it may be inappropriate to send or take flowers, for example, to a Jewish or Chinese funeral. Families who are not used to flowers at a funeral may simply not know what to do with them.

Burial and cremation

Decisions about burial or cremation may be based on personal feelings, cultural traditions or religious teaching. For example, in African-Caribbean communities burial is traditional. Judaism and Islam require burial. Muslim families may want, where possible, to use a Muslim cemetery where religious precepts can be followed. Most Hindus and Sikhs are cremated, and the eldest son traditionally lights the funeral pyre. In response to this wish, many crematoria have adapted their procedures so that family members can help push the coffin into the cremator.

If there is nobody to arrange a funeral, health authorities should ensure that any religious or other wishes the patient might have had are followed. They should also ensure that records of the exact location of the grave are kept so that relatives who may later want to find it can do so.

22 Service planning, management and staff education for a multi-ethnic society

· ·

'The new NHS will have quality at its heart. Without it there is unfairness. This must be quality in its broadest sense. And it must be the quality of the patient's experience as well as the clinical result – quality measured in terms of prompt access, good relationships and efficient administration.' (Department of Health 1997)

For health care to be truly accessible to everyone, the needs of cultural and religious minorities must run as a continuous thread through all health planning, policy making, management, education and practice. Minority needs should not be seen as 'different' or 'separate', or considered only in relation to certain issues or services. There is a limit to what individual health professionals can achieve. It is therefore important that the whole organisation looks at the policy and management issues arising from the responsibility to serve a multi-ethnic population. Individuals should be supported and encouraged by well-informed planners, managers and educators so that they can deliver sensitive, flexible, high-quality care.

A *commitment to equality*

The basic foundation for tackling discrimination, improving care and redressing inequalities is a policy that commits the organisation to providing **equal access to services** for all who need them. The policy should outline the requirements of the Race Relations Act 1976 and its implications for health care provision (see also Chapters 5, 6 and 7). It should include the needs of people of cultural, ethnic and religious minorities, of people who have a disability and of people who experience social deprivation and homelessness.

The organisation's commitment to equality should also be reflected in a policy on **equal opportunities in employment** and in the active implementation of such a policy in all areas. The policy must include strategies for identifying and dealing with harassment, discrimination and victimisation in the workplace (see also Chapters 5, 6 and 7). It is unreasonable and unrealistic to expect staff to be committed to equal access to care if they do not see the principles of equality working in their own organisation.

Identifying local needs and issues

It is important to identify all the different cultural, linguistic and religious groups in the area in order to consult on and plan to meet their needs. This includes groups that are small, isolated or less obvious who often face greater barriers to services than members of larger minority communities precisely because their needs are not recognised (Li 1992).

Ethnic monitoring is an important first step towards identifying different groups within the local population, but it will not give the whole picture. The categories are crude, and individuals rightly have a choice about whether and how they identify themselves. People categorised as the same 'racial group', such as Indian or Black-Caribbean, may be culturally very different (Senior and Bhopal 1994). They are also likely to have differing religious needs. People who do not use the health service will not be identified at all.

Comparing ethnic monitoring data with local census data may help to identify groups who are not using existing services. Their views on how services could be improved should then be sought.

Consultation

Central to the whole process of identifying needs and working out ways of meeting them must be the people for whom health services exist. If the different minority groups are not consulted, services will remain biased towards the needs and preferences of white, middle-class patients and their families. Failure to consult minority service users should provoke as many objections as if a group consisting only of men were to devise and implement policies and practices specifically for the care of women (Alladin 1992).

Consultation should take place from the beginning. It is unacceptable, insulting and pointless to call in people of minority groups simply to 'rubber stamp' the final documents. They must have continuous opportunities to influence the whole process. A clear distinction must also be made between consultation and information-giving. Meetings that are publicised as part of a positive consultation process, but which are really forums for managers to announce firm decisions, cause lasting resentment and suspicion. It is important not to begin a process of consultation without a firm and genuine commitment to making as many of the changes that are needed as possible.

'People keep asking us what we want from the health service and we keep telling them. But nothing ever changes.'
African-Caribbean women's group

Whom to consult

Effective consultation involves building links with people of different communities and inviting them to participate in planning, evaluating and monitoring the quality of services. Care should be taken to consult a broad cross-section of each community and to include people who are less assimilated and more traditional. Interpreters may be needed so that those who face the greatest obstacles in communicating can participate in the consultation process (SHARE 1992).

Consultation may reveal differences of opinion within minority groups. This is to be expected in any group of people. However, variation within a minority group is often seen as a sign of confusion or irrationality and even as a reason for not taking any action. Expecting a level of united opinion on matters that are often difficult and sensitive from people of minority communities where one would not expect the same thing from, for example, a group of English people, is a manifestation of racism (Ahmed, Cheetham and Small 1986).

Religious leaders are a starting point for identifying religious teachings and practices. However, the roles and duties of leaders in different faiths vary. Whilst many will welcome consultation, others may not see it as part of their role. Religious leaders who take a very conservative line on certain issues will not always provide an insight into how people actually live their lives.

Ethnic minority health professionals often have a good understanding of the range of possible needs within their communities and of the problems that people face in getting care. Health advocates, health aides and interpreters can provide a unique view of how services are perceived by the people they work with. Community workers who are in close contact with people of minority groups, and other professionals whose work brings them into contact with people who may not be not using services, such as asylum seekers, refugees and homeless people, may also have useful information and insights into varying needs.

The consultation process

The consultation process must be carefully organised. Arrangements should be made to accommodate people who are not used to voicing their views in public, or who feel uncomfortable talking publicly about sensitive and delicate issues. Meetings in small (and in some cases single-sex) groups are likely to be more effective, especially if service users outnumber policy makers, and if the same group meets several times so that trust and mutual respect can develop. Policy makers must listen actively and with empathy, and must be genuinely and visibly flexible and responsive.

Flexible content

The things that are important to users are not always obvious to the people planning and providing health care. The consultation process should be designed to encourage black and minority ethnic people to raise issues and to set the agenda for discussions. Issues raised by health professionals working at the grass roots, particularly in the community, should also be included; they are often aware of service problems and shortcomings because of their direct contact with clients. Involving professionals from an early stage is also an important way of gaining their commitment to changes and improvements.

'There is a fundamental difference between people who do not come into direct contact with patients and the families and those who do. If one is distanced from the actual human experience, from the immediacy and intensity of the situation and the practical difficulties of providing appropriate care, it is all too easy to devise and implement policies and practices that are either idealistic and impractical or that ignore the actual needs of patients and their families.'
Health care researcher

Commissioning and planning services

A range of issues should be considered when commissioning and planning services (Jamdagni 1996, Gunaratnam 1993). With a few exceptions (such as interpreters and services for people with haemoglobinopathies) separate or special services are not needed (see Chapter 7 *Equal access to care*). Instead, all services should be broad-based and flexible, so that different needs can be accommodated easily as they arise.

The quality standards listed below pull together the key policy and management issues set out in this book and will begin to ensure that services enable people of all communities to benefit equally. Some require a change in awareness or in practice but no extra resources. Others require additional resources in terms of time, training, support or facilities. A few may not be immediately achievable, but all should be regarded as important goals. The process of working out how to achieve and monitor the implementation of each standard should include assessing the resources that will be required and deciding a time scale.

Several of the quality standards listed can be audited. Others can be monitored by checking levels of service use. However, some of those that are most important in ensuring that services are acceptable and accessible are the hardest to measure. This should not be a reason for ignoring them.

Quality standards

- There will be a policy on equal access to services, and steps will be taken to ensure that all staff, including clerks and receptionists, understand the policy and its implications for their work. The rest of the standards outlined below could be incorporated in this equal access policy (see Chapter 7 *Equal access to care*).
- There will be a policy on equal opportunities in employment, and steps will be taken to ensure that it is implemented at every level (see Chapter 6 *Discrimination in employment*).
- Procedures for tackling discrimination, harassment and abuse will be in place and will be well publicised (see Chapters 6 and 7).
- Procedures will be in place to ensure that clients' names are accurately recorded and used, and can be retrieved correctly. Computer systems and all charts, forms and labels will accommodate differing naming systems (see Chapter 30 *Developing appropriate computer systems*).
- Care plans will be used as vehicles for discussing and recording specific cultural and religious needs (see Chapter 8 *Asking the patient*).
- Privacy will be provided in all clinical areas (see Chapters 12 *Modesty* and 13 *Modesty and physical examination*).
- Full-length, long-sleeved gowns with adequate ties, and full-length dressing gowns, will be available in all departments where people are asked to undress (see Chapter 12 *Clothing*).
- People for whom modesty is a particular issue will, whenever possible, have access to staff of the same sex (see Chapters 12 and 13).
- A range of foods will be offered, and menus will include details of ingredients so that all patients can choose foods to suit their religious or cultural needs (see Chapter 11 *Providing food in hospital and other residential care*).
- Relatives will be free to bring in food from home. Adequate storage and heating facilities (within appropriate health and safety guidelines) for such food will be provided (see Chapter 11 *Relatives bringing in food*).

- Privacy and space for families to pray or spend time together or to perform religious ceremonies will be provided (see Chapters 10 *Practical matters* and 17 *Facilities for visitors*).
- Religious items, including religious and wedding jewellery, will be treated with respect and not removed without the consent of the patient or their next of kin (see Chapters 12 *Jewellery and other items* and 20 *The patient's property*).
- Both showers and baths will be provided in all wards (see Chapter 12 *Bathing and showering*).
- Low level taps will be available to enable Muslims to wash their feet before prayer (see Chapter 44 *Worship*).
- Bidets or hand basins will be available in the lavatories. Alternatively, people who clean themselves with running water will be offered their own jug for this purpose (see Chapter 12 *Elimination*).
- The preferences and needs of dependent patients in relation to modesty, personal hygiene and hair care will be identified and met (see Chapter 12).
- People's cultural obligations in relation to visiting will be acknowledged and accommodated whenever possible, especially when a patient is critically ill or dying (see Chapter 18 *The needs of relatives*)
- Discharge procedures will be planned jointly with patients and their families, and will take account of religious festivals and possible constraints (see Chapter 10 *Religious festivals*).
- Written information will accommodate differing religious and cultural issues and will be available in languages appropriate to local community needs, as a back-up to verbal information (see Chapter 29). This will include:
  - letters and appointment cards;
  - important notices and signs;
  - health education material;
  - patient information leaflets.
- Professional interpreters who speak the main local languages will be available, especially for important discussions (eg taking a history, discussing treatment options and obtaining informed consent), and will be on call on a 24-hour basis (see Chapter 27).
- Arrangements will be in place for contacting interpreters who speak languages that are needed less frequently (see Chapter 27).
- Interpreters will receive training on the psychological as well as the practical aspects of optimum care (see Chapter 27 *Training, supporting and managing interpreters*).
- Procedures and practices (including standard infection control procedures) for last offices will accommodate religious and cultural preferences and needs (see Chapter 20 *Infection control issues*).

- After a death, relatives will have complete physical access to the body and will be able to spend as much time sitting with the body, in privacy, as they want to (see Chapter 20 *Spending time with the body*).
- The room set aside for relatives to spend time with the body will have a religiously neutral name and décor, with washing facilities nearby (see Chapter 20 *The chapel of rest*).
- Religious symbols and items appropriate to the main local religious communities will be available and will be stored out of sight. The religious needs of the family will be identified and the appropriate items will be put in place before the relatives arrive (see Chapter 20 *The chapel of rest*).
- Private and comfortable facilities will be available for the family or religious community to sit with the body until it is removed from the unit (see Chapter 20 *Spending time with the body*).
- There will be 24-hour access to the mortuary for those who need to collect the body out of hours (see Chapter 20 *Paperwork and certificates*).
- Arrangements will be in place for issuing Cause of Death Certificates and for registering the death out of hours. If this is not possible, policies will allow the release of bodies out of hours without the 'green form' (see Chapter 20 *Registering a death out of hours*).
- Accurate written information about infection risks and appropriate infection control measures will accompany the body so that anyone who will handle and prepare the body for the funeral can take appropriate precautions (see Chapter 20 *Infection control issues*).
- Discreet property bags will be provided and, whenever possible, relatives will be consulted, before the property is packed, about what should be included and what should be discarded (see Chapter 20 *The patient's property*).
- There will be an accessible, responsive and well-publicised complaints procedure. Information about the complaints procedure will be available in all languages relevant to the local communities.

Implications for service managers

Our own cultural assumptions and beliefs influence our views and actions. Managers too need to reflect on their own attitudes in order to manage a service that is flexible and responsive to everyone regardless of culture, religion or need.

'It has to come from the top. If we as managers are not open and flexible and have not examined our own attitudes and thought through what we need to do to meet minority needs, how can we expect our staff to?'
Director, multi-faith hospice

Service managers also need to take into account that providing culturally sensitive care:

- Takes longer, and it is unreasonable to expect staff to do it well without extra time.
- Requires appropriate resources, such as well-trained interpreters.
- Takes thought and self-awareness, and people cannot be expected to do it well without training. Such training must be skilfully designed and sensitively run so that participants are able to examine their own beliefs and attitudes as a foundation for understanding those of other people. It should not consist of 'facts' about different groups (see Chapters 1 and 2). Training should be available to all grades and to **everyone who has contact with clients, including all front-line staff.** One insensitive or unaware person can easily cancel out the efforts of everyone else.
- Requires flexibility. Once people understand the principles and aims of equal access, they should be encouraged to use their imagination and common sense in devising care that really meets the needs of different clients. Innovations that do not work should be treated as part of the learning process and those responsible for them should not be blamed (Cheung-Judge and Henley 1994).
- Is demanding. Staff should have time with their managers to evaluate their workload and identify their training needs in relation to caring for people of minority cultures and religions. The need for support must also be recognised as normal and healthy rather than as a sign of weakness. People vary in their ability to recognise their own needs for support and have different preferences as to how these should be met. A range of possible support mechanisms should be in place within a culture that clearly accepts staff support as a legitimate need.

'The ultimate purpose of good staff support is to ensure the highest possible standards of care for patients. These standards can only be delivered if there is also high quality staff care.' (Stoter 1997)

Implications for education and training

In a multi-ethnic, multi-religious society it is essential that all health professionals are able to understand, respect and meet a diversity of needs. The necessary information, skills and awareness should be woven into the initial and continuing education of everyone who comes into contact with patients and relatives.

It is important that the cultural and religious needs of minorities are not simply tacked onto the end of the curriculum. This would reinforce the idea that minority needs are extraordinary and abnormal, and that meeting them is optional, while everything contained in the main body of the curriculum is essential. It would help to perpetuate inequalities in provision.

All health professionals and students need training in the subtle skills required to provide health care in a multi-ethnic, multi-religious, multi-lingual society. Lack of training results in an inability to develop therapeutic relationships, which is a source of staff frustration and stress (Murphy and Macleod Clark 1993).

Undergraduate and postgraduate training should include the following (for more details, see Part One and the other chapters (8–21) in Part Two):

- Opportunities for staff to develop awareness of their own personal culture and assumptions as well as the culture and assumptions of the organisation in which they work.
- The effects of racial discrimination and poverty on the health status of minority groups (Culley 1996).
- The implications for health services of the 1976 Race Relations Act.
- Exploration of possible variations in cultural and religious needs in relation to each aspect of physical and emotional care as it arises in the curriculum.

'Awareness of racism and inequality should be a strand throughout the educational curriculum, with positive attempts made to expose learners to all aspects of caring for [patients] from a wide variety of ethnic backgrounds.' (Kroll 1990)

This sort of training requires knowledge, skill and sensitivity. It must be carried out in an atmosphere of trust, respect and safety. Subjects such as inequality and racial discrimination are emotive and difficult to discuss without arousing defensiveness, anger, guilt and resentment. Feelings can run high, especially as the students and health professionals involved are themselves likely to be of different cultures, religions and ethnic groups, and may bring their own, often painful, experiences to the discussion. Health professionals and students can learn a great deal about such issues from each other, but they must first learn to value each other more positively (McGee 1994) and there must be enough safety within the group to make learning possible. However, potential difficulties and awkwardness should not be reasons for inaction. Educators who lack the necessary knowledge, confidence and appropriate skills need further training and support.

References

ACHC (1997) *Hungry In Hospital*. Association of Community Health Councils, London

Age Exchange (1984) *A Place to Stay: Memories of pensioners from many lands*. Age Exchange, London

Ahmed S, Cheetham J, Small J (eds) (1986) *Social Work with Black Children and their Families*. B T Batsford, London

Albery N, Elliot G, Elliot J (1997) *The Natural Death Handbook*. Natural Death Centre, 20 Heber Road, London NW2 6AA

Alladin WJ (1992) Clinical psychology provision: models, policies and prospects. In WIU Ahmad (ed) *The Politics of Race and Health*. Race Relations Research Unit, Bradford University, Bradford, pp 117–37

Altschuler J (1997) Family relationships during serious illness. *Nursing Times* 93 (7): 48–9

American Academy of Dermatology (1997) *Black Skin*. American Academy of Dermatology, Schaumberg, Illinois

Archer CB, Robertson SJ (1995) *Black and White Skin Diseases: An atlas and text*. Blackwell Science, London

Arnold A (1992) Intercultural social work. In J Kareem and R Littlewood (eds) *Intercultural Therapy: Themes, interpretations and practice*. Blackwell Science, Oxford, pp 155–62

Baines MJ (1990) Tackling total pain. In C Saunders (ed) *Hospice and Palliative Care: An interdisciplinary approach*. Edward Arnold, London, pp 26–35

Barrow V (1997) Food for thought. *Nursing Standard* 11 (27): 18

Baxter C (1993) Observing skin. *Community Outlook* Jan: 21–2

Baxter C (1992) Caring for patients' hair. *Community Outlook* Sep: 31–2

Baxter C (1989) *Cancer Support and Ethnic Minority Migrant Worker Communities*. CancerLink, London

Beishon S, Modood T, Virdee S (1998) *Ethnic Minority Families*. Policy Studies Institute, London

Bhakta P, Probert CS, Jayanthi V, Mayberry JF (1992) Stoma anxieties: a comparison of the attitudes of Asian migrants and the indigenous population in the United Kingdom towards abdominal surgery and the role of intestinal stomas. *International Journal of Colorectal Disease* 7 (1): 1–3

Bieri D, Reeve RA, Champion GD, Addicoat L, Ziegler JB (1990) The Faces Pain Scale for the self assessment of the severity of pain experienced by children: development, initial validation and preliminary investigation for ratio scale properties. *PAIN* 41 (2): 139–50

BMA (1993) *Medical Ethics Today: Its practice and philosophy.* British Medical Association/British Medical Journal Publishing Group, London

BMA and RCN (1995) *The Older Person: Consent and care.* British Medical Association and the Royal College of Nursing, London

Bond MR (1980) The suffering of severe intractable pain. In HA Kosterlitz and LY Terenius (eds) *Pain and Society.* Weinheim Verlag Chemie, Germany, pp 53–61

Boston P (1993) Culture and cancer: the relevance of cultural orientation within cancer education programmes. *European Journal of Cancer Care* 2: 72–6

Bowlby J (1980) *Attachment and Loss: Loss, sadness and depression.* Basic Books, New York

Bram G (1983) Breakdown in elderly Polish refugees. In R Baker (ed) *Psychosocial Problems of Refugees.* Refugee Council, London

Breckman B (1981) Psychosocial areas related to stoma care. In B Breckman (ed) *Stoma Care: A guide for nurses, doctors and other health care workers.* Beaconsfield, Beaconsfield Bucks, pp 1–15

Brena SF, Chapman SL (1991) Pain, ethnicity and culture. In WCV Parris (ed) *Contemporary Issues in Chronic Pain Management.* Kluwer Academic, Mass

Brinkley D (1995) *Saved by the Light.* HarperCollins, New York

Buchholz WM (1990) Letter. *New England Journal of Medicine* 323 (19) 1354–5

Buckman R (1996) *How to Break Bad News: A guide for health-care professionals.* Pan Macmillan, London

Buckman R (1984) Breaking bad news; why is it still so difficult? *British Medical Journal* 288: 1597–9

Calanan M, Kelley P (1992) *Final Gifts: Understanding and helping the dying.* Hodder and Stoughton, London

Charlton R (1994) Words of sorrow. *Student British Medical Journal* 2: 42

Cheung-Judge MY, Henley A (1994) *Equality in Action: Introducing equal opportunities in voluntary organisations.* NCVO Publications, London

Chodoff P (1970) The German concentration camp as a psychological stress. *Archives of General Psychiatry* 22: 78–87

Clark WC, Clark SB (1980) Pain responses in Nepalese porters. *Science* 209: 410–12

Cline S (1995) *Lifting the Taboo: Women, death and dying.* Little, Brown and Co, London

Cole WO (1994) *Teach yourself Sikhism.* Hodder and Stoughton, London

Cowles KV (1996) Cultural perspectives of grief: an expanded concept analysis. *Journal of Advanced Nursing* 23: 287–94

Craig KD (1994) Emotional aspects of pain. In PD Wall and R Melzack (eds) *Textbook of Pain*, 3rd edn. Churchill Livingstone, London, pp 261–74

CRE (1993) *The Sorrow in my Heart ... sixteen Asian women speak about depression.* Commission for Racial Equality, London

CRE (1991) *Second Review of the Race Relations Act 1976.* Commission for Racial Equality, London

Culley L (1996) A critique of multiculturalism in health care: the challenge for nurse education. *Journal of Advanced Nursing* 23: 564–70

Currer C (1986) *Health Concepts and Illness Behaviour: The care of Pathan mothers in Bradford* (unpublished PhD thesis). Department of Sociology, University of Warwick, Warwick

Daschner FD (1997) Holy water, tap water or water filters? *Journal of Hospital Infection* 35 (1): 71–2

Davey B (1993) The nurse's dilemma: truth telling or big white lies? In D Dickenson and M Johnson (eds) *Death, Dying and Bereavement.* Open University/Sage, London, pp 116–23

Davidhizar R, Newman Giger J (1998) Patients' use of denial: coping with the unacceptable *Nursing Standard* 12 (43): 44–6

Davies D (1990) The social facts of death. In G Howarth and PC Jupp (eds) *Contemporary Issues in the Sociology of Death, Dying and Disposal.* Macmillan, London

Dawe V (1992) Winning over patient's trust. *Hospital Doctor* 8 Oct: 34

Del Vecchio Good M, Good BJ, Schaffer C, Lind SE (1990) American oncology and the discourse on hope. *Culture, Medicine and Psychiatry* 14: 59–79

Department of Health (1997) *The New NHS: Modern – dependable*, White Paper. Stationery Office, London

Department of Health (1983) *Cadaveric Organs for Transplantation: A code of practice including the diagnosis of brain death*, report of a Working Party on behalf of the Health Departments of Great Britain and Northern Ireland. HMSO, London

Donovan JL (1986) *'We Don't Buy Sickness, It Just Comes': Health, illness and health care in the lives of black people in London*. Gower, Aldershot

Eisenbruch M (1984) Cross-cultural aspects of bereavement. I. A conceptual framework for comparative analysis. *Culture, Medicine and Psychiatry* 8: 283–309

Foster M-C (1988) Health visitors' perspectives on working in a multiethnic society. *Health Visitor* 61: 275–8

Furnham A, Bochner S (1986) *Culture Shock: Psychological reactions to unfamiliar environments*. Routledge, London

Garro LC (1990) Culture, pain and cancer. *Journal of Palliative Care* 6 (3): 34–44

Gatrad AR (1994) Medical implications of Islam for women and children. *Maternal and Child Health* July: 225–7

Gaster TH (1955) *The Holy and the Profane: Evolution of Jewish folkways*. William Sloane Associates, New York

GMC (1998a) *Seeking Patients' Consent*, draft guidelines. General Medical Council, London

GMC (1998b) *Confidentiality: Providing and protecting information* (draft guidelines in preparation). General Medical Council, London

Goldie L (1982) The ethics of telling the patient. *Journal of Medical Ethics* 8: 128–33

Gorer G (1965) *Death, Grief and Mourning in Contemporary Britain*. Cresset, London

Grey A (1994) The spiritual component of palliative care. *Palliative Medicine* 8: 215–21

Gunaratnam Y (1993) *Health and Race Checklist: A starting point for managers on improving services for black populations*. King's Fund, London

Hammick M, Smith J, Corsini L, Hamlyne L, Peirce V (1996) Radiotherapy patients in the United Kingdom: meeting cultural and spiritual needs. *Journal of Cancer Care* 5: 113–15

Hanratty J, Higginson I (1994) *Palliative Care in Terminal Illness*. Radcliff Medical Press, Oxford

Hardy JD, Wolff HG, Goodell H (1952) *Pain Sensations and Reactions*. Williams and Wilkins, Baltimore MD

Haroon-Iqbal H, Field D, Parker H, Iqbal Z (1995) Palliative care services for ethnic groups in Leicester. *International Journal of Palliative Nursing* 1 (2): 114–16

Hart BD, Wells DL (1997) The effects of language used by caregivers on agitation in residents with dementia. *Clinical Nurse Specialist* 11 (1): 20–3

Healing TD, Hoffman PN, Young SEJ (1995) The infection hazards of human cadavers. *Communicable Diseases Report* 5 (5): R61–7

Health and Safety at Work etc Act 1974. HMSO, London

HSE (1994) *Control of Substances Hazardous to Health Regulations: Approved code of practice*. Health and Safety Executive, London

Health Services Advisory Committee (1991) *Safety in Health Services Laboratories: Safe working and the prevention of infection in the mortuary and the post-mortem room*. Health and Safety Executive, London

Higgs R (1999) The diagnosis of dying. *Journal of the Royal College of Physicians of London* 33 (2): 110–12

Hill D, Penso D (1995) *Opening Doors: Improving access to hospice and specialist palliative care services by members of the black and ethnic minority communities*. National Council for Hospice and Specialist Palliative Care Services, Seventh Floor, 1 Great Cumberland Place, London W1H 7AL

Hirschfeld MJ (1977) Care of the aging Holocaust survivor. *American Journal of Nursing* July: 1187–9

Hockley JM, Dunlop R, Davies RJ (1988) Survey of distressing symptoms in dying patients and their families in hospital and the response to a symptom control team. *British Medical Journal* 296: 1715–17

Holmes S (1996) Nursing management of oral care in older patients. *Nursing Times* 92 (9): 37–9

Home Office (1996) *The Work of the Coroner: Some questions answered*. Home Office, London

Horsfield-Gardner J (1987) Asians in Britain: some cultural considerations in stoma care. *Advanced Journal of Clinical Nursing, Nursing add-on* 3 (21): 785–9

Jamdagni L (1996) *Purchasing for Black Populations*. King's Fund, London

Jones R (1992) Primary health care: what should we do for people dying at home with cancer? *European Journal of Cancer Care* 1 (4): 9–11

Kagawa-Singer M (1987) Ethnic perspectives on cancer nursing: Hispanics and Japanese-Americans. *Oncology Nursing Forum* 14 (3): 59–65

Kalow W (1982) Ethnic differences in drug metabolism. *Clinical Pharmacokinetics* 7: 373–400

Karseras PA (1991) Health care for minorities. 2. Improving services. *Care of the Elderly* Nov: 468–70

Katz JS (1996) Jewish perspectives on death, dying and bereavement. In D Dickenson and M Johnson (eds) *Death, Dying and Bereavement.* Open University/Sage, London, pp 199–207

Kiecolt-Glaser JK, Marucha PT, Malarkey WB, Mercado AM, Glaser R (1995) Slowing of wound healing by psychological stress. *Lancet* **346**: 1194–6

Kohner N (1996) *The Moral Maze of Practice: A stimulus for reflection and discussion.* King's Fund, London

Kratiuk-Wall S, Shanley C, Russell K (1997) *Cultural Diversity and Dementia.* Centre for Research and Education on Ageing, Melbourne

Kroll D (1990) Equal access to care? *Nursing Times* **86** (23): 72–3

Kübler-Ross E (1995) *Death is of Vital Importance: On life, death and life after death.* Station Hill Press, New York

Kübler-Ross E (1970) *On Death and Dying.* Tavistock, London

Lennard-Jones JE (1999) Giving or withholding nutrients: ethical and legal aspects. *Journal of the Royal College of Physicians of London* **33** (1): 39–45

Levy RA (1993) *Ethnic and Racial Differences in Response to Medicines.* National Pharmaceutical Council, Reston VA

Li P-L (1992) Health needs of the Chinese population. In WIU Ahmad (ed) *The Politics of 'Race' and Health.* Race Relations Research Unit, University of Bradford, Bradford, pp 105–14

Lister A (1997) Multi-faith hospices. *International Journal of Palliative Nursing* **3** (1): 23–5

Littlewood J (1992) *Aspects of Grief.* Tavistock, London

London Beth Din (1998) *The Really Jewish Food Guide.* United Synagogue Publications Ltd, 735 High Road, London N12

Lowe M, Kerridge IH, Mitchell KR (1995) 'These sorts of people don't do very well': race and allocation of health resources. *Journal of Medical Ethics* **21**: 356–60

Maguire P, Faulkner A (1993) Communicating with cancer patients. 2. Handling uncertainty, collusion and denial. In D Dickenson and M Johnson (eds) *Death, Dying and Bereavement.* Open University/Sage, London, pp 186–91

Maguire CP, Kirby M, Coen R, Coakley D, Lawlor B, O'Neill D (1996) Family members' attitudes towards telling the patient with Alzheimer's disease their diagnosis. *British Medical Journal* 313: 529–30

Mallett J, Bailey C (1996) *The Royal Marsden NHS Trust Manual of Clinical Nursing Procedures*, 4th edn. Blackwell Science, London

Mangan P (1988) Spot the difference. *Geriatric Nursing and Home Care* July: 18

McGee P (1994) Educational issues in transcultural nursing. *British Journal of Nursing* 3 (21): 111–15

Mead GE, Turnbull CJ (1995) Cardiopulmonary resuscitation in the elderly: patients' and relatives' views. *Journal of Medical Ethics* 21: 39–44

Melzak R, Wall PD (1996) *The Challenge of Pain*. Penguin Books, London

Melzack R, Katz J (1994) Pain measurement in persons in pain. In PD Wall and R Melzack (eds) *Textbook of Pain*, 3rd edn. Churchill Livingstone, London, pp 337–51

Moody R (1975) *Life After Life*. Bantam Books, New York

Murphy K, Macleod Clark J (1993) Nurses' experience of caring for ethnic minority clients. *Journal of Advanced Nursing* 18: 442–50

Murray Parkes C (1985) Bereavement. *British Journal of Psychiatry* 146: 11–17

Murray Parkes C (1975) *Bereavement: Studies of grief in adult life*. Penguin Books, London

NCHSPCS (1997) *Ethical Decision Making in Palliative Care: Artificial hydration for people who are terminally ill*. National Council for Hospice and Specialist Palliative Care Services, Seventh Floor, 1 Great Cumberland Place, London W1H 7AL

NCHSPCS (1993) Key *Ethical Issues in Palliative Care: Evidence to House of Lords Select Committee on Medical Ethics*. National Council for Hospice and Specialist Palliative Care Services (see Reference above for address)

Nazarko L (1997) Improving hospital discharge arrangements for older people. *Nursing Standard* 40 (11): 44–7

Ng B, Dimsdale JE, Rollnik JD, Shapiro H (1996) The effect of ethnicity on prescriptions for patient-controlled analgesia for post-operative pain. *PAIN* 66: 9–12

NHS Confederation (1996) *Spiritual Care in the NHS: A guide for purchasers and providers*. NHS Confederation, Birmingham, UK

O'Hara ES, Zhan L (1994) Cultural and pharmacologic considerations when caring for Chinese elders. *Journal of Gerontological Nursing* **20** (10): 11–16

O'Neill J (1994) Ethnic minorities – neglected by palliative care providers? *Journal of Cancer Care* **3**: 215–20

O'Rawe Amenta M (1997) Spiritual care: the heart of palliative nursing. *International Journal of Palliative Care* **3** (1): 4

Open University (1991) *Death and Dying Workbook*. Department of Health and Social Welfare, Open University Press, Buckingham

OUP (1996) *The New Shorter Oxford English Dictionary*. Oxford University Press, Oxford

Patel N, Mirza NR, Lindblad P, Amstrup K, Samaoli O (1998) *Dementia and Minority Ethnic Older People*. Russell House, Lyme Regis

Patel N, Naik D, Humphries B (eds) (1998) *Visions of Reality: Religion and ethnicity in social work*. Central Council for Education and Training in Social Work, London

Patients Association (1996) *Advance Statements about Future Medical Treatment: A guide for patients*. Patients Association, London.

Payne S, Langley-Evans A, Hillier R (1996) Perceptions of a 'good' death: a comparative study of the views of hospice staff and patients. *Palliative Medicine* **10** (4): 307–12

Payne S, Hillier R, Langley-Evans A, Roberts T (1996) Impact of witnessing death on hospice patients. *Social Science and Medicine* **43** (12): 1785–94

Pellegrino ED (1992) Is truth telling to the patient a cultural artefact? *Journal of the American Medical Association* **268** (13): 1734–5

Phillips J (1991) What should happen in the first hours after admission to a hospice. In *Palliative Care: Guidelines for good practice and audit measures*. Royal College of Physicians, London

Phillips DP, Todd ER, Wagner LM (1993) Psychology and survival. *Lancet* **342**: 1142–5

Pickett M (1993) Cultural awareness in the context of terminal illness. *Cancer Nursing* **16** (2): 102–6

Porter R (1997) *The Greatest Benefit to Mankind: A medical history of humanity from antiquity to the present*. HarperCollins, London

Rack P (1991) *Race, Culture and Mental Disorder*, 2nd edn. Routledge, London

RCN and BAAEM (British Association for Accident and Emergency Medicine) (1995) *Bereavement Care in A & E departments: Report of a working group*. Royal College of Nursing, London

Rees JC, Allan KD (1996) Holy water: a risk factor for hospital-acquired infection. *Journal of Hospital Infection* **32**: 51–5

Relatives Association (1997) *As Others See Us: A study of relationships in homes for older people*. Relatives Association, 5 Tavistock Place, London WC1H 9SN

Robinson SM, Mackenzie-Ross S, Campbell-Hewson GL, Egleston CV, Prevost AT (1998) Psychological effect of witnessed resuscitation on bereaved relatives. *Lancet* **352**: 614–17

Rosenbluth V (1997) *Keeping Family Stories Alive: Discovering and recording the stories and reflections of a lifetime*. Hartley and Marks, Vancouver BC

Rutala WF, Weber DJ (1997) Water as a reservoir of nosocomial pathogens. *Infection Control and Hospital Epidemiology* Sep: 609–15

Salem BM (1993) Pakistan Coin Pain Scale. *PAIN* **52** (3): 373–4

Salzer JL, Nelson NA (1983) Health care of Ethiopian refugees. *Pediatric Nursing* Nov/Dec: 449–52

Scanlon C (1989) Creating a vision of hope: the challenge of palliative care. *Oncology Nursing Forum* **16** (4): 491–6

Schott J, Henley A (1996) *Culture, Religion and Childbearing in a Multiracial Society: A handbook for professionals*. Butterworth Heinemann, Oxford

Schull CR (1987) *Medical Problems in the Tropics*. Teaching Aids at Low Cost, Macmillan Education, London

Schweitzer P (ed) (1989) *Across the Irish Sea*. Age Exchange, Blackheath, London

Scrutton S (1995) *Bereavement and Grief: Supporting older people through loss*. Edward Arnold/Age Concern, London.

Senior PA, Bhopal R (1994) Ethnicity as a variable in epidemiological research. *British Medical Journal* **309**: 327–30

SHAP (published annually) *Calendar of Religious Festivals*. SHAP Working Party on World Religions in Education, c/o The National Centre's RE Centre, 36 Causton Street, London SW1P 4AU

SHARE (1992) Purchasing and contracts. *Health and Race: creating social change* issue 4, SHARE, King's Fund Centre, London

Slater M (1993) *Health for All our Children: Achieving appropriate health care for black and minority ethnic children and their families*. Action for Sick Children/National Association for the Welfare of Children in Hospital, London

Soni Raleigh V (1996) Suicide patterns and trends in people of Indian subcontinent and Caribbean origin in England and Wales. *Ethnicity and Health* **1** (1): 55–63

Stanworth R (1997) Spirituality, language and depth of reality. *International Journal of Palliative Nursing* 3 (1): 23–5

Sternbach RA, Tursky B (1965) Ethnic differences among housewives in psychophysical and skin potential responses to electric shock. *Psychophysiology* 1: 241–6

Stoter DJ (1997) *Staff Support in Health Care*. Blackwell Science, Oxford

Torkington NPK (1987) Racism and health. *Women's Health Information Centre Newsletter* Spring: 7

Townsend J, Frank AO, Fermont D, Dyer S, Karran O, Walgrove A, Piper M (1990) Terminal cancer care and patients' preference for place of death: a prospective study. *British Medical Journal* 301: 415–17

UKCC (1996) *Guidelines for Professional Practice*. United Kingdom Central Council for Nursing, Midwifery and Health Visiting, London

UKTCA (1995) *Report of a Two Year Study into the Reasons for Relatives' Refusal of Organ Donation*. United Kingdom Transplant Co-ordinator's Association/MORI Health Research. HMSO, London

UKTSSA (1996) *Ethnic Minorities: Less chance of a match for a kidney transplant?* Information from the UK National Transplant Database 1996. United Kingdom Transplant Support Service Authority, Bristol

Van Steenberg C, Ansak M-L, Chin-Hansen J (1993) On Lok's model: managed long-term care. In CM Barresi and DE Stull (eds) *Ethnic Elderly and Long-term Care*. Springer, New York

Voluntary Euthanasia Society (1998) *An A–Z of Terms*. Voluntary Euthanasia Society, 13 Prince of Wales Terrace, London W8 5PG

Walter T (1996) Facing death without tradition. In G Howarth and PC Jupp (eds) *Contemporary Issues in the Sociology of Death, Dying and Disposal*. Macmillan, London

Walter T (1994) *The Revival of Death*. Routledge, London

Werner D, Thuman C, Maxwell J (1993) *Where There is No Doctor: A village health care handbook*. Teaching Aids at Low Cost, Macmillan Education, London

Wertheimer A (1991) *A Special Scar: Experiences of people bereaved by suicide*. Routledge, London

Wood J (1998) Jewish issues in social work education. In N Patel, D Naik and B Humphries (eds) *Visions of Reality: Religion and ethnicity in social work*. Central Council for Education and Training in Social Work, London

Worden J (1996) *Children and Grief when a Parent Dies*. Guildford Press, New York

Worden JW (1991) *Grief Counselling and Grief Therapy: A handbook for the mental health practitioner*. Routledge, London

Wortman CB, Silver RC (1989) The myths of coping with loss. *Journal of Consulting and Clinical Psychiatry* 57 (3): 349–57

Wright B (1996) *Sudden Death: A research base for practice*. Churchill Livingstone, London

Yee L (1995) *Improving Support for Black Carers*. King's Fund, London

Young EJ, Healing TD (1995) Infection in the deceased: a survey of management. *Communicable Diseases Report* 5 (5): R69–73

Yung YK, Lau BWK, Lai YK (1993) Somatisation in elderly Chinese patients with depression. *Care of the Elderly* Sep: 338–40

Zatouroff M (1996) *Diagnosis in Colour: Physical signs in general medicine*. Times/Mirror International, London

Zborowski M (1952) Cultural components in responses to pain. *Journal of Social Issues* 8: 16–30

PART THREE
Communication

· ·

23 Communication in a multi-ethnic society

'Cross-cultural communication is … far less knowledge than it is a set of skills and an attitude.' (Masi 1992)

In general, the more similar people are in terms of background, culture, experience and outlook the easier it is for them to communicate. They are likely to bring similar expectations, knowledge, perceptions and ways of communicating to the conversation. They are also likely to feel more positive about each other and to assume basic goodwill, overlooking things that could be irritating (Tannen 1992).

Where there are differences in background, culture and experience, smooth communication is more difficult. People may bring different expectations, assumptions and ways of communicating. They may give and expect different cues and have different objectives. They are less likely to persevere or to give each other the benefit of the doubt if things go wrong, and more likely jump to conclusions about each other's abilities, intentions and even personality.

Managing cross-cultural communication well

All the basic principles of good communication apply when working across cultures, but there may be additional considerations.

Possible cultural differences in relation to care

- In some cultures it is important to build a relationship before other matters can be dealt with. Failure to do so may lead to mistrust and non-adherence.

  '[In some cultures] relationship building [is] high on their agenda … In most Western societies, relationship building (except perhaps in the case of courtship) is a long-term objective that regularly loses out to short-term concerns.' (Fisher and Brown 1989)

- In cultures where individualism and autonomy are highly valued, patients are often expected to make their own, largely independent, decisions about medical treatment. In other cultures, decisions about medical treatment may be made by the whole family, or by family members with more authority and experience (eg older people or men). Individuals may be unwilling or unable to make decisions without consultation with their family (see also Chapters 9 *Different families* and 15 *Maintaining patient confidentiality*).
- In some communities, men deal with all public and non-domestic matters. Some men are unused to relating to women in professional roles and expect to discuss important issues with other men. They may be embarrassed and unsure how to relate to women in such situations (see also Chapter 9 *Different families*).
- In many cultures it is unacceptable to discuss intimate matters with a member of the opposite sex (see also Chapters 12 *Modesty* and 13 *History taking*).
- Some people may assume that health professionals deal only with practical matters. They may not feel that it is right to discuss emotional issues with doctors or nurses. In some communities, personal concerns are seen as private and are rarely discussed outside the family.
- Sometimes people have to make difficult choices in a situation in which the professional does not share the cultural or religious constraints or responsibilities that are part of the problem. It is important to respect the person's dilemma and to demonstrate empathy (Masi 1992).
- The way people respond to bad news or difficult situations varies between cultures as well as between individuals. If there is a mismatch between your expectations and those of your patient, you (and they) may feel very uncomfortable (see Chapter 21 *Culture and the expression of grief*).

Patients and relatives who are unfamiliar with the system

- It may be important to explain who you are and what you do, what is happening now and what is likely to happen next. Check if anything is worrying or confusing patients and their families.
- When you ask people what they need, make sure they have enough information to make a decision. Ask specific questions, for example, 'We usually ask people to wear this gown (show it) during this test. Is that all right for you?' rather than 'What are your views about modesty?' If the person does not want to wear the gown, find out why and how their concerns can be accommodated (see also Chapter 8 *Asking effective questions*).

Mutual mistrust

There is extra potential for misunderstanding across cultures. Listen with wide open ears and a wide open mind. Identify and try to put to one side any assumptions you have about the person in front of you. Show that you wish to learn. Notice what you have in common as well as what is different.

Once we have a positive relationship with another person we begin to think about them differently. We have more respect for them and the way they see things, and understand them better. The care we offer becomes more effective as a result.

- People who have experienced rudeness or poor care from others in the past may be suspicious or hostile (see also *Difficult interviews*, below). Try to break the cycle of mistrust by saying that you are aware that they seem angry and asking them to tell you what has caused their anger. Listen to their feelings and accept that these are legitimate. Find out whether you can help. Where appropriate, apologise on behalf of your colleagues or organisation. You cannot communicate effectively if your patient does not trust you, or is distracted by anger or grievance.

  'When I went to the clinic I saw a white doctor who was unbelievably off-hand and rude. He didn't ever really focus on me and my problem, spent the time riffling through his notes and sighing, and at one point implied that I was just a time-wasting hypochondriac. He didn't say "like all you people" but I'm sure that's what he was thinking. At the hospital I saw a different doctor, also white. I told her what had happened last time and that I thought it was racist. She just said, "Well, he was probably very busy you know. We're extremely over-stretched here. I'm sure he's a very nice man. He probably didn't mean anything." I was furious. Why did she automatically take his side like that? She didn't even know him but she automatically took his side.'
  African-Caribbean woman

- For many black and minority ethnic people, questions about family origins or birthplace reinforce the fact that they are often not considered real Britons.

  'When I meet people they often ask me where I come from. So I say "Coventry". And you can see they're not happy with that. "No, but where do you really come from?" they often say. "Coventry", I say. "I was born in Coventry." Sometimes I take pity on them and say, "My parents come from Jamaica", and then they look relieved. But it irritates me being asked where I come from all the time. I'm British, as British as they are, and I wish they'd recognise it.'
  Black British health visitor

Ask only if there is a clear clinical reason, and explain. Try questions such as 'Where does your family originate from?', 'Have you lived in this area all your life?' or 'Tell me about yourself.'

- Asking a patient about their culture can be threatening, especially in the unequal relationship between health professional and patient. Minority cultures are most often discussed in terms of negative stereotypes and problems. Few of us are used to explaining our culture or to seeing our individual behaviour and preferences as cultural. Your patient may feel vulnerable and criticised unless you make it clear that you respect them, their culture and their values (see also Chapter 2).

- Many of the situations in which health professionals meet patients and their families are extremely stressful. In such situations people rarely behave or react as they normally would; family dynamics often change. When working with people of your own culture it is easier to remember this and to suspend judgement. It is harder when working with someone whose culture is unfamiliar to you.

- Good communication across cultural barriers can take time. Time is always a huge problem, but extra time spent on building a good relationship and communicating well can save time, money, frustration and distress, and may even prevent litigation.

> 'One of the major barriers to communication identified by consultants was lack of knowledge of the patient, yet studies have shown that doctors often interrupt patients soon after they get talking.' (Walker 1997)

> 'It is very difficult to open up to doctors and nurses about difficult or important subjects when you do not think they are listening or if they are clearly in a hurry.'
> African-Caribbean patient

Listening with complete respect

The imbalance of power between health professionals and patients can drastically affect communication. Patients are often very much aware of the judgements and assumptions that health professionals are making about them. To try to avoid further disapproval they may conceal important or sensitive items of clinical or personal information. It is then difficult for health professionals to give good practical and emotional care.

To reduce the imbalance in the relationship and to improve care, it is important that health professionals listen to patients with obvious respect. A person who feels respected and listened to is far more likely to communicate well and confidently, and to trust and work with the health professionals caring for them.

Listening with complete respect involves:

- sitting at the same level as the other person;
- looking attentive;
- asking clarifying questions in a style that is not challenging or mocking;
- not joking or trivialising;
- not interrupting or changing the subject;
- not offering platitudes;
- reflecting back a summary of what you have understood, so that the person can either confirm your understanding or help you understand better.

Difficult interviews

Cross-cultural communication can be difficult. It is tiring to listen really well and to keep listening, without resorting to shortcuts and stereotypes. Important questions may draw only a vague and unsatisfying response. They may even offend. It can also be difficult to hide your response to behaviour and ideas that from your cultural perspective are upsetting, unacceptable or simply odd (see also Chapter 8 *Managing negative reactions*).

Some situations are particularly difficult. People who have experienced prejudice and hostility may not wish to expose themselves further and may not be interested in helping you understand them. It is easy in your turn to become uncomfortable, vulnerable and frustrated, and then to turn these feelings against the person or the community they 'represent'. Here is an account by an English health professional of her feelings during a difficult interview with three members of a minority ethnic group. Everyone spoke English as their first language.

'I felt that we were not really making contact, but I did not understand why. So I kept quiet in order not to lose face or look a fool. I just felt I had to plough on and hope for the best, keeping at bay my feelings of discomfort, frustration and being out of my depth.

'When I asked what seemed to me a straightforward question, the reply was often vague and off the point. I am used to getting fairly direct answers to direct questions but with them I didn't. They seemed puzzled by my interest in certain things. In retrospect perhaps I should have found out what they felt about what I was asking, but I didn't.

'Looking back, they were quite different from my stereotype of how they would be. Also their agenda was totally different from mine, though I could not see this at the time. My questions and concerns were a mystery to them. Their ideas about what is important are entirely different. I still don't really know what they were thinking, but I know there are fundamental differences. We were on different planets. The experience was hard because I'm supposed to understand people's needs and wants. It's part of my job and one of the skills I most value.

'Also, they did not seem at all concerned whether I understood or not, they were certainly not falling over themselves to be helpful or to please. I was dismayed to be confronted with my unconscious expectations about how people will respond to me. I had to accept that they were not particularly keen to communicate with me and were certainly not grateful for my efforts.

'It was a challenging, unsettling and exhausting experience. It has taken me two weeks to digest it to a point where I can begin to understand it. I can see why I felt tempted to deal with my discomfort by being brisk and backing off. It would have been easier to dismiss them as unimportant, to think, if they don't want to be clear with me, why should I bother to be clear with them? It would have been easier to give up and to label them as a problem, difficult, uncommunicative, unco-operative, aggressive, all potential steps towards a psychiatric label and excuses for my not listening or persevering.

'In psycho-analytical terms I suppose what tends to happen when cross-cultural encounters between health professionals and patients go badly is that the professionals feel confronted, aggressive or inadequate but cannot tolerate these feelings because 'nice' health professionals shouldn't feel them. So because the health professionals have the power, they project the confrontation and aggression onto the patient. Of course, in reality the patient is not the problem, the communication gap and our inability to bridge it are the problems.'

Beware the slippery slope from cross-cultural misunderstanding to dislike. If we find other people's behaviour unpredictable or odd, especially if we have different backgrounds, we may begin to feel that they are untrustworthy and to question their honesty. Concern about their integrity and character then begins to spread to other areas (Fisher and Brown 1989).

'Several months after I ran a training session on cultural awareness a health professional told me that it had completely changed her attitude to her patients. She explained that now that she understood traditional Asian family structures she realised why some patients had so many visitors on the ward who all said they were close family. "Now I know they are not lying to me about that, I believe other things they tell me. Before, I thought they lied about lots of other things as well."'
English health service lecturer

When things go wrong

Communicating well with people who are ill, anxious and frightened can be extremely difficult. No one gets it right every time. If things go wrong, make it clear that you are not blaming the patient. They are in a far more vulnerable position and it is not in their interests to antagonise you. Try to set aside your own frustration, anger or disappointment for the moment. Acknowledge that the situation is difficult and offer the patient a gentle invitation to say what they are thinking and feeling. Explain, without rancour, how you see the situation. Make it clear that you want to see if you can sort it out between you.

Try also to avoid blaming yourself. Afterwards, find someone who will respect your confidentiality and with whom you can let off steam (see Chapter 8 *Managing negative reactions*). Once you have unloaded your feelings where they can do no harm, take time to reflect on what you did well and on what you would like to do differently next time.

Cultural brokers

If you suspect that you are misunderstanding each other and that this is affecting the care you are able to give, it is often helpful to find a cultural broker. A **cultural broker** is someone who understands both the cultures involved and who can explain to both sides, objectively and clearly, what is preventing full communication and understanding. The best interpreters are also cultural brokers, but to step outside the strictly defined role of interpreter they need support and a degree of autonomy (see also Chapter 27 *What an interpreter does*).

24 Language is more than just words

On the surface, language consists simply of words, linked by grammatical rules to convey meaning. In fact, there are many other devices that also help indicate and support meaning. These include:

- paralinguistic features such as intonation, emphasis, volume and pace;
- non-verbal norms such as physical distance, touch and eye contact;
- cultural features, for example ways of indicating agreement, of being polite.

Although we usually use and interpret these devices unconsciously, they are a crucial part of the message we give (Mares, Henley and Baxter 1985). They are also very important clues for health professionals trying to understand people's physical and emotional needs.

When people learn a second language they usually retain certain paralinguistic, cultural and non-verbal features of their mother tongue. As a result, they may unintentionally offend or give the wrong impression. These misunderstandings can be difficult to sort out because their cause is rarely recognised. We assume that people sound how they mean to sound. Misunderstandings are particularly likely when people are anxious, distressed or under pressure.

Difficulties can also occur when people speak a different variety of English, for example Indian English, Caribbean English or West African English. Each of these has its own particular paralinguistic features – intonation, rhythm, accent and vocabulary – as well as cultural and non-verbal devices. These often differ from those of British English so, even though people who speak different varieties of English use the same words, they may misunderstand each other's intentions or attitudes. British-English speakers also sometimes assume that other forms of English are inferior and that people who speak them are stupid or under-educated. In fact, each is a complete and fully developed language in its own right (d'Ardenne and Mahtani 1989).

'I was simple enough to think that the British people were all the same, all speaking the same sort of language, the language which I learnt at English school in India. I was surprised I couldn't understand the English nurse and was even more surprised because she did not understand English – my English!' Indian man (Ahmed and Watt 1986)

Paralinguistic features

To see how paralinguistic features work, try saying this sentence, 'She says she's been in agony for three hours' in four different ways:

- as a straight statement;
- as a question;
- indicating that you don't believe her;
- indicating that you are shocked that this has been allowed to happen.

Notice how your intonation, emphasis and volume differed each time, so that although you used exactly the same words and grammar, you conveyed very different meanings. In British English, certain paralinguistic features convey the speaker's intentions and feelings, including politeness, apology, anger, sorrow, anxiety, uncertainty, interest or lack of it, disagreement, criticism or urgency. People who do not understand the paralinguistic features of British English may not perceive these messages and may seem insensitive, rude or stupid. Their own use of paralinguistic features may clash with British expectations, and they may be wrongly perceived as angry, resentful, uncertain, excited or uninterested.

Emphasis and pace British English uses emphasis to signal important or new information, or to contradict: for example, 'I told her to take it **three** times a day', 'Mrs Smith **is** coming on Monday'. Emphasis also indicates emotions such as anger or excitement. In other languages, importance may be indicated by speaking faster or more slowly, by adding words or phrases, by repetition or by lowering the voice (Mares, Henley and Baxter 1985). Again, there is a good deal of room for mutual misunderstanding.

Linguistic tunes Each language has its own intonation or tune. In British English it is normal for the voice to rise and fall in friendly conversation. Changing the tune can also modify the meaning of a phrase or sentence. A raised tone at the end of a statement can turn it into a question: 'You've done your urine sample?' And raising the tone of the **whole** sentence is often associated with intense emotion such as anger, shock or excitement: 'You've won the Nobel prize!' or 'You've flooded the whole ground floor!' In other languages a raised tone over the whole sentence may indicate importance or friendliness rather than intense emotion.

British English and other northern European languages use a relatively limited range of tunes in normal speech: speakers of other languages and other forms of English may use a far greater range. To British-English speakers, they may sound excitable and excessively emotional, even unreliable. To other people, British-English speakers may sound uninterested, insincere, bored or condescending.

In tonal languages such as Chinese, Vietnamese and Thai, the tune or tone is part of each word. Changing the tone of a word completely changes its meaning. So, for example, the sound 'ma' in Vietnamese may mean 'ghost', 'horse', 'appearance', 'cheek, 'rice seedling', 'but', 'which' or 'tomb', depending on whether it is said with a high rising, low falling, low rising, low broken, high broken or mid-level tone (Mares 1982). People speaking a tonal language have to get the tone of each word absolutely right in order for a word to mean what they want it to mean. The flexible rising and falling tones that British-English speakers use in a sentence to indicate friendliness are not possible. Friendliness is indicated in other ways. But to British-English ears, the tunes of tonal languages may sometimes sound brusque, imperious or angry.

Volume Normal volume varies a good deal in different cultures. British-English speakers speak very quietly in relation to most of the rest of the world. They often feel disconcerted or upset by people who seem to be shouting. They may feel that the other person (who is speaking perfectly normally in their own terms) is angry, over-emotional, threatening, irrational or simply bad-mannered. In tonal languages (see above), raising the volume is one way in which people indicate the importance of what they are saying.

Structuring conversation In most European languages it is customary to state the main point in an argument first, and then to illustrate or expand upon it. In many other languages it is common to set out the preliminary arguments and illustrations first, working up to the main point as a conclusion. British-English speakers, used to hearing the main point early on, may become bored and impatient when listening to a patient or colleague who uses the other system. They may conclude that he or she has nothing important to say or is stupid and switch off before the key point is reached (Roberts 1985).

Turn-taking and listening signals Conversation requires people to take turns. Different languages use different conventions to indicate when one person has finished and another can begin. For example, person A may lower their voice and slow down to indicate that it is person B's turn; they may begin to repeat themselves; or they may pause for person B to begin. Latin Americans generally take and expect very short pauses; North-American-English speakers take slightly longer pauses; British-English speakers take still longer ones. Problems arise when people use different turn-taking signals. Person B may feel that they are never given a chance to talk; person A may wonder why person B isn't saying anything. They may then label each other pushy, shy, unco-operative or unfriendly (Tannen 1992).

In British English it is considered normal and polite for only one person to speak at a time and for people to pause to allow each other to speak. In some cultures talking at the same time as another person and talking over them ('high-involvement style') is regarded as friendly and polite, and proof that you are really listening; in Northern Europe it is generally regarded as aggressive and pushy (Tannen 1991).

In British English it is also important to indicate that you are listening by nodding occasionally and making encouraging noises. It is also important to make intermittent eye contact. In some languages people show that they are listening by keeping still and remaining completely silent. They may also look away. English speakers used to eye contact and other signals during conversation may feel that they are not being listened to if these are absent (Lago and Thompson 1996).

Silence Silence is tolerated more in some cultures than in others. It also means different things. In some cultures younger and more junior people use silence to indicate respect and affection. In some it is normal for people to sit in silence for long periods before they say anything, or to take long pauses while they are speaking; this indicates that matters are being taken seriously. In English culture silence is generally most acceptable between people who are close; in other circumstances it can feel awkward or rude and people may feel impelled to speak (Lomax 1997).

Misunderstandings and blame

The key point about paralinguistic features is that most of us wrongly assume:

- that the cues and features we are used to and their meanings are universal; and
- that they reliably tell us something about a person's behaviour or their personality.

If a person raises their voice and talks faster, for example, we may conclude that they are angry or hostile. If their voice goes up and down a lot we may conclude that they are excited or over-reacting, or we may simply be puzzled. If they are silent we may think they are disapproving, unco-operative, insolent or withdrawn. But such judgements are unreliable when people speak different first languages or different forms of English (Tannen 1992). The paralinguistic features of a different language are the most difficult thing to learn. Native speakers are generally unaware of them and rarely explain them to people who get them wrong, partly because it is often unclear whether a person is using them intentionally.

'I have been working in Britain for years and my English is pretty good. But I know that in difficult situations, where I have to be sensitive to people's feelings or have to convey something carefully so as not to give offence, I often get it wrong. I can't always pick up the implications behind what they say and I am not sure that I come across as I want to. It's a horrible feeling; you know people have misunderstood you but you don't know how to put it right. In my own language I'm much more confident even after all these years!'
German doctor

Non-verbal signals

Non-verbal signals can also cause problems across cultures, leading people to misinterpret each other's feelings and intentions.

'I shall never forget a misunderstanding when I was a student nurse. Three of us were laughing and joking in the treatment room while sister was doing a ward round with the doctors. She suddenly appeared and told us off for making a noise. I felt really terrible because in my culture we are brought up to respect and obey our elders. My absolute horror must have shown on my face; and she thought I was being insolent and exaggerating, just pretending to be horrified. She berated me for being sarcastic and told me I would certainly never get a job at that hospital. She completely misinterpreted my reaction; there was nothing I could ever do to change her view.'
British-Nigerian nurse

Gestures Some cultures use a lot of gestures and movements when talking; others do not. The significance of different gestures varies. 'Yes' may be indicated by moving the head up and down, by moving it from side to side, or by dipping it sharply downwards (Collett 1993). Gestures such as shrugging the shoulders, making a fist, making a thumbs up sign or clicking the tongue are perfectly acceptable in some cultures but offensive in others. In certain cultures, including those influenced by Islam, it is rude to offer something with the left hand. The left hand is reserved for necessary but dirty chores (see also Chapter 12 *Practical care*).

'I realise that the left hand has no significance for English people, but when someone hands me something with their left hand I can hardly bear to take it. It goes right back to my childhood when if I gave or took something with my left hand I got a real scolding from my mother or one of my aunts for being so rude.'
Somali woman

Facial expressions Health professionals often use patients' facial expressions to help them assess physical and emotional well-being, the need for pain control and so on. Across cultures this can be far more difficult. For example, whereas in English culture a smile may indicate happiness, or an attempt to please, in Japanese culture it may mask embarrassment, anger or grief. In Japan happiness is more commonly indicated with a straight face (Stewart and Bennett 1991).

Eye contact In some cultures, looking people in the eye is assumed to indicate honesty and straightforwardness; in others it is seen as challenging and rude. Most people in Arab cultures share a great deal of eye contact and may regard too little as disrespectful (Argyle 1975). In English culture, a certain amount of eye contact is required, but too much makes many people uncomfortable. Most English people make eye contact at the beginning and then let their gaze drift to the side periodically to avoid 'staring the other person out'. In South Asian and many other cultures direct eye contact is generally regarded as aggressive and rude. This can cause problems, for example, for some overseas-trained South Asian doctors taking oral examinations in Britain. Lowering their eyes as a sign of respect may be wrongly interpreted as a sign that they do not know the answer or are guessing (Sami 1989).

'I trained in Switzerland and I was astonished when a Swiss doctor told me that I would be considered to be telling a lie if I did not look straight into a person's eyes.'
Pakistani doctor

In some cultures and religious groups eye contact between men and women is seen as flirtatious or threatening. Men of these communities who do not make eye contact with women are not usually rude or evasive, but respectful.

Different cultures also vary in the amount that it is acceptable to watch other people. Collett (1993) calls these high-look and low-look cultures. British culture is a low-look culture. Watching other people, especially strangers, is regarded as intrusive. People who are caught 'staring' usually look away quickly and are often embarrassed. Those being watched may feel threatened and insulted. In high-look cultures, for example in southern Europe, looking or gazing at other people is perfectly acceptable; being watched is not a problem. When people's expectations and interpretations clash, irritation and misunderstandings can arise.

Posture Posture that is perfectly normal and neutral in one culture may seem aggressive or withdrawn in another. Most cultures also have gender rules for posture. It may be completely acceptable, for example, for men to sit with their legs apart but not for women. Standing or sitting with folded arms is seen as relaxed and friendly in many cultures but is often interpreted as hostile or defensive in the West.

> 'In Thai culture it is deeply offensive to point the soles of one's feet at people, for example when sitting. Younger people or people of lower status should also try to keep their heads below those of people of higher status, if necessary by bending the knees. It is extremely rude to pass between two adults who are talking without bending down so that one's head is below theirs. In British culture none of this is an issue and most British people in Thailand cause terrible offence without ever intending to or realising it.'
> English teacher

Physical distance In English culture, partners, and parents and children are generally comfortable standing fairly close to each other; friends stand further apart, and acquaintances still further. Northern Europeans tend to stand further apart than people from the Middle East, Greece or Turkey (Morain 1986). Most people try to maintain the distance they find comfortable; if their cultural conventions differ, one speaker may constantly move backwards to try to gain space, while the other 'pursues' them to get closer.

Touch Cultures vary in the extent to which physical contact is allowed and between whom. In low-contact cultures, including British and other northern European cultures as well as Japanese culture, touch occurs only under restricted conditions, such as within the family and in close relationships, sometimes in greetings, and in certain specified settings such as health care. Touch in other situations can cause great anxiety and tension. It is seen as imposing upon a person's privacy (Kagawa-Singer 1987). In contrast, in high-touch cultures, physical contact is seen as friendly and positive. People may touch frequently while they talk. When people from cultures with different touch levels interact, the low-contact person may be seen as aloof, cold and unfriendly, whereas the high-contact one may be seen as intrusive and even perverted (Furnham and Bochner 1990).

Gender also affects the rules of touch. In some cultures it is acceptable for members of the same sex to touch each other in public; in others it is acceptable for members of the opposite sex. The amount of touch expected also varies. In a study of the number of times heterosexual couples touched each other in cafés, it was found that in Puerto Rico they touched 180 times per hour, in Paris 110 times, and in London, about 200 miles away, not at all (Argyle 1975).

> 'You don't always get it right and you have to try to pick up people's reactions. Some of my patients love it when I sit on their bed and have a chat, even put an arm round them. Others just shrink inside or even get angry; they're much more comfortable if I sit in a chair and keep my distance.'
> English staff nurse

Misunderstandings and blame

We rarely notice other people's non-verbal behaviour except when it feels wrong or makes us uncomfortable. However, non-verbal behaviour is learnt in childhood, used unconsciously and hard to change. The rules are rarely made explicit and never taught to newcomers. Because people who use inappropriate non-verbal behaviour are generally assumed to be rude and unpleasant, their non-verbal behaviour is not discussed with them.

Politeness

Cultural rules of polite behaviour enable people to get on together. Some cultures value formal politeness more highly than others. Again, failure to follow the local rules of polite behaviour is almost always assumed to be intentional rudeness.

Please and thank you In British English the words 'please' and 'thank you' are extremely important. Although the amount they are used differs between men and women and in different situations, people who do not say please and thank you are regarded as arrogant and intentionally ill-mannered. Please and thank you are particularly important between people of different status and in formal situations.

In many other languages, including most Asian and African languages, politeness is managed differently. For example, instead of the formulaic please and thank you, politeness may be indicated by a different choice of verb form or pronoun (like *tu* or *vous* in French), or by a different tone of voice. In some cultures please and thank you are not used to people who are doing their job; omitting them is not regarded by either side as at all impolite (Bowler 1993).

> 'In Somali there is no equivalent for please; people usually use relational terms such as brother, sister, uncle etc at the beginning or end of requests. There is an equivalent for thank you but not for the response, the equivalent of "You're welcome".' (Kahin 1997)

Alternatively, gratitude may be indicated non-verbally, by a gesture or a change in facial expression. In some cultures it is common to show gratitude by giving presents or money. People who are used to one particular convention often feel extreme offence or anger when faced by different behaviour. They may find it hard to accept that the other person did not mean to be rude.

> 'While working in a foreign country an Englishman noted that the words please and thank you were seldom used to accompany requests or instructions. Curious about this and not believing that the whole country was rude, he asked someone of the host culture about this.
>
> '"The trouble is, Colin," he was told, "you use please and thank you far too often. How can people believe that you are sincere when you use the words so often that they lose their meaning? If a person of my country says thank you, they really mean it."
>
> "So do I," protested the Englishman.
>
> "Then use them less," said the other man.'
> *Unknown source*

Greetings In many cultures it is extremely important to greet a person every time one meets them, and especially the first time each day. Some cultures also use gestures, for example shaking hands, smiling, bowing or joining the palms of the hands. In English culture greetings are often omitted, especially in work situations. This can seem rude to people used to a more formal system.

> 'In Switzerland everyone shakes hands when they meet and when they part, certainly the first time each day. You always shake hands with the doctor, the nurse, the dentist and so on. Colleagues shake hands when they arrive and when they leave work. Children shake hands with their teachers at the beginning and end of the school day. They also shake hands with each other from the age of about ten. When you shake hands with someone it is very important to look them in the eye. Many Swiss people find the English rude and off-hand even though they don't intend to be.'
> English woman

Saying no In some cultures saying no directly, particularly to a person of higher status or to a guest, is offensive and unpleasant. There are other indirect but polite ways that are normally understood by both sides and which a person can use to refuse a request or answer a question negatively. These include not responding to the request, changing the subject, asking for time to think, making a non-committal reply, or using a special polite phrase that means no but does not explicitly say it. Unfortunately, it can be difficult to translate these phrases into English, and when people try they are often misunderstood.

> 'It is particularly impolite to answer "no" to someone older or of higher status than oneself. In the Vietnamese language there is an expression which avoids this – da khong (South), or thua khong (North). It translates literally as "yes, no" but it is used in the sense of "I'm afraid not" or "I'm sorry to say no".' (Mares 1982)

In some cultures, people who avoid saying no directly are regarded as hypocritical or lying. Directness is valued and is thought to indicate moral integrity. English culture lies somewhere in the middle; there are variations on the basis of class and gender. In general, however, English culture is relatively indirect, expecting people to understand unstated messages, especially when there is any awkwardness. Most English speakers tend to avoid conflict and often try to defuse situations by avoiding or changing a difficult subject, giving a non-committal reply, making a joke or apologising. This can be confusing and even seem deceitful to people of other, more direct, cultures.

Anger English people traditionally avoid showing anger, reserving overt anger for very serious or intolerable situations, often as a last resort. Although it is thought to be sometimes necessary, it often leaves deep scars. In Chinese and Japanese cultures, the expression of anger is traditionally regarded as completely unacceptable and destructive. The idea that it is important to express anger, and that unexpressed emotions are harmful, may be seen as ridiculous or even dangerous (Kagawa-Singer 1987). In some other cultures anger is more lightly expressed, received and forgotten. Fierce argument and confrontation may be seen as a positive sign of friendliness and engagement. Here again there is a good deal of opportunity for misunderstanding and mutual resentment.

> 'I find the English deceitful. If you say that you are angry about something they all agree, but when you want to go and confront the person responsible they melt away.'
> Belgian woman

Embarrassing words Every language has a range of polite and impolite words for most different bodily functions and parts of the body. In British English, words of Latin origin are generally more acceptable in polite conversation than words of Anglo-Saxon origin. There are also a large number of euphemisms and words regarded as bad or derogatory, which may vary in different parts of the country. Certain words, such as stool, urine and intercourse are used mainly in medical contexts. All this poses major problems for people whose first language is not English. It can be extremely embarrassing and difficult to find out the acceptable words for these things in a new language. People may also unintentionally cause offence by using an offensive lay or slang word in a medical context.

'When my son started school he came back with all these new English words. Then the old lady next door came and told us she had heard him using some words that were extremely rude. Did we know? We didn't even know what the words meant, and nor did he. All his friends used them. But they knew where not to use them, and he didn't!'
Croatian woman

Suspending your automatic responses

'Try to remember that they may not mean what you heard them say.' (Tannen 1991)

Misunderstandings about other people's personality or intentions are inevitable when we have different linguistic and cultural conventions. Our reactions to the way people speak and behave are largely automatic and often very strong. There are no easy solutions. It is, however, always important:

- to be aware of the reasons why things may go wrong;
- to monitor and try to suspend your automatic responses; and
- to assume, at least until other clear evidence emerges, that the other person does not wish to irritate or offend you.

If you know each other well, it may be possible to discuss your reactions tactfully, find out whether the other person realises how they appear, and possibly and with great respect suggest modifications in their approach. Try to find out about other cultures' conventions of non-verbal behaviour and politeness. There may be things that you automatically do that cause offence to others; try to find out if you are being misunderstood and whether it would be helpful to adapt some aspects of your approach.

25 The consequences of the language barrier

Patients and relatives

The NHS Patient's Charter stresses patients' right to the health care they need and to information about facilities, proposed treatments and alternatives, and possible risks (DoH 1996). But if patients and relatives cannot discuss symptoms, problems and prognoses, ask questions, understand replies, outline choices or raise anxieties, health care is often unavailable or is reduced to the most basic physical minimum.

Reduced information, consultation and support

Patients who speak little or no English are generally given less information and offered fewer choices (Bowler 1993, Currer 1986, Homans and Satow 1982). They are often unable to understand what is done to them and why. They cannot ask questions, voice worries, discuss important issues, ask for what they need or receive support. They cannot give genuinely informed consent (Windsor-Richards and Gillies 1988). When patients and relatives cannot communicate with the health professionals caring for them, their fear and sense of helplessness are likely to increase.

> 'I never realised that my husband would die. I thought he would get better. Maybe the doctor told me many, many times, but I did not understand, I didn't know the words and I never saw anybody so ill before.'
> Tamil woman

The medical treatment given to people who speak little or no English may also be affected by lack of communication. Watson (1986) quotes a doctor who said she had prescribed a contraceptive method to a non-English-speaking woman, 'not because she judged it to be the most efficacious or the most suitable medication for the patient, but because the others were too complex to describe'.

In some cases non-English-speaking people may become the targets of anger and resentment from professional staff.

> 'I don't think the staff respect our people. Once there was a lady next to me who didn't speak English. The nurse was making fun of [her] and laughed at her for not being able to explain something.'
> Bengali woman (Slater 1993)

> 'Please understand us better and don't shout at us so much. Some staff are really rude to us.'
> Somali woman

Clinical dangers

Health professionals base their decisions about care and treatment on the patient's account of their illness and medical history as well as on clinical signs. If the patient speaks little or no English the required information may be either unavailable or inaccurate. This is bound to affect clinical care (Parsons and Day 1992). It must also mean that professionals sometimes fail to identify problems or symptoms and that the necessary action is not taken or is taken too late. Expensive but unnecessary tests and even inappropriate treatments may be carried out because patient and professional cannot understand each other. Patient adherence is bound to be affected.

> 'I saw a woman the other day who had been all round the hospital departments. She had severe headaches and she'd had every test under the sun. Finally the doctors decided it must be psychosomatic so they sent her to me. I was the first doctor who'd been able to speak to her directly, without her husband being present to interpret. It turned out that the headaches were caused by her husband hitting her. She hadn't been able to tell anyone before.'
> Italian psychiatrist (Shackman 1984)

Unless special efforts are made, general attempts to improve communication between professionals and patients, such as better complaints and suggestions systems, do not benefit people who speak little or no English (Audit Commission 1993). Their needs are not fed back into the system and so may be ignored by planners and managers.

Health professionals

Although they are not in the same dependent and vulnerable situation as their patients, language barriers are also extremely frustrating and difficult for health professionals. Most professionals feel that they cannot give the care they want to give or use their skills properly. They are forced to compromise and lower their standards, treating patients without explanation or discussion. Many miss the rewards of a good relationship with patients and relatives, and know that they are unable to give the same level of care, support and comfort. Many feel guilty, furious, ineffective and stressed (Bowler 1993, Murphy and Macleod Clark 1993).

'I know I couldn't give him the emotional care I wanted to and he needed. There were so many times when he was crying and you could see he was frightened and I just couldn't help. It was like there was this wall between us. I felt so bad and there was nothing really I could do except the physical care. I got so frustrated and sometimes angry, angry with him and with myself and with the whole situation.'
Scottish nurse

Working across a language barrier also takes a good deal more time. For professionals who are already very hard-pressed this may feel like the last straw. Some turn their frustration against their patients. Occasionally anger, frustration and pressure can lead to panic and to extraordinary and unprofessional behaviour.

'If women can't speak English they cannot communicate their fear and must be left with some degree of emotional trauma. I've seen [staff] being rough and brutal and shouting at women who are terrified of being examined, often because they don't understand what is going on.'
English health professional

Managing our own reactions

Take a moment to ask yourself the following questions:

* When a patient who does not speak much English arrives at a clinic or surgery, how do you feel?
* How do you react?

Most professionals feel dismayed, irritated, angry or inadequate, or all of these. They know that to do this patient justice they will have to give them more time, and time is always short. Some feel angry that the patient has not learnt English, especially if they have been in Britain for some years (see below). If there is no interpreter, useful discussion will be almost impossible. Professionals simply have to 'get by' and do the best they can, knowing that it is not enough.

However much we try to hide our internal reactions, they always influence how we approach and care for patients. Non-verbal signals are hard to conceal, and people who do not understand what is being said are often particularly sensitive to them. Patients easily sense discomfort, anger or resentment on the part of professionals. These add to their own feelings of inadequacy, vulnerability and frustration.

> 'I speak five languages. In my own language I can say what I want in the way that I want it. I am also a poet. I have eight grandchildren and I have cared for and supported my family all my life. I am a good cook. I grow beautiful roses in my garden. But in this clinic, because I do not speak good English, I am nothing. They do not see me – just a stupid old Indian man who "cannot speak".'
> Elderly Gujarati man

A patient in such a situation may assume that you do not like them or that the diagnosis is worse than they feared. They may simply decide that you are a racist. In some circumstances they may also decide not to accept any advice or treatment, or not to come back again until their condition has become much worse, by which time it may be harder or impossible to treat.

Many health professionals, especially those who themselves speak more than one language, understand the problems facing adult immigrants who speak little or no English. However, some see learning English as a simple moral duty, and regard a patient's failure to do so as evidence of idleness and stupidity. They may see the provision of interpreters as an unfair and unnecessary cost. Some vent their frustration on non-English-speaking patients. A few cases have been reported of professionals refusing to treat patients until they learn English (Watson 1986).

There is no doubt that caring for people across a language barrier is frustrating, very difficult and time consuming. It is also clear that non-English-speaking patients would get better care if they spoke English and so it is in their own interests to learn the English they need for encounters with the health service. However, most patients are only too aware of this. They understand very well the problems caused by their lack of English. They would speak it if they could. Adding to the pressure they already feel in this situation by showing your frustration and anger only makes matters worse.

Who speaks English?

A survey in 1994 looked at the level of English among adults in the main black and minority ethnic groups in the UK whose community first language is not English: Indian, Pakistani, Bangladeshi, East African Asian and

Chinese. Each respondent's level of English was assessed by a bilingual interviewer (Modood, Berthoud et al 1997). **Everyone born in Britain spoke fluent English.**

Among people who had migrated to Britain, ability in English was linked mainly to age on arrival in the UK and to gender. People who arrived in Britain aged over 25 were least likely to speak English well:

- Among 16- to 24-year-olds, almost everyone (over 96 per cent) spoke English well. Slightly fewer Pakistani and Bangladeshi women in this age group (about 80 per cent) spoke English well.
- Among 25- to 44-year-olds, most people (over 70 per cent) spoke English well. Again, Pakistani and Bangladeshi women were the exception. Only about half of all Pakistani women and about a quarter of all Bangladeshi women spoke English well.
- Among 45- to 65-year-olds, over 50 per cent of men in all the groups spoke English well. Half or more of the Chinese, Indian and East African Asian women interviewed spoke English well. Only 28 per cent of Pakistani women and 4 per cent of Bangladeshi women in this age group spoke English well (Modood, Berthoud et al 1997).
- Among people over 65 in these communities, levels of English are generally lower than among younger immigrants (HEA 1994, South Glamorgan Race Equality Council 1994, Tang 1994).

Among immigrants in other communities whose first language is not English, levels of English depend similarly on age, length of time and age of arrival in Britain, and level of education before migration, as well as on their circumstances and opportunities in Britain.

Why do some people not speak English?

Learning a language as an adult

Many adult immigrants who arrive in Britain speaking little or no English find it very difficult to learn more. Precisely because their English is poor, they are unlikely to develop the kinds of relationships with English speakers that will help them learn (Li 1992, Currer 1986). Most people's domestic and work responsibilities leave them little or no time. Women with small children and a home to look after, for example, are very unlikely to have any chance to learn English informally, to practise it or to get out to English classes. In any case, they often see learning English as selfish and not as a priority in terms of their duties: the day-to-day needs of their family and their home come first. Men and women in paid employment tend to get jobs that require little English and may have no opportunity to learn more. They often work unsocial hours and shifts.

> 'In fact, most [Pathan] women did express a desire to learn English and most saw that it would be an advantage to them. Their husbands were even more keen that they should do so, as they bore many of the burdens of their wives' lack of ability to communicate when necessary. But the incentives were not sufficient to overcome the difficulties of an overbusy daily routine of housework and childcare' (Currer 1986).

Language is a tool. Research into adult learning shows that most adults learn only what they need urgently to fulfil their short-term responsibilities (Rogers 1989). Simply living in a country where a different language is spoken does not mean that one learns the language. The key issue is whether one needs to use the language frequently.

> 'My husband goes out to work so he speaks English much better than me. I speak very little English and I am very shy about it. So when I have to go anywhere I always try to take him with me and he can do all the talking. I would feel a fool speaking my bad English when he can say all the things much more clearly for me. Especially when it's really important and the people are so busy and in such a hurry always.'
> Punjabi woman (Mares, Henley and Baxter 1985)

In the day-to-day lives of many non-English speakers in Britain there is very little need for English. Most have also developed strategies for managing without. If they live in an area with other members of their own community they can generally get help when necessary from people who speak English better than they do. They can shop in supermarkets where English is hardly needed, or in shops run by people who speak their language.

> 'Although some were more sympathetic, in one case [an official] stated that, considering the length of time East European migrants had been living in the UK, they ought by now to be able to speak English and communicate with other English speakers. If they did not … they had no one but themselves to blame. Seen through the eyes of a local official whose experience had not been one of exclusion, this statement may have some logic. But seen in the context of the history of the East European refugee – stateless, living at the economic, social and political margins of British society – the inability to speak the language of the "host" community looks rather different.' (Bowling 1990)

Language is also situational. A new situation or a new topic demands new vocabulary. People who speak quite enough English to cope with the normal demands of living may become completely lost when they need to discuss a medical problem or a family crisis.

Motivation and confidence

A major factor in learning is motivation, in this case the wish to learn English in order to speak it to people. The experience of hostility, racism or impatience from English speakers can destroy people's confidence and their wish to speak English. People with little formal education may also lack the confidence to attend language classes and may find it difficult to learn in an academic environment (Mares, Henley and Baxter 1985).

'Language learning in Vietnam is still seen as an academically oriented pursuit, and something to be done at school, while young. Many adult refugees feel that they have a mental block on learning English, believing they are too old to learn. Even those who are in their early twenties say this is their reason for giving up. Inadequate, or inappropriate, English language class provision further hinders those who try to overcome these difficulties.' (Tang 1994)

Table 25.1 Factors that help or hinder people learning English

Factors that help	Factors that hinder
Completed secondary or higher education, confident learner	Little formal education, little confidence in ability to learn
Relatively new in the country	In the country for several years
Younger	Older
Arrived in Britain under age 25	Arrived in Britain over age 25
Responsibilities that require contact with English speakers	Heavy domestic or work responsibilities, little opportunity to talk to English speakers
Self-confidence	Low self-confidence and shyness
Important role and responsibilities outside the home	Largely domestic role and responsibilities
Accessible, suitable classes	Inaccessible classes, unsuitable approach, irrelevant vocabulary
Urgent, frequent need for English	English rarely needed except in occasional, stressful situations
Lots of opportunities for practice	Few opportunities for practice
Nobody available to interpret or speak English	Family member who speaks better English
Frequent positive contact with English speakers	Little contact with English speakers, fear of hostility and racism

Paradoxically, the longer that people have been used to operating and fulfilling their daily responsibilities without English, the more going to classes seems irrelevant and even pointless. People may then only really need English in exceptional and particularly difficult circumstances for which it is unlikely that any classes can equip them. This is when health professionals usually encounter them. In such situations both professionals and patients should have access to trained interpreters who can help them overcome the language barrier (see also Chapter 27).

26 Communicating across a language barrier

Stress, language and behaviour

Stress and language

Illness, confusion, pain, stress and anxiety can all temporarily or permanently prevent people speaking or understanding English.

> 'My father spoke four languages fluently all his life. But when he was really ill he could only speak Polish, his mother tongue. His sister, who also speaks Polish, was the only person who could communicate with him.'
> British man

Even people whose English is normally excellent may find themselves lost for words, unable to ask simple questions or to express themselves at all.

> 'My English is excellent and people say I don't even have an accent, but when my son was seriously ill and had to be taken to hospital my English suddenly disappeared. I could hear what they were saying but my brain didn't seem to work any more. My thoughts were racing in Italian but I couldn't say what I wanted in English. It was like a nightmare.'
> Italian nurse

Judgements across the language barrier

Trying to communicate across a language barrier, especially with people in authority or in frightening situations, also affects the way many people behave. Beware of the judgements you make about people who are on the other side of the language barrier.

> Think back to a time when you were having difficulty under-standing and being understood by someone in authority, possibly in a language you did not speak well.
>
> - How did you feel? Physically? Emotionally?
> - How did you cope?
> - How did you react to that person at the time? If you met them again later?

In situations like this people commonly find that they:

- feel nervous and less able to think clearly, get upset easily, get frustrated, tense and angry;
- become very sensitive to people's non-verbal signals: body language, tone of voice, gestures;
- smile a lot and try to show that although they cannot communicate they want to be helpful;
- quickly become exhausted and understand less and less;
- remain passive and silent, avoid eye contact and avoid initiating or pro-longing conversations;
- give simple, though inaccurate, answers or explanations because they cannot explain things as they want to;
- try to give the impression of understanding more than they do in order not to irritate the other person;
- avoid situations and discussions they feel they can't cope with. With health professionals they may, for example, describe specific physical symptoms rather than attempting to explain intangible chronic com-plaints or complex emotional problems.

Conversations across a language barrier are wearing for both sides. You may have noticed how hard you have to concentrate to try to understand someone whose English is not very good, how tiring it is, and how tempt-ing it is to give up. You may also have found that you feel like reducing the amount you communicate and settling for the minimum.

Ways of reducing stress

Reducing stress can dramatically improve people's ability in English. Try to find ways of reducing unnecessary stress. You will still need a professional interpreter for all important conversations (see Chapter 27). To reduce stress:

- Make sure you have the person's name right and are using and pro-nouncing it correctly (see also Chapter 30).

- Allow more time. Try not to show that your time is short. Signs of pressure or impatience increase stress and may further reduce the amount you can achieve.
- Kindness, a sympathetic manner and a reassuring tone of voice help even if people do not understand what you say. Most non-English-speaking patients and relatives are only too aware that many professionals are irritated and frustrated by them.

> 'The women did not even look for success in communication. They did, however, notice whether or not people tried and whether or not they seemed to care.' (Currer 1986)

Try to convey support through non-verbal signals such as touch, a smile and eye contact, bearing in mind cultural conventions (see Chapter 24).

> 'Sometimes when she was feeling sick I would sit down with her and wait till she stopped being sick. By the end of the week she just wanted me to stay there. She would grab hold of my arm and she used to stroke my face. She'd talk in her language and I couldn't understand but she was smiling. Even though you couldn't communicate, there was just something there.' (Murphy and Macleod Clark 1993)

- Watch for signs of weariness in the other person and do not carry on too long. The level of concentration required is tiring for both of you.
- When carrying out any procedure always say what you are doing or going to do next. Never maintain total silence or give the impression that you are ignoring the person. A reassuring tone of voice is much better than silence.
- Do not discuss the patient or say things you don't want them to hear in their presence. Everyone understands more of a foreign language than they speak.

> 'The two doctors discussed my results beside my bed. I could understand some things but not the detail. I think one doctor said things were very serious and they should operate the next day, the other said they should do more tests and wait. I was too upset and frightened to tell them I could follow what they were saying.'
> Chinese man

- Try to ensure continuity of care. The difficulties of establishing relationships are even greater across a language barrier. For patients and relatives, getting to know individual health professionals helps reduce stress and makes communication easier. Keep good notes so that different professionals don't have to keep asking the same questions.

- Try to learn a few words of the other person's language. 'Good morning', 'good-bye', 'yes', 'no' and other helpful words can make a great difference to your relationship. Trying to speak their language also puts you on the same footing and enables you to understand some of their feelings of embarrassment and the difficulty of remembering even simple words and phrases in a foreign language.

> 'One patient who neither spoke nor understood English attended an appointment for an endoscopy. She was met by a nurse who was able to say, "Hello, how are you?", "Are you OK?" and other odd phrases in Gujarati. [Her son] said that although his mother knew she could not have a conversation with the nurse, she felt much more relaxed and at ease throughout.' (Haroon-Iqbal 1994)

- Non-English-speaking patients often find that health professionals spend less time with them because they cannot communicate easily with them. Although this is understandable it is also hurtful. On a ward or in residential care, try to spend time with non-English-speaking patients as well as with those who speak English. If there are two patients who speak the same language ask whether they would like to be in neighbouring beds. Loneliness is often a major problem.

> 'Some days nobody speaks to me for hours. I cannot understand English but I am still a person. I feel better when somebody greets me, even a wave or a smile or "Good morning". You would be surprised what a difference it makes.'
> Greek patient

Simplifying your English

There may be ways in which you can adapt your language to make it easier to understand. The guidelines below offer some ideas. It is important to use them sensitively. Never assume on the basis of a person's name or appearance that they do not speak English.

Speak plain English

- Speak slowly and clearly. Try not to speed up. This is the single most helpful thing you can do.
- Try not to speak louder than normal.
- Avoid hospital and clinical jargon and euphemisms. Expertise generates its own jargon and nowhere more than in medicine (Buchanan 1995).

Use plain, everyday words as far as possible. Be aware that the special clinical meaning of certain words, for example, 'positive' and 'negative' when talking about test results can be very confusing.

'Terms such as "waterworks", "down there", "the other end", "tummy" and "dizzy" are difficult even for those Asian women who are competent in English'. (Bowler 1993)

- Listen for the words the person uses and understands and try to use the same words.
- Do not use 'pidgin' English; it is not easier to understand and sounds patronising. Instead, make sure the most important words in each sentence are clear.
- Be succinct and clear but do not condense what you want to say. This simply makes it denser and more difficult to understand.
- Wherever possible, demonstrate things or point them out on a picture rather than simply relying on the spoken word. It is generally more acceptable and respectful to use pictures of clothed rather than naked human figures (see also Chapter 14 *Pain-measurement tools*).
- Everybody understands more of a foreign language than they can speak. People may therefore understand what you are saying but may be unable to answer your questions properly or discuss things in the necessary detail.

Always check that the other person understands

Encourage people to stop you if they don't understand what you are saying. Make it clear that you really want to know and that you will not become impatient.

When you are checking if the other person has understood, try to avoid questions that can be answered with 'yes'. 'Yes' is probably the first word that anyone learns in a new language, but it does not necessarily mean one has understood or is agreeing. It often means something like:

- 'Yes, I'm listening and I'm trying to understand.'
- 'Yes, I want to be helpful even though I don't understand.'
- 'Yes, I am listening, I don't understand but I know you mean well.'
- 'Yes, I'm listening, I don't understand but I don't think I ever will and if I say yes we might be able to end this conversation.'

It is humiliating and upsetting not to understand what someone says to us, and difficult to admit, especially to busy health professionals, that we have not understood. Most people trying to communicate in an unfamiliar language say 'yes' a lot, to show that they are really trying. It is dangerous to assume that 'yes' under these circumstances indicates understanding and agreement.

Try to ask questions that actually check out whether the person has understood. For example, ask them to show you or to tell you what they will do. Or ask a question to which the desired answer would be 'no'.

Say things in the right order

If you have a complicated matter to explain, stop and think first:

- plan what you are going to say and in what order;
- stick to one subject at a time;
- choose the words you are going to use;
- if you need to give instructions, give them in the order in which they need to be done;
- when you have dealt with the subject, pause and check that the person has understood.

Then introduce a new subject as necessary.

Avoid overestimating the amount a person understands

Many people who have picked up English through hearing it spoken are very good at social conversation and everyday topics. They seem fluent but may get completely stuck when trying to discuss unfamiliar topics with, for example, special medical vocabulary.

'Often I know what the doctors are talking to me about but I can't actually understand what they are saying. I can pick up "blood pressure" for example but then I don't understand what they are saying about it. Is it good or bad? I keep listening, trying to understand and look intelligent but really I'm lost. I don't think they realise; I hope not.'
Brazilian patient

If a person does not fully understand what is said to them, they cannot remember it. Write down important points about treatment, drugs and so on in simple English as an aide mémoire. Even if the patient or relative cannot read it themselves, they will usually have someone who can.

Observe the other person's reactions carefully

It is sometimes possible to tell from non-verbal signals when people don't understand or are becoming exhausted. It is usually best to wind up the interview and to try to fix another time to talk. Alternatively it may be possible to give the patient a short break and come back to them in half an hour or so.

It is almost impossible to give good practical and emotional care across a language barrier. You should have a professional interpreter for all important conversations.

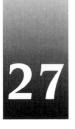

27 Working with professional interpreters

· ·

'No agency can provide an effective service to people with whom it cannot communicate.' (Shackman 1984)

When health professionals and patients do not share a common language, someone is needed to interpret. In order to ensure good two-way communication and clear mutual understanding this person must:

- be trained and experienced;
- be fluent in both English and the patient's mother tongue;
- understand medical terminology and what the health professional is trying to achieve;
- be someone whom both the health professional and the patient can trust.

Terminology Many titles are used to describe people who help non-English-speaking patients and their families to communicate with health professionals and vice versa. These include interpreter, health aide, bilingual support worker, linkworker, language aide and health advocate. The variety of terms reflects the current lack of clarity about the responsibilities of the job and its generally low status. In this book the term interpreter is used, with full recognition of the breadth and complexity of the role of health interpreters, the responsibilities they carry, their importance in ensuring that patients and families get the care they need, and the status that should be accorded to them.

Interpreters are also referred to here as she, though it is recognised that a male interpreter may be needed to discuss personal issues with male patients. For grammatical simplicity this chapter also focuses on communication with patients. However, in many cases interpreters are needed to assist communication with relatives, and often with patients and relatives together.

'Without an interpreter we are both virtually deaf and dumb. It's awful for me and awful for my patient. We both feel powerless, inadequate and frustrated. The interpreter is crucial. She's like a fuse box in an electrical circuit. Everything goes through her. But I don't imagine it's easy being the fuse box either.' English health professional

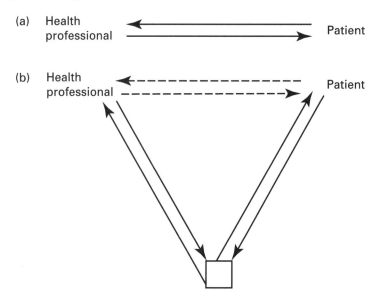

Figure 27.1 (a) Direct communication vs (b) communication through an interpreter

Professional interpreters: the benefits

Evaluations show that the provision of trained, professional health interpreters and health advocates has major benefits for patients, families, professionals and for the service. These include:

- better and more accurate communication;
- improved outcomes;
- shorter hospital stays and reduced interventions;
- better-informed patients, a shared understanding of the problem and the purpose and manner of treatment;
- greater continuity of care and emotional support for patients, opportunities to express needs, concerns and opinions;
- reduced stress on both sides;
- improved practical provision to meet patients' cultural needs and preferences – for example, facilities for private prayers, more appropriate

hospital food, longer dressing gowns in clinics, and information leaflets in appropriate languages
- greater job satisfaction for professionals (Leather and Wirz 1996, Warrier 1995, Rocheron and Dickinson 1990).

'Every time I see a patient who does not speak English I have to spend three or four times as long with her as with my other patients. And I don't achieve much. It can't cost more to employ a competent interpreter than to waste my time like this.'
Hospital doctor (Consumer Congress Trust 1996)

Under section 20 of the 1976 Race Relations Act (see Chapter 6) it is illegal knowingly to provide an inferior quality of care to a particular racial minority group. The failure to provide interpreters for a minority group many of whose members are known to speak little English could be construed as unlawful.

Working well with a professional interpreter

For health professionals, working well with an interpreter involves a difficult balance between:

- retaining overall responsibility for the discussion;
- ensuring that the patient gets the care they need and want; and
- helping the interpreter to work effectively and to use her skills to the full.

All this requires conscious and careful management.

Beforehand

- If this is the first time you and the interpreter have worked together, and especially if the interview may be difficult, discuss how you will work together.
- Make it clear to the interpreter that you value her as a colleague. Explain the purpose of the session. Ask her to alert you to any cultural or other issues that arise, and to stop you if she or the patient have difficulties. Encourage her to tell you if you talk too fast or don't pause often enough. Check that she understands the importance of keeping both you and the patient fully informed of what is going on. For example, if she needs to have a longer conversation with one of you, she should summarise what she is saying to the other person.
- Check with the interpreter how to pronounce and use the patient's name correctly.

- Discuss how the interpreter should respond if the patient becomes very upset or does not want to be interrupted. It is very difficult and even counter-productive for an interpreter to ignore a patient's distress and continue translating mechanically. It may be better for her to concentrate on supporting the patient, summarising what has been said to you when the right moment comes.

'I was with this patient and she was crying. She was so devastated, we cried together, I held her. I needed to be close to her and to be myself, to try to comfort her. The doctor was great. She let us hug each other. She let the patient hug her, and she just waited and stayed with us. Before the interview, which we knew was going to be so hard, she said to me, "If there's anything you need to do or say, or I need to say, please tell me".'
Iraqi interpreter

At the beginning of the interview

- Check, if necessary, that the interpreter really speaks the patient's language and (if appropriate) dialect. Not all the South Asian languages spoken in Britain are mutually comprehensible (see Table 41.2). People who speak one Chinese dialect do not necessarily speak another.
- Try to check that your patient feels able to talk openly to the interpreter, though this is hard. Ask the interpreter if she knows of any reason why the patient may be reluctant to talk to her. It is important that you can honestly assure the patient that everything they say will be treated in total confidence (see Chapter 15 *Maintaining patient confidentiality*). There may be issues of security if the patient is a refugee or asylum seeker and is at risk of political violence (see Chapter 35 *Interpreters*).
- Allow more time. You need at least twice as long because everything has to go through the interpreter in both directions. If the subject is complicated or new, or involves unfamiliar words, procedures or ideas, the interpreter may have to do a lot of explaining. The patient may also raise other issues and queries that need to be discussed.
- The patient and the interpreter may need time to get to know each other. People in many cultures find it discourteous to go straight into the content of a discussion, even (or especially) a medical one (see also Chapter 23 *Possible cultural differences in relation to care*). Your patient may need to talk to the interpreter and feel comfortable with her before revealing intimate personal information. With a family group, the interpreter may need to take time to establish credibility with each generation (Ahmed, Valentine and Shire 1982). If you can, introduce people and leave them alone for a few minutes.

During the conversation

- You are still responsible for the care and well-being of the patient. Do all the things you normally do. Greet the patient. Sit facing them, and speak directly to them using normal gestures and expressions. Look at them most of the time (bearing in mind possible cultural conventions about eye contact – see Chapter 24 *Non-verbal signals*). Try not to draw back physically or emotionally from the patient because you are communicating through an interpreter.
- Use all your normal communications skills, listening, observing, responding, explaining and checking. Try to keep your English simple and jargon-free so that it is easy for the interpreter to translate. Break up what you say into manageable chunks. Ask the interpreter to stop you if there is anything she doesn't understand or if you go too fast.

> 'I found initially talking to the Vietnamese through an interpreter extremely difficult. The first … meeting I held was an ordeal of fire. A totally unreal situation. I couldn't work out how much I should say before stopping for the interpreter … I would say a sentence and they would wink, OK, stop. Or they would tell me when to stop. After a while I realised that both Vietnamese and Chinese don't say what they are going to say in one sentence. They will explore a concept for two or three minutes. People complain that you ask a question and it takes half an hour to answer. I was fortunate in having two experienced people who educated me.'
> Refugee worker (Shackman 1984)

- Everyone always understands more of a foreign language than they can speak. The simpler and clearer your language, the more likely the patient is to understand some of what you say. If the patient's English is fairly good, you could agree to converse in English, asking the interpreter to listen for and help with any misunderstandings.
- Beware of putting a clinical burden on the interpreter. Except in very exceptional circumstances and with a clear protocol, never leave an interpreter alone to give clinical advice. Interpreters are not responsible for the care of the patient and are not normally qualified doctors or nurses. It is your responsibility to check that the patient understands, that they are not left with any unanswered questions and that they know what will happen next.
- If a patient is given any written material or instructions, the interpreter may need to translate them. This is a time-consuming task. If it happens regularly, you need to discuss with the interpreter's manager arranging time for her to do the translation.

- Although most of your attention should be on the patient, remember the interpreter's need for acknowledgement and support. Give her the time she needs. Try not to look impatient while she and the patient are talking together. Show that you respect her expertise and judgement.
- At the end of the interview, encourage the interpreter to talk generally to the patient to find out if they have any other worries or problems.

Afterwards

- Talk to the interpreter about how the session went. Ask for any insights or information she was unable to give you at the time. Ask if there is anything you can do to make her job easier next time. Be prepared to spend time listening to her if she has had to give bad news or to deal with a difficult situation. An interpreter always bears the brunt of the patient's emotions.
- In hospital or other residential care, try to ensure that an interpreter visits each of your non-English-speaking patients at least once a day to find out how they are and if they have any unmet needs or worries. Make sure the interpreter knows where to refer anything that needs action, and that all staff recognise her importance as the patient's advocate and supporter.

If you are not satisfied with the interpreter provision you have, discuss this with the person in charge and ask for improvements. Trust between professional and interpreter is central to successful interpreting (Pharaoh 1995). You should have access to a competent, trained, professional interpreter whom you respect and trust whenever you need one.

The need for more black and ethnic minority health professionals

Communication through an interpreter, however good, is never likely to be as effective as direct communication between a health professional and a patient who share the same language and cultural understanding. It is important, therefore, that health authorities and trusts serving a multi-ethnic population also employ black and ethnic minority health professionals at all levels and in all fields. The recruitment and use of interpreters must go hand in hand with an effective equal opportunities employment policy (see also Chapter 7 *How to tackle racism and racial equality*) (Shackman 1984).

What an interpreter does

Imagine that you are an interpreter working in a busy outpatients clinic in north-eastern China where there are a large number of Europeans who do not speak the local Chinese language. The doctor is a middle-aged Chinese man. You have to interpret in the following situations. What would you do in each situation?

Mrs Hayes has late-onset, non-insulin-dependent diabetes that is poorly controlled. She is also obese and hypertensive. The doctor advises her to cut down on fried noodles and eat more steamed vegetables and durian. She says yes but you think she probably eats an English diet and that this advice is irrelevant to her. He also tells her to take some gentle exercise but you know she lives on the thirteenth floor on a run-down and violent estate.

- What do you do? What are your responsibilities in such a situation?

Mrs Brown comes for a check-up 18 months after a mastectomy. After examining her, the doctor tells you she needs to be scanned as soon as possible as she has axillary and cervical nodes and a palpable liver.

- How do you feel? What do you say to Mrs Brown? What are your responsibilities in such a situation? What will your responsibilities be during and after the scan? How will you manage?

Mr Jackson returns to outpatients. The doctor is concerned because, despite treatment, he is still grossly hypertensive. Mr Jackson admits to you that he stopped the tablets because they made him sleepy and dizzy, but he does not want to tell the doctor for fear of annoying him.

- How do you feel? What are your responsibilities in such a situation? What do you do?

Mr Buonomo is breathless and has blood-stained sputum. He is anxious and distressed. You do not speak Italian. There is no Italian interpreter. When you tell the doctor you cannot translate for Mr Buonomo he says, 'Come on, it's important. I know you Europeans all understand each other's languages. Please have a go.' Mr Buonomo is obviously very upset and pours out his worries to you in Italian. You don't understand what he is saying but you can't stop him.

- How do you feel? What do you say? What are your responsibilities in such a situation?

Health care interpreting is never straightforward. In none of the situations above will the patient get good care if you simply translate words from one language to another, even when that is possible. Often the interpreter is the only person who has the complete picture of what is going on and the only one who can communicate with and help both sides. She understands more than the patient about the health care system, how it works and what kind of care it should provide. She understands more than the health professional about the patient's personality, situation, feelings, needs, culture, religion and likely expectations. She has responsibilities to both parties and she alone is in a position to assess the situation.

> 'Our job as interpreters is often not to translate just the words but to explain what the patient actually means so that the professional understands the whole message, not just the words.'
> Iraqi interpreter

The interpreter's tasks include:

- Translating as accurately as possible everything that the health professional and the patient say.
- Helping to establish a relationship of trust and a rapport between all three parties.
- Helping the professional make a full and accurate assessment of the situation.
- Ensuring that both the health professional and the patient have the information they need to make informed decisions, and that both feel fully involved.
- Explaining treatments, tests and other aspects of health care that the patient is not familiar with, encouraging the patient to ask questions if they do not understand or need more information.
- Providing emotional support and encouragement for the patient, helping to ensure that they get the treatment and care they need.
- Explaining cultural factors that may be important for both sides to understand.
- Challenging negative stereotypes, racism and discriminatory practices.

The interpreter has to make continual on-the-spot decisions about each speaker's intentions and meaning and to convey these as best she can. The more complex the ideas, and the more difficult or upsetting the issues are, the harder her task. At the same time, she must keep pushing the responsibility and the control of the discussion back to the health professional and to the patient.

Translating words

Given such a list of responsibilities, the translation of words from one language to another could be seen as the easiest part of a health interpreters' job. In fact, even this is rarely straightforward. No two languages have exactly the same grammatical structures, or express things in exactly the same way. Word order and the sequencing of ideas differ. Sometimes an interpreter needs several sentences to translate a single word; sometimes a single word conveys several sentences. The more different the roots and structures of the two languages (eg Bengali and English), the more difficult the interpreter's job.

- Sometimes there are **no equivalent words or expressions**. The vocabulary and concepts in each language reflect the culture and key concerns of the people who speak it. Many words are untranslatable from one language to another because they express concepts that are culture-specific.

  Western medical and health-care terminology can cause particular difficulties because there may be no equivalent in the patient's language. One health survey team found that a wide range of the English health-related terms they wanted to use had no equivalent in some South Asian languages, and were not generally understood in some communities. These included 'stress', 'personal space' and 'healthy foods' as well as many medical terms such as 'gangrene', 'diabetes' and 'degenerative illness'. In many languages there is no word for 'depression'. South Asians who were familiar with these concepts tended to use the English word for them (HEA 1994).

  In the same way, English has adopted words from other languages and cultures for many concepts that had no real English equivalent, such as angst, karma, yin and yang. Some words simply do not exist and have to be expressed in round-about ways. For example, English only has words to describe the closest family relationships. In South Asian and many other Eastern languages there are precise single words for relationships that are important in these cultures, such as 'my mother's elder brother' 'my mother's younger brother', 'my father's elder brother', and 'my father's younger brother'.

- In many languages there are **no socially acceptable words** for female or male genitalia or for sexual activities. In western Europe such words have developed only since the nineteenth century, with the medicalisation of sexuality and of sexual behaviour (Khan 1994) (see also Chapter 34 *Difficult words*). Interpreters may have to develop and explain their own translations for such words to patients. They may have to find other acceptable ways of explaining what they mean. They may also have to deal with their own and the patient's embarrassment and reticence.

- Sometimes the **words are unfamiliar to the patient.** Even if words exist in the patient's language, he or she may not know them. Specialist terms and medical jargon may all need explaining, just as they would to many English-speaking patients. An interpreter may have to choose between simply translating the word, knowing that it makes no sense to the patient, or giving a detailed explanation and checking that the patient has understood.

Even if the words are clear and appear to be the same, there may be important **differences in meaning.**

'At the height of the cold war, the Soviet General Secretary proclaimed in a major speech, 'We will bury' the Western capitalist countries. Most Americans and other Westerners saw this as a clear threat to bomb the USA and western Europe into oblivion. The speech greatly increased public fear and hostility towards the Soviet Union. Later it was pointed out that in Russian the phrase did not imply a threat but simply expressed the belief that the Soviet system would outlive the Western system. A healthy young Russian might say, 'I will bury my father,' meaning that he expected to outlive him. Nevertheless, most Westerners remembered the threat, not the explanation. The misunderstanding sowed lasting suspicion.' (Fisher and Brown 1989)

The interpreter's other tasks

As well as translating what each side says, an interpreter must make difficult decisions all the time about what and whether to explain, whether and how to intervene, and how to help both sides manage the consultation as well as possible.

'It's very pressured. The [professional] wants me to translate everything as fast as I can, to make the interview go well and to make the patient comply. The patient wants to make sure I understand her situation, explain it fully to the [professional], and get her the care she needs. Both of them want me to solve their problems, and if things go wrong I'm often the one who gets the blame.' Interpreter

From the patient's point of view, the interpreter's **advocacy and guidance** are often crucial. The interpreter can encourage the patient to ask questions, or can ask on the patient's behalf. She has the experience to know how the consultation should go and to help steer it so that the patient gets the care they need.

Doctor to 70-year-old patient: *'I think we need to do a prostatectomy.'*

Interpreter to patient [in patient's language]: *'He wants to do a prostatectomy. Ask him why and what it might mean for you.'* (Adapted from Ahmad 1989)

The interpreter must also act as **supporter and companion** to patients who are anxious, distressed, frightened or vulnerable. She feels and understands the patient's emotion most directly, it is to her that the patient often turns for support, especially if they share a cultural or religious heritage. When bad news has to be broken it is mainly the interpreter, rather than the professional, who has to prepare the patient to receive it, to translate it and to support the patient and their family. As a member of the patient's community, the interpreter must be able to show her concern and sympathy in a way that is culturally appropriate if she is to retain credibility and trust and to do her job properly.

> 'We have to keep boundaries, we have to be impartial, but sometimes other people's situations really get through to us. Things remind us of our own losses, we get involved because we can see the person's situation, they are so frightened and lost, we care so much that this person should get the care they need. And they see me as a friend, they expect me to care, to help and to grieve, to mourn with them. You can't just cut them off; that would hurt them terribly.'
> Iraqi interpreter

To ensure a fully satisfactory consultation, interpreters also have to compensate for the patient's lack of knowledge and their dependence in the medical situation. They need to ensure that each patient is able to participate as far as they wish in their own care and to make their own informed decisions. Sometimes, however, interpreters have to decide whether they should translate something that they know is culturally inappropriate or unacceptable to their patient, or that could have disastrous long-term consequences.

> 'I was interpreting in court in a maintenance case. The families of both the wife and the husband were there. The husband's lawyer was trying to whittle down the amount of alimony by suggesting that she was partly responsible for the divorce. He told me to ask the wife whether she had had intercourse with anyone before she married. I had to refuse to ask that question. In a public court before members of her own family and community even to ask her such a question would be to label her a prostitute. She would be publicly destroyed. Of course she hadn't been with another man before she married. Nobody believed she had. So I told the judge I couldn't ask the question and explained why. I was shaking with fear.'
> South Asian social worker (Shackman 1984)

Translating for ill and dependent patients and their families poses major problems for interpreters of many communities. The value placed on patient autonomy, the patient's right to know and to make informed decisions, and the importance of telling the full truth depend very much on culture. At present, British and North American professional thinking on these issues is out of step with that of most of the rest of the world (Pellegrino 1992). In such cases, an interpreter may be caught between her duty to interpret everything and to act as a neutral channel of communication between professional and patient, and her knowledge of what is culturally acceptable (see also Chapter 15 *Telling patients the truth*).

> 'If a doctor or nurse asked me to tell a patient that they were going to die it would depend. Sometimes I would say, "I can't, it's not on, this is not what we do in our culture, I cannot do it and the patient does not want or expect to hear it". Or sometimes I would translate it, but I would add other words to soften it, to make it less cruel. I would say "God forbid", or "I tell you this but I hope it never happens".'
> Iraqi interpreter

The power structure and culture of the health service, and the low status that patients are often accorded, especially if they are black and speak no English, add to the pressure on interpreters. If there is **rudeness or racism** from either side, the interpreter bears the brunt of it, and also has to decide how to handle it, and whether and how to take it further.

> 'Linkworkers frequently heard comments made by staff which revealed a remarkable degree of insensitivity and intolerance towards linkworkers and their clients. Racist stereotyping was not infrequent.' (Rocheron and Dickinson 1990)

If managers and policy makers do not hear the views of non-English-speaking patients, they cannot respond to them. Interpreters have a unique knowledge of the care that these patients are receiving and the problems they face. They should be able to feed **comments and criticisms** back to service providers so that provision can be improved. Unless there is a formal route for such feedback, interpreters inevitably absorb and, in effect, silence the legitimate demands and complaints of non-English speakers about the service they receive (Shackman 1984).

Interpreters should also be able to **help individual patients and families make complaints**. If patients themselves are reluctant, the interpreters need ways of feeding back to managers gross cases of poor service with confidence. They require strong support.

Training, supporting and managing interpreters

Selection

Health interpreting requires interpersonal skills and sensitivity as well as linguistic ability. In general, interpreters are likely to be most acceptable to patients and relatives if they have a similar background in terms of life experience, class and religion. Because an interpreter's work requires patients to talk about sensitive and personal matters, it is important to ensure that, in her own community, she is considered mature enough and completely trustworthy. A calm personality, a non-threatening approach and ease in discussing emotional topics are essential (City and Hackney CHC 1988, Ahmed, Valentine and Shire 1982).

Training

Interpreters are expected to convey clinical information simply and clearly, a task that even doctors and nurses often find difficult. Without special training there is a danger that they will piece together their own understanding of medical procedures and vocabulary, and pass this partial understanding on to patients (Audit Commission 1993). Simply knowing how to speak two languages is therefore not enough. **In terms of communication, interpreters face exactly the same demands as health professionals and must have similar training** (BHAN 1991).

In addition, interpreters' training should include discussion of their role and responsibilities and of confidentiality; practice in the linguistic and other skills needed to interpret accurately; experiential training in dealing with difficult interpreting situations, including, for example, breaking bad news, supporting people who are distressed or frightened, interpreting when there is conflict, and handling racism assertively. Interpreters, like other health professionals, also need time to examine their own attitudes and feelings in order to be able to provide more effective support, as well as regular opportunities to discuss difficult issues and incidents away from the workplace.

Managing and supporting interpreters

Experience shows that interpreters are often most effective if they are managed by someone with status and power who is not part of the nursing or medical hierarchy, or who is outside the organisation altogether (Warrier 1995, City and Hackney CHC 1988). The inevitable conflicts can then be openly discussed and resolved in the interests of patients and the community. The manager must also be of sufficient seniority to sort out practical problems and to ensure that the best possible use is made of the interpreters. Waiting for hours with a patient in a clinic, for example, is extremely wasteful and costly. Using the same interpreter for a patient each time, provided the patient is satisfied, increases the benefits. It is also important to ensure that interpreters are called when they are needed. In some places, resistance by staff has meant that interpreters were not used even when they were available.

> 'Many of my colleagues resent the interpreters. They feel that the patients should have learnt English and if they haven't that's their problem. They resent the expense. To me the benefits and cost effectiveness of interpreters are very clear, which is more than you can say for some of the tests and treatments we carry out!'
> English doctor

Lack of clarity about the interpreter's role and responsibilities, as well as the conflicts and pressures inherent in the job, often lead to difficulties. Sometimes patients and relatives ask interpreters for additional help, for example with personal matters or housing and financial problems. This is particularly likely in communities that are deprived and struggling and have little or no access to other sources of help or to help in their own language. Although understandable, it can place an intolerable burden on the interpreter, especially if she lives in the community. Sometimes professionals also ask interpreters to do things that are outside their remit. A clear job description and supportive management can help interpreters refuse such requests and keep their job to manageable proportions. Interpreters also need personal support, someone to listen who understands the conflicts that are part of their daily work and the pressures they experience.

> 'The patient was a young boy. I visited him every day and talked to the family, interpreted for them, tried to help, tried to support them. When he died I needed someone to listen to me, to hear my sorrow, to share the problem and to tell me I did a good job. I am a professional but I am also a human being. But there was nobody.'
> Iranian interpreter

The challenge for professionals

Many health professionals who work with interpreters understand and value their contribution, involving them fully in the care of the patient (Warrier 1995). However, others feel strongly that interpreters should act only as word-for-word translators. They find it frustrating and difficult to work with an interpreter. They feel de-skilled, out of control, insecure, inadequate and embarrassed. They may not know how to handle the session or may feel redundant. They may find it hard to be dependent on someone with lower professional status. They may feel threatened if the interpreter acts as an advocate or supporter for the patient. They may not be sure whether what they want to say is really getting through and whether what they are hearing is accurate and complete. They may fear that she is inserting her own views into the translation or that she is becoming too emotionally involved.

> 'We have an interpreter. But I am never quite sure that she tells the women everything I say. She seems to make a lot of decisions for them. She wears a white coat and feels, I think, very much one of us. Her husband is a teacher and sometimes I feel she looks down on the women as uneducated and stupid, and feels she knows better than they do.'
> Scottish health professional

Often these fears are reasonable. Interpreting is a very difficult job. Interpreters who have received no professional training or guidance and who have merely been selected because they speak several languages frequently make mistakes that cause problems. Some interpreters also become marginalised and disempowered. Some may distance themselves from their patients and may identify more with higher-status health professionals. Good selection and training and strong management should help prevent some of these problems.

> 'I feel useless because I can't use my normal communication skills. At the same time, if it weren't for the interpreter I couldn't communicate at all with some of my patients. It's always a compromise, but we're getting better at it. I'm coming to trust her judgement and that she will tell me what's going on. I couldn't do it if she weren't so good.'
> White British senior registrar

Training for professionals

> 'Training staff in how to make use of interpreters' time and skills will minimise costs, time and skill wastage.' (Slater 1993)

All professionals who work with interpreters should receive training. This should include an understanding of what is involved in health interpreting; an understanding of the pressures and difficulties affecting each party in the interpreting triangle and how to help manage the conversation as well as possible; dealing with difficulties and conflicts; maintaining a good relationship with patients when an interpreter is present; and supporting the interpreter. Training should also include discussion of cultural issues and working across cultural barriers, and of racism, how it works and how to challenge it (see Chapter 7 *How to tackle racism and racial inequality*).

28 Using informal interpreters

Using friends and relatives to interpret

'Wherever I went my husband was with me. When he couldn't accompany me a lady member of the family used to go with me to explain things to me. But it was not always possible for them to accompany me, so I had to skip two appointments. I was scared to go on my own because of the language.'
Bengali woman

In most situations, even when there is a clear need for a trained interpreter, none is provided. Health professionals and patients have to struggle through, with stress and frustration on both sides, and achieving very little. Often, patients are asked or expected to bring someone to interpret for them. But a relative or friend is unlikely to be familiar with clinical procedures or to understand the terms used. The translation is likely to be inaccurate and unreliable.

'No one would expect an untrained nurse to take on skilled nursing care of a patient, and neither should responsibility for crucial medical interpreting rest on untrained interpreters.' (Hilton 1997)

Take a minute to think about how you would feel if you had to talk to a doctor through an interpreter about your symptoms. Suppose you had had a biopsy and needed to discuss the results and treatment options.

Who would you prefer to translate for you and why?

- your husband/wife/partner?
- your son or daughter?
- a friend?
- a hospital cleaner?

- a man or woman waiting in the surgery?
- a neighbour?
- a trained interpreter?

Accuracy A study of four consultations with Gujarati-speaking patients using family 'interpreters' who were thought to be fluent in both languages, found an alarmingly high proportion of mistranslations, misunderstandings and omissions. In each interview the English-speaking doctor thought it had gone reasonably normally.

'In the 143 questions and answers, there were more than 80 words or phrases which were mistranslated, misunderstood or not translated by at least one interpreter. These included anatomical terms – for example, leg used for ankle; back teeth for jaw; neck for tonsil; and chest for ribs. Symptoms caused more difficulties – such as laxative used for diarrhoea; watery faeces for passing water; and getting fat for swelling. Technical terms were often mistranslated, with breathlessness used for asthma and being mad for epileptic fit. Words such as gynaecological, waterworks and gallstones were not translated at all ... Children found it embarrassing to translate questions about menstruation or bowel movements to their parents, and there was a general tendency for questions about bodily functions to be ignored.' (Ebden, Bhatt et al 1988)

The study also found that simple questions were translated best, though still with mistakes. Complex questions proved more difficult, and serial questions (when the doctor asked several questions together) the most difficult of all. In one interview over half the serial questions were mistranslated or not translated.

'Some people used as interpreters do not understand exactly what you want them to do, or that they are supposed to translate everything that is said in both directions. They may just have a conversation with the client and relay what seems useful. They may answer a lot of your questions themselves. This often happens with family members since they usually know many of the answers to your questions without having to ask your client. They may see no point in asking when they already know the answer perfectly well.' (Shackman 1984)

An informal 'interpreter' is also unlikely to be able to explain important cultural issues in either direction, or to guide the patient through the system. In addition, if family members or friends need to take time off work to accompany patients to appointments, their own job and the family's income may be put at risk (Shackman 1984).

Bias and distortion Depending on the relationship between patient and 'interpreter' there may also be bias and distortion in the interpreting. Different family members may each have their own ideas about the situation and may give these rather than translate the views of the patient. The 'interpreter' may not feel happy translating some of what is said; the patient may not feel able to answer questions honestly or voice any worries.

Embarrassment Both sides may be very embarrassed by certain questions or procedures. In one study over a third of female patients who used informal interpreters reported difficulties. These included inhibitions about discussing health issues via their husband, son or daughter (see below), as well as problems with inaccurate interpretation (HEA 1994). For older people it may be specially embarrassing to discuss intimate matters through a junior family member or a relative of the opposite sex. In cultures where men discuss intimate topics only with men, and women with women, even husbands and wives may not feel able to discuss these issues together. In some cases partners may know very little about such matters and may not know the relevant words either in English or in their first language.

> 'I went to the doctor and took my grown-up son but he wouldn't interpret personal things. He said, "How could you ask me to interpret that?".'
> Elderly South Asian woman

Confidentiality Patients need to be absolutely sure that everything they say will be kept totally confidential and that nothing will be repeated to anyone outside. Many patients do not want their spouse, their children (even if adult) or other family members to hear distressing information. There may also be personal information that they do not wish the rest of the family to know. Confidentiality is even more problematic with non-family members, particularly in small communities where most people know each other and news travels fast. If there is a social stigma attached to a particular condition, confidentiality is particularly crucial. Breaches of confidentiality can have serious consequences not only for the patient themselves but also, in some cases, for the whole family (see Chapter 13 *Illness and stigma*). Confidentiality can be ensured only if a professional interpreter is used when discussing diagnosis, prognosis and treatment options with the patient.

Children

In some cases children are used as interpreters. This is always completely unacceptable.

'Under no circumstances should children be asked to interpret medical details for their parents. It appears to us to be unethical, unprofessional, uncivilised and totally unacceptable.' (Rack 1991)

Nevertheless, this is still common practice and seems to be widely regarded as acceptable. A recent survey of the handling of sudden deaths in accident and emergency departments indicated that 33 per cent of departments commonly used children to interpret (RCN and BAAEM 1995).

All the problems outlined above apply in the case of children, but are likely to be even more acute. Using children to translate matters that are distressing, confidential or personal can cause serious long-term damage both to the children and to family relationships. Parents are placed in a dependent role and children are given knowledge, responsibility and power that they should not have. Most parents try to shield their children as far as they can from distressing or sensitive information and so are unlikely to answer difficult or sensitive questions honestly or to tell you everything you need to know. Parents are unlikely to be prepared to talk through a child about sexual or other intimate matters. Most children anyway do not speak both languages equally well. They do not understand adult communication and are unlikely to be able to translate important medical terms accurately or reliably. In addition, using children to interpret usually means keeping them away from school.

'Many English-speaking professionals believe that ethnic-minority parents do not mind using their children to interpret in such cases. Our experience indicates that they generally mind intensely but do not know what else to do.' (Shackman 1984)

Staff lists

Non-professional staff Some hospitals use lists of staff who speak one or more other languages to interpret, sometimes paying them a small fee. While this may be useful in emergencies and in other exceptional situations, it is inadequate and undesirable as part of a general communications policy. In the case of staff who are not health professionals (eg cooks and cleaners), many of the same issues arise as with relatives and friends, in particular suitability, confidentiality and trust.

Health professionals When black and minority ethnic health professionals are used as interpreters, confidentiality, professional standards and the accurate translation of medical terminology are not a problem, but other factors need to be considered. Taking health professionals away from their normal work on a regular basis may adversely affect them and their work and put them under serious pressure. It also wastes and ignores their professional skills, places them in a subordinate position to their colleagues, and may affect their career development and prospects (Shackman 1984). Where it is policy to use health professionals to interpret on a regular basis, it is important to discuss the implications for everyone concerned and to make sure that the minority ethnic professionals concerned are happy with the situation (see also Chapter 7 *How to tackle racism and racial inequality*).

Working with informal interpreters: minimising problems

Because there are currently so few interpreters, it is often impossible to avoid using an informal interpreter. Occasionally, patients may prefer to have a close family member to translate for them, rather than expose themselves to a professional but unknown interpreter.

The following are some ideas to help manage communication as well as possible through an informal interpreter.

- **Listen carefully to the person's command of English and decide how much you can expect him or her to translate.** Many people with patchy English end up having to interpret for friends and relatives because there is no one else. You may need to modify your language to make it easier to translate (see Chapter 26 *Simplifying your English*). You may decide to communicate only the essential details for now and to leave the important issues until you can get a trained interpreter. You may even decide that you can communicate better directly with the patient than through the interpreter you have available.
- **Find out what the interpreter's relationship is to the patient.** It is often very difficult for patients to find sympathetic people who speak good English, whom they feel comfortable using as interpreters, and who are able to accompany them to clinics or spend time with them in hospital. The person the patient brings to translate may be a spouse, partner, child, close relative, distant relative, friend, acquaintance, neighbour, community worker, or someone who charges a fee for interpreting. The interpreter's relationship with the patient will affect what you can ask them to translate and what the patient is willing to say.

'There are no interpreters at this hospital and patients who don't speak English have to resort to desperate measures to get treatment and to communicate with professionals. In the Oncology Department a woman brought

her six-year old daughter to translate for her. The girl had to tell her mother that she had to have both breasts removed. A Portuguese couple brought a man to help them discuss what kind of breast prosthesis the wife might have after her operation. It later emerged that he just worked in the local electrical shop. They didn't know him at all well but he had kindly agreed to come along and help them because they were desperate.'
White British researcher

- **Be aware that your patient may not want the interpreter to know everything about them.** If a patient does not feel comfortable with the person acting as an interpreter, needs to discuss intimate and personal matters, or does not trust the interpreter to keep the discussion confidential, they may not wish to discuss things fully or truthfully. Will using this person to interpret put your patient at risk in any way? Might the things you need to discuss affect family relationships or the patient's reputation in their community?
- **Find out whether the interpreter feels able to interpret everything you need.** A relative, friend or stranger may be too embarrassed to discuss some things with the patient, may disagree strongly with some of what you want translated, or may find the information so distressing that they cannot bear to tell it to the patient. A non-professional interpreter may become upset when seeing or discussing medical procedures and may themselves need support. If the interpreter is part of the family and will themselves be closely affected by what they translate, you may need to give them additional care and support. Bear in mind that your interpreter's language ability may be also affected if they become distressed.
- **Help the interpreter to do as good a job as possible.** Find out if the interpreter is worried about translating in this situation. Spend time explaining what you want and finding out if there are problems. Try to give the interpreter the confidence to tell you if there are things they do not understand or are not sure how to translate. **Make it clear that you are grateful for their help and realise that the situation is not ideal. Do not blame them for having come along to translate nor resent the fact that they cannot do it better.**

Mistranslations can have serious or even fatal consequences and can cause great distress to patients and their families. Unless you are completely happy with your interpreter's accuracy, suitability and reliability, **you need to find a professional interpreter as soon as possible to check out what has been said.**

29 Written materials

Written information can be extremely helpful in helping patients and families remember and build on what they have been told. Written material also helps people prepare for hospital admission, operations and other treatments, understand pain relief and cope better with other aspects of their care. It is available as a reminder long after any verbal information has been given (Crawford 1997, RCP 1997).

Written information can be particularly important for people who speak little or no English. They may find it even more difficult to remember what was said (see Chapter 26 *Ways of reducing stress*) and are often cut off from other sources of information. But written material is effective only if:

- it takes into account the values, knowledge and way of life of its target audience;
- the information it contains is useful and relevant;
- the language is easy to understand and the message clear;
- it is respectful and non-patronising.

In a multi-ethnic community it is important to consider these criteria in relation to a wide range of communities and lifestyles, and to take different expectations and attitudes into account. Material must not imply, for example, that English or Western ways are 'better'. The language must be very clear, accessible to as many people as possible but not condescending. It is important to consult professionals working in the community, minority ethnic community workers and representatives, and consumers themselves, to ensure that money and time are not wasted on producing materials that are irrelevant, incomprehensible or offensive.

Sometimes the information or advice to be presented is very specific. When communities have different cultures and traditions, it may be most useful to produce separate leaflets. For example, advice on preparing suitable food for African-Caribbean or Somali patients who have difficulty swallowing may need to be different from that for patients who eat a traditional English diet. Advice on intimate matters such as stoma or colostomy care, or how to manage after an operation, may need to take different cultural and religious concerns into account.

Materials in other languages

In most minority communities there are people who can read their own language but cannot read English. Even people who speak English fluently may be unable to read it, as speaking and reading a language are different skills. Levels of ability in English vary: many people who can read about everyday topics in English find the language of medical or health information leaflets very difficult and need translated or bilingual materials.

What languages do people read?

In all communities, most people can read their first language. However, in some communities older people are less likely to read at all, and in others they may read their own language but not English. If women have traditionally had little access to formal education, they are also less likely to be literate.

Younger people in almost all communities are more likely to have been educated in Britain and to have English as their main language of reading and writing. Table 29.1 shows levels of literacy in English within the South Asian communities. Levels of literacy in English in other communities varies, depending largely on their history and on their circumstances in Britain.

Table 29.1 Levels of literacy in English in the South Asian communities (%)

Age group	Women			Men		
	16–29	30–49	50–74	16–29	30–49	50–74
Indian	88	67	34	96	83	71
Pakistani	77	31	7	91	77	54
Bangladeshi	64	15	4	90	60	38

(Adapted, with permission, from *Health and Lifestyles: Black and minority ethnic groups in England*, 1994, Health Education Authority.)

- The mother tongues of most people from India (and of Indian origin from East Africa) are Punjabi and Gujarati:
  - many Punjabis of Indian origin in Britain read and write Punjabi, usually in the Gurmukhi script;
  - people from Gujarat, or of Gujarati origin from East Africa, are most likely to read Gujarati written in the Devnagri script;
  - one national survey (HEA 1994) found that only 2 per cent of people of Punjabi and Gujarati origin prefer to read Hindi.

- Most Bangladeshis in Britain speak Sylheti, a dialect of Bengali. Sylheti has no written form; the language of education in Bangladesh is Bengali written in the Devnagri script. Seventy-nine per cent of all Bangladeshi people in the UK read Bengali; literacy levels are lower among Bangladeshi women aged over 50. The Health Education Authority 'Health and Lifestyles' survey used Bengali to communicate in writing with Bangladeshi respondents but was careful to use 'the terms closest to those which would be used by Sylheti speakers wherever possible'. (HEA 1994).

- The mother tongue of most Pakistanis in Britain is Punjabi. But the language of education in Pakistan is Urdu, written in the Arabic script. Although Punjabi can be written in the Arabic script, it rarely is. The most useful language for material intended for the Pakistani community is therefore Urdu (HEA 1994).

- Chinese is written in ideographs. Vietnamese is written in the Vietnamese script. In the Vietnamese community in Britain, most people of ethnic Vietnamese origin read Vietnamese. Many people of ethnic Chinese origin read both Vietnamese and Chinese. A small survey of older people in a Vietnamese community found that only a fifth read English (South Glamorgan Race Equality Council 1994).

Producing materials in other languages

'Producing material which is culturally relevant to the target group will not come naturally to someone who does not share that culture.' (Lovell 1990)

Good written material is based on the needs of the people for whom it is intended. It takes into account what they are already likely to know, what they need or want to know more about, which terms they are familiar with and which require explanation, and their likely main concerns. Decisions on language and content should be based on local research, working closely with members of the group or community for whom the material is intended. In some cases it may be possible to translate an existing English text, being careful to modify the text to take cultural, religious and other possible differences into account. In others it may be better to start from scratch, producing information in the target language from the beginning.

Sometimes bilingual materials, in English and the community language, are most useful. People can then read whichever language they find easiest. English-speaking professionals also know exactly what is in any material that they hand out. If the material is not bilingual it must at least state somewhere, in English, the title and subject. An English version should be available for professionals who cannot read the translation.

Will written materials be really useful?

If reading levels are low in the target group, or if the content is difficult to convey simply in writing, it may be better to produce audio-tapes in other languages. Like written materials (see below), they must be acceptable and comprehensible. It is extremely important to work closely with community workers and other members of the target community.

In cultures where oral traditions are more highly valued than visual traditions, or where what happens in relationships carries more weight than impersonal facts, face-to-face conversations may be more effective than either written materials or tapes, and, given the production costs of high-quality materials, may be no more expensive.

Points to bear in mind when translating existing material

- The meaning of the English original must be absolutely clear and the language as straightforward and simple as possible. A complicated, unclear or badly worded English text will be made even worse by translation.
- The overall message must also be very clear, and must be understood by everyone involved in the translation. An unclear message can easily be obscured or lost altogether in the long and complex process of drafting, consulting and checking across cultural and language barriers (Lovell 1990).
- Choose translators who write well and colloquially in the target language. Someone who speaks a language fluently may not be able to write it well. In some languages it is customary for writers to use a very formal elaborate style; in health-related materials for a wide readership an accessible, colloquial style is required (Mares 1982).
- Good translation is difficult. Try to use experienced translators with a portfolio of past work that can be assessed, and to be prepared to pay them a professional fee. Faulty or inappropriate translation can render materials useless or incomprehensible. BHAN (1991), for example, cites an example of an HIV/AIDS leaflet in which the phrase 'oral sex' in the English original was translated into 'verbal sex' in Hindi. In a leaflet about screening, 'smear test' was translated as 'fat test' (Naish, Brown and Denton 1994).

Points to bear in mind when producing materials from scratch

Producing good written material about health matters always requires careful thought and skill, even more so in a different language and across cultural barriers.

- Work closely with community members and/or translators who understand the needs, expectations and concerns of the people for whom the material is intended. Once everybody is absolutely clear about its aims and message, the topics to be covered, and possible cultural or religious factors to be taken into account, ask them to draft the material from scratch in their own language, discussing any difficult decisions or uncertainties with you.
- In some subject areas either suitable terms do not exist or the terms that do exist are offensive or unacceptable (see Chapter 27 *Translating words*). Detailed explanations or new words may be needed.
- Get someone to translate the material into English so you can check the technical content.
- Find one or more people who were not involved in producing the material to comment on the clarity, style and content of the material, and whether they are appropriate for the target group, before you go ahead with the final printing.

Illustrations and pictorial conventions

Consider any illustrations carefully and seek the views of users. Cartoons and drawings of people of different communities frequently cause unintentional offence. Pictorial conventions and symbols such as ticks, crosses, arrows, bolts of lightning, things crossed out, outline maps and so on, are often assumed to be a way of communicating on paper with people who cannot read. In fact they are linked to literacy; people who cannot read may not understand them (Mares, Henley and Baxter 1985).

Producing the materials

It is essential to get the materials re-checked at every stage of production. Be particularly careful if the designers and typesetters cannot read the text and spot mistakes themselves. Labels under illustrations in Urdu materials, for example, have sometimes been transposed because the Arabic script runs from right to left.

The personal and clinical importance of names

Recording each person's name correctly and consistently is vital to effective and safe care. Lost, confused and duplicated records cause delays and frustration and waste money. In some cases they are also dangerous: the results of tests or treatments may become attached to the wrong set of notes, important clinical information may be missed, the wrong patient may be treated or not treated for a serious illness. Sometimes poor notes lead to litigation.

Addressing people correctly and in such a way that they recognise their own name is also fundamental to good care. Our names matter to us. Wilful or careless misuse of names is alienating and insulting and can affect caring relationships.

> 'It upsets me really. I can pronounce English names – why is it so difficult to get a Vietnamese person's name right? What if I always called you by the wrong name. How would you feel?'
> Vietnamese man (Mares 1982)

The British naming system

There are many different naming systems in the world, of which the British system is only one, but it is the one that health professionals use automatically and the one on which records are based. British records rely on the following assumptions:

- everyone has a personal name and a surname;
- the order of the names indicates their usage: the surname always comes last and the personal name first;
- surnames are not male or female; they are gender-neutral names handed down within families through the generations;

- in formal situations most people give their first and last names, or title and last name.

Also:

- some people have a number of middle names, which are less important;
- most personal names are recognisably either male or female.

In addition, to help link members of the same family:

- most women take their husband's surname when they marry;
- most children share their surname with one, if not both, of their parents;
- in most families all the children share the same surname.

Based on the British naming system, the primary identifying point in health service records is the last name, followed by first and middle names, and date of birth.

Other naming systems are often very different:

- Although everyone has a personal name it does not always come first.
- The title may come after the name, rather than before it. Sometimes the title is part of the name.
- In some systems the family name comes first instead of last. However, not all systems have a family name. In many systems no one in a family shares a name.
- Some people have a religious name, which must never be used on its own.

Retrieval systems based mainly on last name and date of birth (see below) do not work in all naming systems. As a result, the records of people whose names do not fit in with the conventions of the British naming system may become confused, lost or duplicated.

Other naming systems

Here are some examples of other naming systems common in Britain:

- In the **traditional Chinese naming system** the family name comes first, followed by a two-part personal name always used together (or occasionally a single personal name). There are only about 100 common Chinese family names, so the personal name is very important for identification. In many families the first part of the personal name is shared by all the children of the same sex. A woman does not change her family name on marriage. She usually adds her husband's family name before her own (see Table 30.1). Chinese Christians may have a Christian personal name as well, which usually comes first.

Table 30.1 Example of a Chinese family using the traditional naming system

Family member	Name
Husband	Cheung Koon-Sung
Wife	Cheung-Ng Wai-Yung
Sons	Cheung Chi-Wah
	Cheung Chi-Kong
Daughters	Cheung Mee-Ling
	Cheung Mee-Tuan

- The **traditional Vietnamese naming system** is similar to the Chinese. There are only about 25 common family names in Vietnam.
- In the **traditional South Asian Muslim naming system** (used in Pakistan, Bangladesh and India), there is no family name shared between men and women (see Table 30.2); all names are either male or female.
  - Most **South Asian Muslim women** traditionally have a two-part name: a personal name followed by a title (such as Bano, Bi, Bibi, Begum, Khanum, Khatoon, Sultana) or a second personal name (eg Akhtar, Jan, Un-Nessa and Kausar). Women do not traditionally have a family name or share a last name with their husbands, fathers or children.
  - Most **South Asian Muslim men** traditionally have a religious name (the most sacred are Mohammed, Allah and -Ullah). The religious name usually comes first (except -Ullah, the form of Allah which follows another name). The religious name is often regarded as the most important part of the name. Among South Asian Muslims the religious name should **never** be used alone.

Everyone also has a personal name. This usually comes second. The religious name and the personal name are generally used together in formal situations; in some cases separating them makes nonsense of the name. Many men have only these two names. Some men have a two-part personal name instead of or as well as a religious name; again these parts should not be separated.

Some men have another name, which usually comes last but may sometimes come first. This may be a male title (eg Miah), or a clan or village name (eg Chaudry, Khan, Ansari) or their father's first name. These names are sometimes shared with other male members of the family but this is a matter of family custom and personal choice. Because clan and village names are male names, they are not traditionally used by women.

Table 30.2 Example of a Pakistani family using the traditional naming system

Family member	Name
Husband	Abdul Rahman
Wife	Fatma Jan
Sons	Mohammed Ra'uf
	Mohammed Riasa
	Mohammed Rashid
Daughters	Salamet Bibi
	Mehr-un-Nessa

- The naming systems of **Muslims** in other parts of the world vary. For example, in **the Middle East** the personal name traditionally comes first, usually followed by the father's and paternal grandfather's personal names, and then, sometimes, by a family name. Women use the same system. They do not, traditionally, change their names when they marry. It is perfectly acceptable to use Muhammad, alone or with another name, as the personal name of a Middle Eastern Muslim man. Traditional polite usage is title plus first name, first two names, or first plus family name (if there is one).
- In the **traditional Somali naming system** everyone has a personal name, which comes first, followed by their father's personal name, then their paternal grandfather's personal name, then their paternal great-grandfather's personal name and so on. Some people know their paternal lineage for up to 25 generations.

  Most people, however, use only the first two or three names for day-to-day purposes. Women retain their own names on marriage. Children are given a personal name, followed by their father's and paternal grandfather's personal names as outlined above. Thus Shadia, the daughter of Ibrahim and granddaughter of Osman is called Shadia Ibrahim Osman. Her husband is Mohammed (his personal name) Abdullahi (his father's personal name) Omar (his paternal grandfather's personal name). Their son Hamza's name is Hamza Mohammed Abdullahi.

  In the traditional system there is therefore no last name linking a married couple or their child. In the West, some Somali people adopt their father's or husband's second or third name as a family surname to try to fit in. Mohammed Omar Abdullahi's wife thus may become Shadia Omar and or Shadia Abdullahi, their son Hamza Omar or Hamza Abdullahi. Somalis who are unfamiliar with the British records system may not realise the importance of a consistent 'surname'.

Women are more likely to stick to the traditional system. In addition, there is a high rate of marriage breakdown among Somalis in the UK (see also Chapter 40 *Traditional family structure and relationships*) and women who have adopted their husband's name to fit the British system are likely to revert to their own names when they separate or divorce.

It is generally acceptable to use title plus last name to address someone formally.

- The **traditional Sikh naming system** is based on a historical religious ruling that requires Sikhs not to use a family name. Instead, most Sikhs use only a first name plus a male title (Singh) or a female title (Kaur) (see Table 30.3). Devout Sikhs may find it unacceptable to use a family name. Most Sikh first names can be used for both men and women.

Table 30.3 Example of a Sikh family using the traditional naming system

Family member	Name
Husband	Kushwant Singh
Wife	Daljeet Kaur
Sons	Ranjeet Singh
	Jaswinder Singh
	Joginder Singh
Daughters	Dilvinder Kaur
	Davinder Kaur

- In the **traditional Greek Cypriot naming** system most people have two names. Some women use their husband's last name as a surname; some use their husband's first name instead. But the male name is traditionally changed to the female form, for example, the wife of Mr Marcos is Mrs Marcou, the wife of Andreas is Mrs Andreou.
- In the **traditional Turkish naming system** most people have two names: their personal name and their father's or husband's personal name. Women take their husband's first name as their last name when they marry. Children take their father's first name. The father does not, in the traditional system, share a last name with his wife or children.
- Most Hindu families in Britain originated in north-western India. In the **traditional Hindu naming system** used in this area, most people have three names: a personal name, a complementary name and a family name. Because most of the Hindu families in the UK originated in Gujarat, certain Gujarati family names, such as Patel, are very common.

The complementary name is always used with the personal name and does not stand alone. The most common female complementary names are Behn, Devi, Gowri, Kumari, Lakshmi and Rani. The most common male complementary names are Bhai, Chand, Das, Dev, Kant, Kumar, Lal, Nat and Pal. Occasionally, people's complementary names are changed, for example when they marry.

Men and unmarried women sometimes use their father's personal and complementary name as a middle name. Married women may use their husband's personal and complementary name (see Table 30.4).

Women traditionally take their husband's family name when they marry, and children use their father's family name. But the family name is not traditionally used when talking to people. Instead people may give only their first and their complementary names. Sometimes a complementary name is incorrectly recorded as a family name by someone unfamiliar with the Hindu naming system.

Table 30.4 Example of a Gujarati Hindu family using the traditional naming system

Family member	Name
Husband	Vijaykumar Jayantilal Patel
Wife	Lakshmidevi Vijaykumar Patel
Son	Subashbhai Vijaykumar Patel
Daughter	Neeshagowri Vijaykumar Patel

- The **Yoruba** and **Ibo (Nigerian)** naming systems are similar to the British one: each person has one or more personal names followed by a shared family name. Women take their husband's family name on marriage and the children take their father's family name.

A child's personal name may be chosen by senior family members. New parents in Britain may have to wait some time to hear from the family 'back home' before they can name their baby. In some communities several family members each give the child a name; some people may have nine or ten personal names. However, they are likely to use only two or three for official purposes. Many Nigerian Christians have a traditional Nigerian personal name and an 'English' personal name; for example, Mrs Ade Victoria Abosede. Some younger Nigerians associate English personal names with colonial rule and prefer to have two Nigerian personal names.

The Nigerian personal name always has special significance. Many are standard names to indicate position in the family or other characteristics. For example, in Yoruba tradition, the first set of twins in a family are always given the names Taiwo (the first baby) and Kahinde (the second) in addition to their other personal names. There are also special names for each of a second set of twins, for the third and fourth children born after twins, and for a child born after infertility problems. A child may also be given a name to indicate the return of the spirit of a person who has died. For example, Iyabode means 'mother who has come back' and may be given to the next baby girl born into a family after the death of the grandmother.

Because a person's first name is often a standard name, indicating their role or position, it may not be sufficient to identify them. It is important to record both personal names in full to prevent confusion in records etc. Traditionally, as a sign of respect, a younger person never addresses an older Nigerian person by their personal name. Once a woman becomes a mother she is called Mama followed by the name of her first child. For example, a woman who names her daughter Sarah will be called Mama Sarah. Younger people may address people who are only a few years older (including health professionals) as Auntie or Uncle. They may use the titles Brother and Sister for their older siblings.

In some Nigerian families, therefore, younger people do not know their parents' personal names and the parents may not wish them to. It is important to find out how each person wants to be addressed, particularly in the presence of younger family members. Some accept the widespread modern English practice of using personal names on almost all occasions, others prefer not to (see also Chapter 9 *Names*). If in doubt, it is safest and most respectful to use title plus family name. It is customary and polite to address an older Nigerian man as Sir.

Spelling

English spelling is complicated and offers many ways of indicating the same sound. However, there is a limited range of conventional spellings for common British names (eg Taylor or Tailor but not Tayllor). The same does not apply to names that have been transliterated from other alphabets. A search in one set of hospital records, for example, found 15 ways of spelling the South Asian Muslim name that is pronounced K'reshi and is normally written in the Arabic script. These included Qureshi, Kuraishi, Kureshi, Qurayshi, Qrashi, Qureschi and Qurraishy; all were attempts to write down the sound correctly, but filed in different places. Some languages have sounds that English does not have; it is then impossible to spell the name in English in a way that indicates its correct pronunciation.

Because there is no single correct spelling for transliterated names, a name may be spelt in different ways on different documents. Asking people for passports to help sort out the problem is more likely to damage relationships and to make them feel that they are being checked up on than to provide a definitive spelling, since the passport reflects only one possible way of spelling the name. In some cases a name has been misspelt by the official who issued the document.

Dates of birth

Birthdays and their celebration are an extremely important part of modern Western culture, and a person's date of birth is part of their official identity, used as a way of double-checking records. But in many cultures birthdays are not traditionally celebrated. In less bureaucratised countries, births and deaths are not always registered, or have not been until recently. People born in these countries may never have had their date of birth recorded and may not know it. They may also not realise that their date of birth matters for British records and that they must give a consistent date of birth in all official situations.

Many people who are required to give a date of birth but do not know it, choose, for ease of memory, the first of January of the year in which they were, or think they were, born. As a result, there may be a large number of patients whose 'date of birth' is January 1st. Health professionals do not always understand this.

> 'One midwife, in all innocence, remarked how surprising it was that "all these women" are born [on January 1st]. This reflects how incomprehensible it is to Western people that someone should not know their birthday; it is more likely [to them] that a high percentage of Asian women should be born on the same day.' (Bowler 1993)

Changing names and adopting a family name

Many people change their names to try to fit in with the British system once they realise that the British records system requires a consistent, identifiable last name. But for most of us our name is part of our identity and culture. People are often very reluctant to change their names, especially if the new name sounds wrong, offensive or silly to them.

People whose name does not include a shared family last name have the greatest problems in relation to the British records system. To try to fit in, some women use their husband's last name as a British-style surname. (Occasionally they are simply assigned their husband's last name by a clerical officer or health professional.) But in some naming systems there is no suitable 'surname' available. Simply adopting or assigning the husband's or father's last name as a surname may be unhelpful in terms of identification. Sometimes it is unacceptable:

- If a Bangladeshi woman whose husband's 'last name' is the male title, Miah, adopts this as a surname, she becomes Mrs Miah, equivalent to Mrs Mister. This is both ridiculous and not helpful for identification. Similarly, many Sikh women object to being called Mrs Singh.
- If Fatma Jan, in Table 30.2 above, adopts or is given her husband's last name, Rahman (in fact his personal name) she becomes Mrs Rahman. This is like calling the wife of John Brown, Mrs John. It may be unpleasant and unacceptable for many women, particularly in a community where gender differences are clearly delineated.

Practical problems and hostility From a practical point of view, changing one's name is not always easy. For example, Leung Kar-Po, who is Chinese, changed her name to Kar-Po Leung, so that her family name now comes last, fitting in with the conventions of the British naming system. But she was not able to explain what she was doing, and ended up with several unconnected sets of records, some under Po and others under Leung.

People who try to change their names often encounter suspicion and hostility, especially if they are members of black or ethnic minorities or speak little English. Their legal status in Britain may be questioned if their documents contain different names.

In some families, some members have changed their names and adopted a British-style surname, others have not. For example, in some Sikh families some members use a family surname. For other family members this may be out of the question on religious grounds (see Chapter 48 *Guru Gobind Singh*). In South Asian Muslim families it may be more acceptable for the sons to take on their father's personal name as a surname than for the wife and daughters. In some families, members born in the UK are registered under a family surname, overseas-born members are not.

Recording people's names correctly

With so many variations in naming systems, health professionals cannot rely on everyone producing a personal first name, a final surname and a date of birth. It is essential to record enough information to enable records to be retrieved with absolute accuracy, and to ensure that the patient is always addressed in a way that is recognisable and acceptable to them (see *Addressing people correctly*, below).

Recording the name

For each patient, ask:

- What is your full name?
- What would you like us to call you?

In each case it is very important to note the full name. Identify the personal name and the family name, if there is one. If there is no family name, identify a 'key name' under which you will file the patient's records. This will almost always be the last name. Explain to the patient, if necessary, the importance of giving this name in all contacts with the health service. If the key name is a title or is very common in your area you may need to record extra identifying information. For example, it may be helpful to note, purely for records, the names of other family members:

Fatma Jan (wife of Abdul Rahman)

Mohammed Ra'uf (son of Abdul Rahman)

Salamet Bibi (daughter of Abdul Rahman)

When a name is 'wrong'

Sometimes health professionals who are familiar with other naming systems recognise that a patient's name is clearly wrong in traditional terms. It is then important to find out whether the name has been mis-recorded by mistake and should be altered, or if this is now the patient's accepted official name for records. Some people whose names became altered by mistake have come to terms with the new form of their name and now use it in all contacts with health and other services. Others find the altered name unacceptable and do not use it, especially if it goes against the conventions of their own naming system.

In such a complicated situation it is important not to be too purist – for example, refusing to accept a name that appears to be the result of earlier misunderstandings. **The important thing for records is consistency.** In some cases, a patient may need sympathetic help with sorting out different names in their different records.

Developing appropriate computer systems

Once a name has been recorded correctly, make sure that it is used correctly on all records, notes and labels with the key name clearly indicated. It may be necessary to redesign forms to provide extra spaces and to alter computer programmes to provide sufficient fields to help identify individuals with different naming systems. For example, booking forms, notes and computer packages could be amended as shown in Figure 30.1.

FULL NAME

Preferred form of address

File under **(key name)**

NAME OF NEXT OF KIN (incl. relationship to patient)

Figure 30.1 Sample form for recording patients' names correctly

Computer-generated material In the British naming system, where the most important names come last and first, it is common on labels and letters to omit middle names or reduce them to initials. Sometimes only title, one initial and last name are used. In some naming systems this can cause serious confusion, especially when the last name is a title or a very common name and the middle name is the key identifier. If the three sons of Abdul Rahman in Table 30.2 (above) use the second part of their father's name, Rahman, as a family name, their key identifying name will be lost if their 'middle names' are reduced to initials. They will all be Mohammed R. Rahman. In South Asian culture it is also unacceptable to use Mohammed alone to address someone.

Computer programmes that generate letters and labels must be modified to ensure that patients' vital identifying information is not lost and that names are used acceptably.

Addressing people correctly

'When I go to the doctor and a name is called I watch to see if anyone else moves. If no one else gets up, then I go and ask if it's me they've called. Otherwise I could sit there all morning and never find out. People are always getting the wrong bit of your name, or pronouncing it so you can't recognise it.'
Vietnamese patient (Mares 1982)

Differences in how names are used often cause problems and frustration to both patients and professionals. Not everyone can be addressed by Mr or Mrs plus their last name. For example, with patients whose last name is a title, such as Singh, Kaur, Begum or Miah, the traditional British system of address, Mr Singh, Mrs Kaur, Mrs Begum or Mr Miah, is meaningless. Even if a woman does not mind being called Mrs Kaur, her husband or her son are certainly never Mr Kaur.

It is important to note how to address each person correctly. As a general rule, it is safest and most courteous to use the full name until you have had an opportunity to ask the person. Do not use the first name alone unless you have checked that this is acceptable. In some cases, the first name is not the personal name or cannot be used alone. In some cases people use a nickname or a shortened form of their first name and feel very uncomfortable being addressed by their official first name. With older people in particular, the automatic use of first or personal names in institutions can increase the effect of creating a kind of second childhood and lower their status.

If a name is pronounced very differently from the way it is spelt, note the correct pronunciation in brackets. Underline the stressed syllable(s) if necessary.

Jahanara Bibi (Jahanara Bibi – use full name)

Dilvinder Kaur (Dilvinder Kor – use full name)

Lew Sapieha (Leff Sapiayha – Mr Sapieha)

Mohammed Yunus Miah (Muhamad Yoonus Meeah – use full name, or first two names together)

Cheung-Ng Wai-Yung (Use Mrs Ng or full name)

Shahida Begum Ditta (Shaheeda Baygum Ditta – use full name or first two names, not Mrs Ditta)

References

Ahmad WIU (1989) Policies, pills and political will: a critique of policies to improve the health of ethnic minorities. *Lancet* **1**: 148–50

Ahmed G, Watt S (1986) Understanding Asian women in pregnancy and confinement. *Midwives Chronicle and Nursing Notes* **99** (May): 98–101

Ahmed S, Valentine S, Shire S (1982) Translation is at best an echo. *Community Care* **22** (Apr): 19–21

Argyle M (1975) *Bodily Communication.* International Universities Press, New York

Audit Commission (1993) *What Seems to be the Matter: Communication between hospitals and patients*, National Health Service Report No 12. Stationery Office, London

BHAN (1991) *AIDS and the Black Communities.* Black HIV/AIDS Network, London

Bowler I (1993) Stereotypes of women of Asian descent in midwifery: some evidence. *Midwifery* **9**: 7–16

Bowling S (1990) *Elderly People from Ethnic Minorities: A report on four projects.* Age Concern Institute of Gerontology/Kings College, London

Buchanan M (1995) Enabling patients to make informed decisions. *Nursing Times* **91** (18): 27–31

City and Hackney CHC (1988) *Experiments in Health Advocacy.* City and Hackney Community Health Council, London

Collett P (1993) *Foreign Bodies: A guide to European mannerisms.* Simon and Schuster, London

Consumer Congress Trust (1996) *Now We're Talking: A report setting out how public services in London are breaking through the language barrier, and pointing the way ahead.* Consumer Congress Trust, 20 Grosvenor Gardens, London SW1 0DH

Crawford H (1997) Patient information for pain control in palliative care. *Nursing Standard* **11** (48): 42–4

Currer C (1986) *Health Concepts and Illness Behaviour: The care of Pathan mothers in Bradford* (unpublished PhD thesis). Department of Sociology, University of Warwick, Warwick

d'Ardenne P, Mahtani A (1989) *Transcultural Counselling in Action.* Sage, London

DoH (1996) NHS: *The patient's charter and you.* Department of Health, London

Ebden P, Bhatt A, Carey OJ, Harrison B (1988) The bilingual consultation. *Lancet* 1: 347

Fisher R, Brown S (1989) *Getting Together: Building a relationship that gets to yes.* Century Hutchinson, London

Furnham A, Bochner S (1990) *Culture Shock: Psychological reactions to unfamiliar environments.* Routledge, London

Haroon-Iqbal H (1994) *Palliative Care Service use by Black and Minority Ethnic Groups in Leicester.* Leicestershire Health Trust, Leicester

HEA (1994) *Health and Lifestyles: Black and minority ethnic groups in England.* Health Education Authority, London

Hilton C (1997) Global perspectives: a sensitive view. *Elderly Care* 8 (6): 12–15

Homans H, Satow A (1982) Can you hear me? Cultural variations in communication. *Journal of Community Nursing* Jan: 16–18

Kagawa-Singer M (1987) Ethnic perspectives of cancer nursing: Hispanics and Japanese Americans. *Oncology Nurse Forum* 14 (3): 59–65

Kahin M (1997) *Educating Somali Children in Britain.* Trentham Books, Stoke-on-Trent

Khan S (1994) *Contexts: Race, culture and sexuality.* NAZ Project, Pallingswick House, 241 King Street, London W6 9LP

Lago C, Thompson J (1996) *Race, Culture and Counselling.* Open University Press, Buckingham

Leather C, Wirz S (1996) *The Training and Development Needs of Bilingual Support Workers in the NHS in Community Settings.* Centre for Child Health/Department of Health, London

Li P-L (1992) Health needs of the Chinese population. In WIU Ahmad (ed) *The Politics of 'Race' and Health.* University of Bradford, Bradford, pp 105–16

Lomax B (1997) Learning to understand a patient's silence. *Nursing Times* 93 (17): 48–9

Lovell S (1990) *Health in any Language*. North East Thames Regional Health Authority, London

Mares P (1982) *The Vietnamese in Britain: A handbook for health workers*. National Extension College, Cambridge

Mares P, Henley A, Baxter C (1985) *Health Care in Multiracial Britain*. National Extension College, Cambridge

Masi R (1992) Communication: cross-cultural applications of the physician's art. *Canadian Family Physician* May: 1159–65

Modood T, Berthoud R, Lakey J, Nazroo J, Smith P, Virdee S, Beishon S (1997) *Ethnic Minorities in Britain: Diversity and disadvantage*. Policy Studies Institute, London

Morain GG (1986) Kinesics and cross-cultural understanding. In JM Valdes (ed) *Culture Bound: Bridging the cultural gap in language teaching*. Cambridge University Press, Cambridge

Murphy K, Macleod Clark J (1993) Nurses' experience of caring for ethnic minority clients. *Journal of Advanced Nursing* 18: 442–50

Naish J, Brown J, Denton B (1994) Intercultural consultation: investigation of factors that deter non-English speaking women from attending their general practitioners for cervical screening. *British Medical Journal* 309: 1126–8

Parsons L, Day S (1992) Improving obstetric outcomes in ethnic minorities: an evaluation of health advocacy. *Journal of Public Health Medicine* 14 (2): 183–91

Pellegrino ED (1992) Is truth telling to the patient a cultural artefact? *Journal of the American Medical Association* 268 (13): 1734–5

Pharoah C (1995) *Primary Health Care for Elderly People from Black and Minority Ethnic Communities*. Age Concern Institute of Gerontology/Department of Health/Stationery Office, London

Rack P (1991) *Race, Culture and Mental Disorder*. Routledge, London

RCN and BAAEM (British Association for Accident and Emergency Medicine) (1995) *Bereavement Care in A & E Departments: Report of a working group*. Royal College of Nursing, London

RCP (1997) *Improving Communication between Doctors and Patients*. Royal College of Physicians, London

Roberts C (1985) *The Interview Game and How it's Played*. BBC Publications, London

Rocheron Y, Dickinson R (1990) The Asian Mother and Baby Campaign: a way forward in health promotion for Asian women? *Health Education Journal* 49 (3): 128–33

Rogers J (1989) *Adults Learning.* Open University, Buckingham

Sami AR (1989) Eye, eye [letter]. *British Medical Journal* **298**: 1523

Shackman J (1984) *The Right to be Understood: A handbook on working with, employing and training community interpreters.* Available from Jane Shackman, 28 The Butts, Chippenham, Wilts, SN15 3JT

Slater M (1993) *Health for All our Children: Achieving appropriate health care for black and minority ethnic children and their families.* Action for Sick Children/National Association for the Welfare of Children in Hospital, London

South Glamorgan Race Equality Council (1994) *Towards a Good Old Age?* South Glamorgan Race Equality Council and South Glamorgan Social Services Department, Cardiff

Stewart EC, Bennett MJ (1991) *American Cultural Patterns: A cross-cultural perspective.* Intercultural Press, Yarmouth ME

Tang M (1994) *Vietnamese Refugees: Towards a healthy future.* Deptford City Challenge, c/o UK Programme Department, Save the Children, Cambridge House, Cambridge Grove, London W6 0LE

Tannen D (1992) *That's Not What I Meant.* Virago, London

Tannen D (1991) *You Just Don't Understand: Women and men in conversation.* Virago, London

Walker G (1997) Give it straight to the patients. *Hospital Doctor* 22 May: 48

Warrier S (1995) *Consumer Empowerment: An evaluation of linkworker and advocacy services for non-English speaking users of maternity services.* Maternity Alliance, London

Watson P (1986) Towers of Babel. *Nursing Times* 3 Dec: 40–1

Windsor-Richards K, Gillies P (1988) Racial grouping and women's experience of giving birth in hospital. *Midwifery* **4**: 171-6

PART FOUR
Specific Health Issues

• •

This section examines a few key health issues that have special relevance to certain religious and ethnic minority groups or which affect them in particular ways.

31 Other medical systems

Although allopathic Western medicine is generally held in high regard, for many people it is not the primary or sole source of information on how to maintain health, nor the only system that they turn to when they are ill. Many people use other medical systems and consult other practitioners instead of or as well as allopathic medical practitioners.

Historically, Western medicine has generally viewed other medical systems and approaches to health care with suspicion and scepticism. Ahmad (1992) points out that there has been a tendency to use value-laden language (such as, for example, 'folk' or 'traditional' medicine) in discussions about other systems and practitioners, especially those that originated outside Europe. Nevertheless, in many Western countries there has recently been a dramatic growth in the use of what are more acceptably called complementary and/or alternative medical systems. These include homoeopathy, herbalism, osteopathy, acupuncture and aromatherapy, as well as other medical systems with their origins in the Caribbean, the Far East and South Asia. One attraction of complementary and alternative systems can be the more personal and detailed holistic approach taken by many practitioners. (For more details about specific systems, see Chapters 37, 38 and 41.)

'There are implicit assumptions that Western medicine is rational, scientific and safe ... But these assumptions are not beyond criticism.' (Ahmad 1992)

Other medical systems and minority groups

Systems of diagnosis and treatment vary throughout the world. Ideas about the maintenance of health and the treatment of illness are handed down from generation to generation and often maintained when people migrate. Most people prefer the system that they are used to and which offers methods that they regard as tried and tested. Each system also influences the way people think about the body and its functions, and their beliefs about illness and treatment.

Many people, especially older people, use self-prescribed home remedies and tonics based on herbs and other substances for minor symptoms. These may be in the form of tablets, capsules, powders, poultices, teas or soups. Some also use self-prescribed dietary remedies (see also Chapter 11 *Food and illness*). People are particularly likely to turn to complementary or alternative systems for intractable illnesses, for conditions that they feel are not treated or recognised in Western medicine, or where they do not know of a Western over-the-counter equivalent. Some may also prefer to consult a complementary or alternative practitioner of their own community if they speak little or no English, especially on matters that are embarrassing or difficult to explain. Some may take complementary or alternative remedies in conjunction with pharmaceutical preparations.

Benefits and risks

Although few complementary or alternative remedies have been scientifically evaluated, many people experience benefits from them. Some have ingredients similar to their Western equivalents. There is a growing interest in complementary and alternative remedies among Western pharmaceutical companies, many of which send researchers to other parts of the world to identify effective remedies and to isolate the active ingredients.

Despite the undoubted value of many complementary and alternative remedies, there can sometimes be problems. People whose first choice is a complementary or alternative medical system may delay seeking advice from a Western doctor until their disease is well advanced. Some medicines can be toxic (Graham-Brown 1992, Penharic, Walton and Murray 1992). Some interact with certain Western medication and cause unexpected and often unrecognised problems (Atherton 1994, Healy and Aslam 1989).

In addition, because most complementary and alternative medical systems are not regulated, the contents, packaging and labelling are not always standardised. Ingredients may not be listed at all, may be incomplete, or may be written in languages that health professionals in Britain cannot read. Some herbal medicines contain a number of different plants, each of which may contain up to 30 active ingredients. Some contain plant toxins, toxic minerals or chemicals. Some contain additional drugs that are available only on prescription in the UK or have been withdrawn from sale.

Implications for practice

It is important not to assume that all complementary and alternative medicines are harmful or ineffective. However, if a patient deteriorates unexpectedly, or develops signs and symptoms that cannot be explained, it may be helpful to consider the possibility of adverse reactions or toxicity from complementary or alternative remedies. It is important not to make any assumptions about who is or is not likely to be taking such remedies.

Finding out if a person is taking complementary or alternative medication requires tact and sensitivity. Many patients and families are reluctant to tell health professionals. Some do not realise that it may be important. Others realise that they are likely to meet with disapproval and criticism. Many find it impossible to believe that what they are taking could be harmful, especially if they and their family have been using similar remedies all their lives. Indeed, they may have chosen a complementary or alternative system because they know that allopathic treatments and medicines sometimes produce severe side effects and adverse reactions.

Simply telling people never to take complementary or alternative remedies is usually counter-productive, especially if they have always used them. Rather than giving the impression that you consider all complementary or alternative medicine harmful, it may be more helpful to explain tactfully why you are concerned in this particular case. People are also more likely to be open about taking complementary or alternative medication if, from the beginning, they have experienced respectful and non-judgemental care from those looking after them, and their individual cultural and religious needs have been met.

Identifying contents

If the patient has had an adverse reaction, samples can be sent for analysis to the Traditional Medicine Surveillance Group (see below). A complete daily dose should be sent, ideally accompanied by the packaging, the written prescription, the practitioner's name and address, the source of the ingredients, details of the dose and duration of use. If a patient is taking unlabelled medication, or if there is reason to think that the contents list is incomplete, ask for permission to contact the practitioner who prescribed it in order to find out what it contains.

Useful address

The Traditional Medicine Surveillance Group
Medical Toxicology Unit
Guy's and St Thomas' Hospital NHS Trust
Avonley Road
London SE14 5ER
Tel. 0171-635 9191 or 0171-955 5095

Provides specialist information to the medical profession.

32 Female circumcision – female genital mutilation

Female circumcision is increasingly known as female genital mutilation (FGM) because:

- it involves removing healthy tissue;
- it has no health benefits;
- in its more radical forms it results in significant long-term morbidity.

It is estimated that over 100 million girls and women throughout the world have been genitally mutilated (RCN 1994).

FGM in varying degrees is common in half the countries of Africa, particularly across central Africa from west to east. In some African countries it is traditionally carried out on all women, in others it is performed on fewer than 5 per cent. FGM is also practised to some extent in a few areas of the Middle East and south-east Asia (Hosken 1994, Jordan 1993). It is not practised in Saudi Arabia. In countries where FGM is traditional, many members of the educated elite are abandoning it (Hedley and Dorkenoo 1992). Nevertheless, in many communities there are powerful beliefs that reinforce the value and benefits of FGM (see below).

What does FGM involve?

There are three types of FGM:

- Removal of the clitoral hood. This is the only type that can correctly be called circumcision.
- Excision of the clitoris and part or all of the labia minora (clitoridectomy).
- Infibulation, the most extensive form of FGM in which the clitoris and the labia minora are removed. The labia majora are reduced and then stitched together, leaving a small opening so that urine and menstrual fluid can escape. Occasionally infibulation is performed over an intact clitoris.

FGM is carried out on babies or young girls, usually before the onset of puberty, often by older women or traditional birth attendants. In certain communities, FGM marks a girl's transition to womanhood. It is usually done without anaesthetic, using a range of implements that are often unsterilised. Surgery under such conditions carries a considerable risk of infection, haemorrhage, damage to surrounding organs and even death. Even the less severe forms of mutilation can cause heavy scarring, especially if there have been additional infections (Ladjali, Rattray and Walder 1993).

Infibulation also causes numerous long-term medical problems. A woman who has been infibulated may be left with an orifice no bigger than the diameter of a pencil. As a result, it can take some women up to 20 minutes to empty their bladders, leaving them prone to recurrent pelvic and urinary tract infections and often with irregular, prolonged and painful periods. Women who have undergone infibulation may also suffer from keloid scarring, cysts and abscesses. Intercourse is impossible. When they marry, some women may have to be cut open to make intercourse possible. This may result in infection.

'Some women would rather be divorced than have to have sexual intercourse.'
Somali woman

Infibulation can also cause major obstetric problems. These include prolonged and difficult labour, possibly leading to fetal brain damage and even fetal death. Women may require an episiotomy to allow the baby to be born and this can damage the urethra, rectum and perineum. Infertility may also be a problem, due to persistent infections.

The law

Under the Prohibition of Circumcision Act 1985, it is illegal to perform FGM in Britain (Jordan 1994). Performing FGM is punishable by a fine or imprisonment. Nevertheless, the practice is known to continue. In some cases girls are taken abroad for FGM to be carried out. In 1993 the French courts convicted and imprisoned a woman who paid for her two daughters to be circumcised, and a man who ordered his wives to circumcise their daughters.

Infibulation is also illegal in the UK. Consequently, complete repair of the vulva after birth so that it is restored to its infibulated state is illegal (Schott and Henley 1996, Jordan 1993).

Understanding why

FGM is deeply embedded in certain cultures. It is believed to ensure chastity and sexual continence, to be more aesthetic and hygienic, and to make women pure and marriageable. In some languages the word for female circumcision means purification, cleaning or ablution. In certain communities it is commonly believed that if a woman is not circumcised her clitoris will grow and block her vagina. In some other communities the clitoris is seen as a male organ that must be removed for a woman to become truly female (McConville 1998). Women who have not undergone FGM may be unable to find a husband in a society in which marriage is highly desirable and may also be their only option. They may be assumed to be promiscuous and sexually voracious, and excluded from their community.

FGM continues because people feel it is the right thing to do and because they want their daughters and granddaughters to be marriageable, acceptable and happy in their own community. Many see FGM as a positive and normal part of their heritage and identity. In some communities, young women who have not undergone FGM may feel abnormal, unattractive and ashamed.

'Circumcision is honoured in our homeland. We do it because we love and cherish our daughters. When people talk about abuse and mutilation I feel confused and very full of pain.'
Egyptian woman

Many people also cite religious requirements as a reason for performing FGM. A few Muslim scholars argue that Islam requires FGM, though it is not practised in the Middle Eastern Muslim states and is known to pre-date Islam (Dorkenoo and Elworthy 1994). In Egypt, the Sudan and some other countries it is also practised by Christians, and in sub-Saharan Africa by Animists as well. However, there is increasing awareness in some communities, for example in the Somali community, that FGM is a local cultural tradition rather than an Islamic requirement. There is no reference to female circumcision in the Qur'an, the Muslim holy book, nor in the Christian Bible.

In some countries midwives and doctors are now trained to perform FGM. The rationale for this is that health professionals working in hygienic conditions are much safer and less likely to cause either immediate or long-term damage to women than traditional practitioners. Opponents of this view, including the World Health Organization, argue that this practice institutionalises FGM and seems to justify it, thus making eradication more difficult.

FGM and implications for care

Physical examination

It is important not to subject women who have or might have undergone FGM to repeated questioning about it or to physical examination. However, in some cases it is important for staff to know in advance. In such cases, the degree of mutilation should be assessed and an agreed plan for care recorded.

If a woman has been infibulated, it will be difficult or impossible to perform any examination or procedure via the urethra or vagina. Women who have undergone any form of FGM are very likely to be embarrassed about exposing their genitals, especially in a society that openly disapproves of what has been done to them. Women may also be unwilling to be examined by male doctors for religious or cultural reasons (see also Chapter 13 *Modesty and physical examination*). In addition, many women who have undergone FGM are extremely frightened about having to open their legs and being touched during vulval or vaginal examination, as this can evoke terrifying flashbacks of being mutilated. It is therefore very important to build a calm, trusting relationship beforehand, to minimise the number of examinations and always to give careful explanation about what will and will not be done. It is essential to be gentle and understanding if a woman is reluctant, resists examination or finds it difficult to co-operate. If she does not speak English, a female professional interpreter must be available.

Women in communities where FGM is practised are often concerned that medical students and student nurses might be called in during examinations 'to have a look'. Some have heard stories of women being photographed during examination for research purposes. Such fears add to women's reluctance and fear of examination. Properly informed consent must be obtained before any non-essential staff are allowed to be present, and before any action is taken that does not directly benefit the woman.

Personal hygiene

Women who need help with personal hygiene should be treated with sensitivity and respect to avoid adding to any feelings of humiliation and distress. As with any other patient, ask how the woman wishes to be washed and what help she needs after using a bedpan, commode or toilet.

Language

Many people find it embarrassing and difficult to discuss the parts of the body involved in FGM. They may not know acceptable words even in their own language (see Chapter 27 *Translating words*). The Western term 'female genital mutilation' may not be understood and is also insulting to many people who firmly believe that the practice is benign and valuable. It is important that health professionals use language that is respectful and does not insult individuals, their culture or traditions. In English it is generally respectful to use the terms circumcised and circumcision with patients.

Managing negative reactions

Health professionals are often deeply shocked or disgusted on finding that a woman has undergone FGM. Some convey this to women in their care.

'I am appalled by some of the things health professionals say to women who have had FGM. After all, it is not her fault this was done to her. We don't express shock, horror or disgust when we see a grossly obese woman even if we do have strong views about her size and the implications for her health.'
Irish gynaecologist

It is unacceptable for women who have undergone FGM to be treated in any way differently or seen as oddities. Their feelings and self-respect should be considered at all times.

'We know that people here think that it is wrong and we are beginning to see that it is not a good idea. But all the publicity is terrible for us. Every time someone looks at us in the street we feel as though they are wondering what our genitals look like. It is very humiliating.'
Somali refugee worker and mother of five

It is most important that health professionals give every woman sensitive and respectful care. Those who are understandably distressed by what they see need to postpone their reactions and to deal with their feelings in a confidential setting, well away from the women they care for (see also Chapter 8 *Managing negative reactions*).

Breaking the cycle

In the UK, 10,000 girls are estimated to be at risk of FGM (Dorkenoo and Elworthy 1993).

There is much debate on how to end the practice. Although it is illegal both to perform FGM and to ask someone else to perform it, it will take time to stop a practice that is deeply rooted in culture and history. Many health professionals and others hesitate to encroach on cultural practices and fear being seen as interfering or racist. Some believe that a non-confrontational approach puts them in a better position to inform women about the law, where appropriate, and to help women realise how their daughters will benefit both physically and psychologically if they remain intact. Others believe that encouragement and education are too difficult and too slow. They believe that FGM must be stopped immediately by prosecuting those responsible, even at the risk of antagonising the communities concerned and driving the practice further underground.

Encouragement and sensitive support from outsiders can help those people within communities that practise FGM to stand out against it. In contrast, self-righteous statements and ethnocentric condemnation from outside are more likely to increase communities' defensiveness and feelings of injustice and so to be counter-productive. Community leaders and women them-selves need to decide that FGM should stop. This is already happening among some groups of African women.

For individual parents, the decision not to carry out FGM can be very dif-ficult. They need strength and courage to believe that their uncircumcised daughters will not become lonely, stigmatised outcasts. They have to with-stand family and social pressures to do with cleanliness, womanliness and morality. In the West, some parents may feel that it is even more important to maintain the practice of FGM because of the 'flagrant sexual behaviour' of Western youth (Hussein 1995).

> 'Female circumcision is our tradition, part of our history and our way of life. We have always done it. If our community rejects it simply because outsiders say we should, we may be once again giving up our birthright for the illusory promises of Westernisation. Economic and cultural imperialism have damaged us severely in the past; we have learnt not to trust all those Europeans who come and tell us what to do. We have to think very carefully about their moti-vation and be sure before we act.'
> Ghanaian woman

In addition, a mother who thinks through the reasons for not allowing her daughter to undergo FGM is likely to have to face the enormity of what she herself has experienced. Psychologically, this is asking a great deal. FGM is carried out at the request of parents and is sometimes performed by an aunt or a grandmother. Although the motives are clearly very different, coming to terms with FGM can be compared to trying to come to terms with the experience of incestuous abuse and family violence.

Parents who are caught between strong tradition and a growing awareness of the long-term trauma that FGM can cause need continuing help and support. Health professionals can have the greatest impact if they understand the cultural and historical bases of FGM and the dilemma that faces individuals in communities where FGM is practised. (For more information about initiatives in Britain contact FORWARD – see below.)

Useful address

FORWARD
(Foundation for Women's Health and Development)
38 King Street
London WC2 8JT

Works to raise awareness of female genital mutilation, and offers support and counselling to those who are affected by it.

33 Haemoglobinopathies

The haemoglobinopathies are a group of autosomal, recessive, inherited disorders of haemoglobin. The most common are sickle cell disease and thalassaemia. There are mild and severe forms of both conditions. In the UK, the haemoglobinopathies mainly affect black and minority ethnic groups. However, no specific haemoglobinopathy is confined to a single ethnic group. As more and more people have mixed heritages, the distribution of the haemoglobinopathies is likely to increase.

Health service provision

Although there have been significant numbers of people in Britain with thalassaemia and sickle cell disease for over 40 years, health services have been slow to acknowledge and respond to their needs. The number of people with haemoglobinopathies is similar to the numbers with cystic fibrosis or haemophilia, but haemoglobinopathy services are more haphazard and less well funded. Although treatment, screening and counselling are now good in some places, they are poor and patchy in others, especially where there are relatively few black and minority ethnic people (Streetly, Maxwell and Mejia 1997). Inadequate resources and provision, as well as lack of information and training among health and other professionals, mean that patients who are having an acute sickle crisis or who need a blood transfusion are not always treated appropriately or sympathetically. The counselling, information and support that they and their families need are often lacking.

Many patients with haemoglobinopathies are members of already disadvantaged minorities. In addition to serious and sometimes fatal disease, they are more likely to experience poverty, poor housing, discrimination in employment and racial hostility (see also Chapter 5 *The effects of racism*) (Department of Health 1993, Davies 1986). They often live in areas where health, social services and other resources are most stretched.

Support for families

The physical, practical and emotional consequences of loving someone who has a haemoglobinopathy are enormous. Every family member has to adjust emotionally, and to learn how to help and support the person with the condition. Parents of affected children commonly feel shocked, guilty, angry, fearful, helpless and ashamed (Sickle Cell Society, undated). Their difficulties are compounded if services are inadequate and if health professionals lack information and understanding (Eboh and Van den Akker 1994).

As with all hereditary conditions, there is sometimes a stigma against people who carry a haemoglobinopathy. People who do not have accurate information and who know nothing about genetic inheritance may also believe that haemoglobinopathies are infectious, or may put a child's illness down to inadequate parental care.

'We have been supporting a mother in a middle-class Bangladeshi family. She is living in a traditional household with her in-laws. Her one-year-old has beta-thalassaemia, which does not need regular treatment but does need careful monitoring. When he began to fail to thrive, the family blamed her for being a bad mother. They did not want to accept that it was a genetic disease that implicated the father as well as the mother. So the family held her entirely responsible.'
Haemoglobinopathy support worker

Stigma may limit the support available from the wider family network and from the community, and may make some people feel very isolated. Fear of stigma may lead some families to hide the fact that they have an affected member. Confidentiality is clearly very important.

'We know of two brothers who both have a child with sickle cell anaemia, but neither of them knows about the other. The children are treated at different hospitals and neither family wants anyone, including their extended family, to know that they have an affected child.'
Sickle Cell Society worker

Thalassaemia

Thalassaemia indicates either partial or no production of a globin chain that is vital to the structure of the haemoglobin in the red blood cells (Anionwu 1993).

Alpha-thalassaemia major

This is the most severe form of thalassaemia and is incompatible with life. The affected fetus develops hydrops fetalis and dies, usually during the second trimester.

The trait for alpha-thalassaemia major occurs in people of Chinese, Vietnamese, Cypriot, Greek and Middle Eastern heritages (Anionwu 1993, Department of Health 1993) and in people with south-east Asian or southern Chinese heritage

Beta-thalassaemia

A person with **beta-thalassaemia major** does not make enough of the beta-haemoglobin chain that is essential for the production of adult haemoglobin A. This results in a life-threatening haemolytic anaemia, which must treated with regular blood transfusions and with a chelating agent to prevent iron overload. People with beta-thalassaemia major are likely to have growth retardation and delayed puberty, and may be infertile. Without regular iron-chelating treatment, frequent blood transfusions lead to iron overload, which damages major organs such as the heart, liver, pancreas and pituitary gland. Frequent transfusions also increase the risk of infections such as hepatitis C. However, with early diagnosis and regular treatment, life expectancy in the industrialised countries is now about 40 years.

Carriers of beta-thalassaemia are sometimes described as having **beta-thalassaemia minor** or thalassaemia trait. They may have mild anaemia, which should not be treated with iron. Beta-thalassaemia trait occurs in varying rates among people of Cypriot and other Mediterranean, South Asian, southern Chinese, Vietnamese, Middle Eastern, West African and African-Caribbean heritages. It also occurs very rarely in people of white British heritage (Department of Health 1993).

Thalassaemia in Britain

There are about 600 people with beta-thalassaemia major in the UK (Department of Health 1993) and several thousand carriers. The main affected groups are the Cypriot community and certain South Asian communities. Levels of awareness and the uptake of premarital and antenatal screening are generally high in the Cypriot community, which is relatively small and concentrated (Anionwu 1993). As a result, although the carrier rate is high in this community, the number of babies born with beta-thalassaemia major is relatively small.

However, South Asian communities, which are considerably larger and spread more widely throughout the UK, are generally less well informed. Studies indicate that many South Asians know little about the disease and how it is inherited, or about the possibility of screening (UK Thalassaemia Society 1995, Anionwu 1993). This makes informed choice impossible and means that the shock of having an affected child is immense.

> 'It is really difficult to cope with a child with thalassaemia. When you know absolutely nothing about it beforehand it is a tremendous shock. Of course you love your child, but the illness affects the whole family. It's a whole lot of effort and heartache with nothing to show at the end. People need to know what it will be like so they can decide whether to go ahead or have a termination. Most people who have an affected child ask for screening in their next pregnancy and if the child is affected they have a termination.'
>
> Thalassaemia specialist

A campaign to raise awareness of thalassaemia among South Asians began in 1997 (UK Thalassaemia Society 1998). The purpose of the campaign was to begin discussion and debate among the South Asian communities. Because the concept of genetic disease is not well understood in some South Asian communities, the campaign explained genetic inheritance and encouraged screening, preferably before conception or at least antenatally so that people could make an informed choice about continuing with a pregnancy. The cultural and religious diversity within the South Asian communities meant that the campaign had to be targeted differently in different areas, and had to recognise that the choices that people might make about screening and termination would vary. The campaign also aimed to increase knowledge and awareness among health professionals and health and social policy makers.

Practical care

Identifying carriers People of reproductive age whose heritage indicates that they might carry thalassaemia should be offered screening and counselling before starting a family. There should be efficient and effective screening policies.

Treatment and provision for people with thalassaemia Treatment involves regular blood transfusions every three to six weeks, and subcutaneous administration of an iron-chelating agent via a syringe driver for six to eight hours continuously at least five or six nights every week. Regular chelation requires personal discipline and routine. It interferes with people's freedom and their ability to be spontaneous, and can cause practical as well as emotional stresses.

'When she got married one young woman decided to have her chelation treatment during the day rather than at night.'
Specialist nurse

Teenagers, in particular, may need special help and support to continue with regular iron-chelating treatment. The daily reminder that they are different from their peers can be hard to tolerate. Some get into the habit of skipping treatments and by the time this is discovered they may already have organ damage, sometimes irreparable.

'We make it very clear to them that they must have all their treatments even though at first they feel no ill effects from missing some of them. We show them their blood results and the results of any other tests we do so that they can see for themselves that missing treatments does matter and is affecting them.'
Thalassaemia specialist

Regular admission to hospital for transfusion is disruptive for the individual and for their family. People who do not live near a specialist centre have to spend additional time and money travelling, sometimes long distances, for treatment. Extra stress is caused if patients are cared for on general wards by staff who have little or no knowledge of thalassaemia and its effects, and if there are delays because nobody is available to set up the infusion.

Ideally, people with thalassaemia should be admitted to a dedicated unit so that they can gain support from others with the disease and can be cared for by specialist staff. Admission times should be flexible, offering treatment in the evening, overnight and at weekends so that patients' schooling, work and family life are disrupted as little as possible.

Sickle cell disease

Sickle cell disease (SCD) is among the most common inherited disorders in Britain. Streetly, Maxwell and Mejia (1997) report that there are about 10,000 people in the UK with SCD, of whom about 9,000 live in London. The national figure is projected to rise to 12,000 by the year 2011. In addition there are many thousands more who carry the trait (Anionwu 1994, NHS Management Executive 1994).

The different kinds of sickle cell disease include sickle cell anaemia, haemoglobin SC disease and sickle beta-thalassaemia, and can vary a good deal in their severity and symptoms. Sickle cell anaemia and one form of sickle beta-thalassaemia are usually the most severe.

SCD *carriers in different ethnic groups*

Sickle cell trait (Hb AS) occurs in varying rates in people of West African, African-Caribbean, Cypriot and other Mediterranean, South Asian and Middle Eastern heritages. C trait (Hb AC) occurs in varying rates in people of Ghanaian and African-Caribbean heritage. D trait (Hb AD) occurs in varying rates in people of Chinese, Cypriot and South Asian heritage and, very occasionally, in people of white British heritage (Department of Health 1993).

Sickle cell crises

Sickle cell disease is caused by an abnormality in the structure of the globin chain of red blood cells. This results in a tendency for the red blood cells to change temporarily into a spiked sickle shape when they are deprived of fluids or oxygen. The sickle-shaped cells block peripheral venous blood flow, causing venous occlusion and pain that is often excruciating. This is known as a sickle cell crisis. Between crises and when their pain is under control, most people with sickle cell disease remain well.

Sickle cell crises may be brought on by many factors, including infection, dehydration, fever, sudden changes in temperature, anaesthesia, acidosis, hypoxia and physical stress. They can be precipitated by physical factors often linked to poverty such as cold, an inadequate diet and the exertion of carrying shopping or children up several flights of stairs. Crises can also be caused by emotional stress to which incidents of racial hostility and discrimination may contribute.

Affected individuals can try to minimise the likelihood of crises by avoiding precipitating factors. However, sickling is often unpredictable. Some people go through long periods with few or no crises, and then periods with frequent, severe crises, for no apparent reason (Anionwu 1994).

Frequent painful crises requiring a lot of time off work may lead to unemployment: because they often seem well between crises, people with SCD are sometimes labelled lazy or exploitative. The provision of benefits to patients who are severely affected by SCD and who cannot work seems to be patchy and to depend on the level of information and the assumptions of the individual making the assessment (Sickle Cell Society, personal communication 1998).

In addition to painful sickle crises, people with the more severe forms of SCD may be grossly anaemic and are particularly vulnerable to infections. The cumulative effects of infections, persistent chronic anaemia and infarctions caused by sickle cell crises result in progressive organ damage and eventually in organ failure. Life expectancy is shortened, men living to an average of 40 years and women to 45 years. Children are at risk of strokes: the highest death rate due to SCD occurs in children under the age of five because of their susceptibility to infections, especially pneumococcal infections.

Practical care for people with sickle cell disease

Prophylactic antibiotics are given to children and some adults to reduce the incidence of pneumococcal infections. Pneumococcal infections are a major cause of death in early childhood. Some hospital units also give folic acid. Some patients require blood transfusions which, if they are frequent, must be combined with iron-chelating therapy.

Managing pain During a crisis, a patient urgently needs rest, support and reassurance, as well as warmth, fluids and analgesics of appropriate strength. Most people can manage painful crises at home and only go to hospital when they have tried everything and are desperate for help.

The best way of managing severe vaso-occlusive pain has not been established and more research is needed. Opiates are commonly used and some specialists advocate the use of approaches borrowed from the management of cancer pain (Davies and Oni 1997, Brookoff and Polomano 1992). However, a number of studies have shown that people with sickle cell crises are often thought to be exaggerating and so are given lower levels of pain relief than they need (Anionwu 1983). This may be due in part to prejudice against black and minority ethnic people and assumptions about high levels of drug abuse in black communities. It may also be because prescribing is based on the assumption that crises are short term, when in fact the pain may be due to irreversible infarction (Brookoff and Polomano 1992). Sometimes inadequate pain relief is given because health professionals find it hard to distinguish between the behaviour of people who are addicted to street drugs and that of people in severe, untreated pain.

'While the addict takes the drug to get "high" and largely to avoid life, the patient with pain takes the drug to get on with living life.' (Vallerand 1994)

Insufficient pain relief causes fear, resentment and desperation, especially in patients who have had frequent experiences of inadequate care. Some may be thought to exaggerate their distress to try to persuade health professionals to give them the relief they need (see also Chapter 14 *Pain and pain relief*). Patients who feel that their pain relief is wearing off may also become very insistent. This phenomenon has been described as 'opiate pseudo addiction ... an iatrogenic syndrome of abnormal behaviour that develops as a consequence of inadequate pain management' (Weissman and Haddox 1989, cited in Vallerand 1994).

Whilst it is true that doctors need to be very careful about prescribing controlled drugs, frequent doses of opiate analgesia are not in themselves sufficient evidence of iatrogenic addiction. The patient's description of the pain and of the precipitating factors are important in assessing the situation. It is much easier to elicit these if the patient is given pain relief first (Oni and Bent 1998). A strict protocol should ensure that patients with sickle cell crises receive appropriate levels of analgesia without delay (Department of Health 1993).

> 'Imagine having a heart attack – you know, when not enough blood is getting to the heart muscle. Well, sickling means that not enough blood is getting to the part of my body that's affected. You give an injection for heart attack pain without loads of questions and delay, why not for sickling?'
> Man with sickle cell disease

The psycho-social aspects of managing the pain of a sickle cell crisis are often neglected. A paternalistic approach to pain management tends to create a sense of dependency in some people, which may then begin to permeate other aspects of their lives. Some people need support to develop a range of strategies for managing their pain themselves, using approaches such as massage, relaxation and transcutaneous electronic nerve stimulation as well as analgesics. Patients and their families also need information about drug-seeking behaviours so that they can avoid behaviour that could lead to addiction (Brent Sickle Cell and Thalassaemia Centre, personal communication 1998).

Repeated admissions

Although over 90 per cent of hospital admissions of people with sickle cell disease are for painful crises, nearly all sickle pain is coped with in the community. However, some patients may have to make frequent visits to hospital for painful crises and other urgent needs: about 10 per cent of sickle cell patients account for 90 per cent of all hospital admissions (Brent Sickle Cell and Thalassaemia Centre, personal communication 1998). People who attend frequently should not be stigmatised as 'non-copers' and implicitly blamed or given inferior or slower treatment. Some people attend frequently because they lack social support and the strategies to manage pain themselves. However, many are simply more severely affected by the disease: frequent visits to hospital for severe pain have been shown to correlate with early death in patients over the age of 20 (Davies and Oni 1997). It is important that frequent attenders are met with understanding and that everything possible is done to make them feel comfortable. This avoids adding to the stress and emotional pressure they and their families are experiencing and may reduce the need for anxiolytics.

Choice of hospital

Many sickle cell patients develop a good rapport with a particular hospital and prefer to receive care there even though it may not be the closest to their home. This is especially likely if the hospital has a dedicated department or day unit to which people can go directly for prompt and specialist treatment without having to wait in the accident and emergency department (and then wait again for admission to a general ward). It is important to consider these issues when planning services and placing contracts. Many ambulance drivers are prepared to take patients to their preferred hospital provided that this will not lengthen their journey unreasonably. There have been instances of patients taking their own taxis to ensure admission to their chosen hospital (Streetly, Maxwell and Mejia 1997, Department of Health 1993).

SCD *and general anaesthesia*

People with SCD are at particular risk during general anaesthesia and need careful management. Although people with sickle cell trait are otherwise healthy and have a normal life expectancy, there are also implications for their management during general anaesthesia. Patients whose inheritance indicates that they might have SCD or carry sickle cell trait should be tested before being given a general anaesthetic unless their medical records clearly show that they have already been tested (Streetly, Maxwell and Mejia 1997, Department of Health 1993).

Useful addresses

Brent Sickle Cell and Thalassaemia Centre
122 High Street
Harlesden
London NW10 4SP

A walk-in centre providing information, screening and counselling to people who might be affected by sickle cell disease or thalassaemia.

UK Thalassaemia Society
19 The Broadway
Southgate Circus
London N14 6PH

Works to raise awareness of thalassaemia, and provides information and advice to people who might be affected.

34 HIV/AIDS and minority groups

Attitudes and assumptions

Whilst people with most life-threatening diseases attract sympathy and support, people with HIV/AIDS can suffer an almost unique degree of prejudice, hostility and rejection. Negative attitudes, especially when combined with racism, place an unendurable burden on people who are coping with a fatal disease and who may already have watched loved ones die of the infection.

Health professionals caring for people with HIV/AIDS must therefore examine their own attitudes and feelings about the illness and about the ways in which it can be acquired. They also need to avoid possible assumptions and stereotypes about people of black and minority ethnic groups (see Chapters 1 and 2).

> 'If staff do not explore their own subjective value system and culturally based preconceptions and assumptions, they cannot give accurate, objective information and therefore cannot meet the client's potential needs.' (Aston 1993)

Methods of transmission

HIV/AIDS is stigmatised partly because it is infectious and ultimately fatal, but mainly because of the ways in which it is transmitted. The behaviours that carry a risk of acquiring HIV are generally disapproved of by mainstream society, and are openly condemned by some religious and conservative communities.

Homosexual transmission

World-wide, only 5–10 per cent of HIV is transmitted through homosexual contact. However, this is one of the most common methods of transmission among the majority population in the West (Panos Institute

1992). Although generally tolerated, homosexuality remains unacceptable to many people in most Western countries. Gay men and women still experience prejudice, discrimination and rejection.

Attitudes to homosexuality elsewhere vary a good deal. 'Homosexual' as a description of identity, sexual orientation or sexual practice is largely a late twentieth century Western concept and not one that people from other parts of the world necessarily identify with. In many countries, sexual activity between men is not generally perceived or described as 'homosexual'. In relation to anal intercourse, distinctions are sometimes made between the man who penetrates and the man who is penetrated: the former may not be regarded as homosexual while the latter may be (The NAZ Project, personal communication 1998). In many parts of the world it is customary for men with a primarily homosexual orientation to marry and have children. In some countries, sexual intercourse between men is ignored provided it does not interfere with family and community stability. In others, it is highly stigmatised and/or illegal, and incurs severe penalties, even death. All these factors make it likely that male-to-male transmission of the HIV virus world-wide is under-recognised and under-reported.

In the UK, homosexual behaviour raises particular dilemmas for people in conservative and religious communities where it is forbidden or unacknowledged, and where everyone is expected to marry and have children (see Part Five). Adult children who do not wish to marry are often very aware that they are causing shame and sorrow to their families and especially to their parents. Many homosexual men and women feel unable to resist family and community pressures and agree to marry. Others feel unable to do this. However, if they wish to live openly as homosexuals, they are often forced to move far away from home and to cut themselves off from their families and communities. This can be particularly hard for black and minority ethnic people who may never be completely accepted by white society. The conflicting and irreconcilable pressures they face may become intolerable.

'A young gay Bengali man came under great pressure from his mother to marry and have children. She could think and talk of nothing else and said that if her son loved her he would agree to get married. People in the community were beginning to talk and she was ashamed among her friends, all of whom had married sons. The young man's partner, who was white, wanted him to leave home so that they could live openly together. He could not understand why the young man didn't just make up his mind and do what he wanted. If his mother didn't understand, that was her problem. Both the mother and the partner become more and more insistent. Eventually the young Bengali man committed suicide.'
South Asian HIV/AIDS worker

Constrained by time and the necessity for secrecy, homosexual men who marry may seek fleeting sexual satisfaction in situations where the danger of infection is particularly high. Even if they become HIV-positive or know that they are at risk, it is very difficult for them to practise safe sex with their wives. In many communities, having children is one of the main purposes of marriage and precludes the use of condoms. Some religions prohibit condoms. Using a condom would also require a man to admit his homosexual activity to his wife, risking discovery and placing everything at risk (Khan 1994).

'I know of many cases where a married man is HIV-positive or even has AIDS and his family does not know.'
South Asian AIDS worker

'If you live with family it's hard to keep your illness a secret when you have to take 18 tablets five times a day.'
Minority group AIDS worker

Intravenous drug use

Another common method of transmission in the West is through intravenous drug use. However, this accounts for only 5–10 per cent of transmission world-wide (Panos Institute 1992). Intravenous drug use is almost universally unacceptable and is therefore usually covert. It is always a shock to discover that a family member is using drugs. People in conservative and religious communities who are found to be taking drugs may be particularly likely to face ostracism and rejection, and may find it hard to get the support they need without leaving their community.

Heterosexual transmission

World-wide, 70–75 per cent of HIV transmission is through heterosexual contact. In sub-Saharan Africa, for example, HIV/AIDS mainly affects heterosexual men and women and babies (Panos Institute 1992). Some people in the West with HIV/AIDS who have travelled to other parts of the world may therefore have acquired the infection through heterosexual contact.

It is often assumed that people who live in, or come from, areas with high rates of heterosexual transmission are promiscuous and that this is somehow part of their culture. However, promiscuity and casual sex occur everywhere. The key factors that increase rates of heterosexual transmission of HIV in developing countries are linked primarily to socio-economic conditions, including extreme poverty. At national levels this limits the amount that can be spent on health, education and other services. At an individual level it constrains people's choices and opportunities. For example:

- In the West, treatment is readily available to people with curable sexually transmitted diseases. Such services are too expensive for most developing countries. People with untreated genital lesions are more vulnerable to infection with HIV.
- Lack of money may also mean that there is little public health information about HIV/AIDS and how to prevent them. In some countries the existence of HIV/AIDS is not acknowledged by the authorities and there is little or no emphasis on public education.
- Many people have no access to public information media such as radio and television, which are taken for granted in the West. Insufficient money for education results in low literacy levels; information about HIV/AIDS and prevention cannot be disseminated easily.
- In some countries, the use of condoms is forbidden by religious or other authorities. Even where condom use is permitted, condoms are often not available or affordable.
- Communities and families become dislocated and societies break down when poverty forces large numbers of people to leave home to find work. In many developing countries, men, and sometimes women, have to leave their homes and live in city slums to seek a source of income for themselves and their families (Panos Institute 1992). Such dislocation is even greater when there is violence, war or famine. Loneliness, unhappiness and vulnerability may lead people in these situations to turn to casual sex for comfort and solace. Refugees who are in a state of shock and who often see no hope for the future are also particularly vulnerable, both physically and emotionally (UNAIDS 1997) (see also Chapter 35).

Casual heterosexual sex, which would involve some risk in a Western industrialised country, thus often carries a high risk in many developing countries.

'It makes me very angry when people in the West casually blame the rapid spread of HIV/AIDS in Africa on promiscuity. While promiscuity plays a part, it is clear that it is only one of the many complex factors fuelling the spread of the epidemic. Moreover, having lived and worked as a health promoter in various Western countries for the last 15 years, I know that people in the West are just as likely to be promiscuous as people anywhere else. If there is a difference it is that Westerners are generally better informed about the risks of HIV/AIDS and other sexually transmitted diseases; they are richer and have more access to condoms and better health care.'
Health promotion worker

Women in countries where there are high rates of heterosexual transmission often face additional risks.

- Male-to-female transmission is twice as efficient as female-to-male transmission. In developing countries, inadequate nutrition may make the female genital tract more vulnerable to damage, which further increases the risk of transmission (Panos Institute 1992).
- Most women do not feel able to refuse sex or to insist on using a condom, especially if they (and their children) are economically dependent on their husband or partner.
- Female refugees are particularly at risk of violence and rape, both while fleeing and in camps (UNAIDS 1997).

Transmission through blood transfusions

Attitudes towards people who acquire HIV/AIDS through blood transfusion have been markedly different from those towards people who acquire the infection through other routes. Blood for transfusion is now screened in many parts of the world and the numbers of people infected via this route are decreasing. In 1992 they represented about 3–5 per cent worldwide (Panos Institute 1992). However, many hospitals, especially in the developing countries, have no resources for testing donated blood. People who have received transfusions in countries where testing is not available may be at risk.

Vertical transmission

Globally, 5–10 per cent of HIV is transmitted from mother to child. In poor countries, drug treatment is not available to pregnant women who are HIV-positive, increasing the risk to their babies. Most mothers who are HIV-positive have to breast feed because they cannot afford powdered milk.

HIV/AIDS and minority groups in Britain

Double jeopardy

People with HIV/AIDS who also belong to a black or minority ethnic group are often doubly disadvantaged. They are often poorer and more isolated, and may find it harder to access services, especially if they also face language barriers. Africans with HIV/AIDS are particularly vulnerable because many of them are also asylum seekers and are coping with the aftermath of persecution and the trauma of dislocation (see Chapter 35 *Understanding the experiences of asylum seekers and refugees*). People who have acquired the infection through heterosexual contact are more likely to have children who may also be infected.

'The white gay community has had a 15-year learning curve. They have got used to talking openly about sexual matters. Many of them are very articulate in English, well informed and are able to be very effective advocates. In contrast, Africans with HIV in the UK are at the start of a learning curve. Many are unfamiliar with the British system and do not know how to access good care. They may not speak much English. Many are struggling with cultural differences and with social and economic deprivation coupled with anxiety about what will happen to their children who may also be HIV positive.'
Black HIV/AIDS worker

AIDS *awareness*

In some communities and religious groups, sex is seldom discussed openly and there is a high level of denial about HIV/AIDS. Little or no information about sexual health is available and people may be lulled into a false sense of security. They may not regard themselves as being at risk and therefore tend to be diagnosed and offered treatment at a much later stage.

Information and sexual health programmes must be precisely targeted, taking into account the language, culture, attitudes, traditions and religious beliefs of each community. Labels such as 'homosexual' or 'gay' may be meaningless to some people (see earlier in this chapter). It may also be important that information and education are given by people who share the culture or ethnicity of the people they are working with.

'We can often get the message across better because we are black and they are black. It is much harder when it is a white person, especially if they are talking about what to do, what not to do and how to behave. People may just think that they are judgmental and racist.'
Black HIV/AIDS worker

Family and community attitudes

Many people with HIV/AIDS in all communities experience prejudice, hostility and rejection, not only from society in general but also from those closest to them. Families with strict moral or religious codes may find it especially difficult or impossible to accept a family member who is HIV-positive or has AIDS. In some communities, individuals may keep their illness secret for as long as possible for fear of being dishonoured, shamed and rejected. A married person with the infection may, however, find it impossible to practice safer sex with their spouse (see above).

Even where families themselves are supportive, they may suffer from hostility and rejection by others. Some families are therefore particularly anxious about secrecy, especially in communities where shameful or unacceptable behaviour by one member can drastically affect the lives and marriage prospects of other members.

Most black and minority people are also very aware of the prejudice and hostility towards their community among wider society, including sections of the media. Black and minority ethnic people, especially older people, often feel particularly anxious that no breath of public dishonour should touch their families or their communities. In such circumstances it can be particularly difficult for issues such as HIV/AIDS, homosexuality and drug abuse to be discussed openly and for some people to admit that they occur.

Attitudes towards women

Despite moves in some societies towards equality between the sexes, all societies still have very different standards for men and women, especially in relation to sexual behaviour. As a result, women with HIV/AIDS are likely to experience even more disapproval and less support than men, regardless of the fact that they might have been infected by their partner rather than as a result of their own behaviour. Women with children attract extra censure and hostility because they are seen as particularly irresponsible. Concern for infected women is often overshadowed by apprehension about the fate of their children (Levine and Dubler 1990). In many communities, gender roles also place a greater burden on women to care for immediate and extended family members affected by HIV/AIDS, often at the expense of their own health.

Black and minority ethnic women face additional prejudice, in some cases from their own community as well as from society at large (Positively Women 1994). Rather than receive the care and support they need, they are often burdened with stigma and discrimination. They are likely to find it more difficult to get access to services, and are more likely to be poor, isolated and unsupported.

Discussing HIV/AIDS

Difficult words

The advent of HIV/AIDS means that we all have to learn to talk about things that were formerly taboo and secret. We have had to develop a new, socially acceptable language. Terms such as 'penetrative sex', 'anal sex', 'safer sex' and 'condoms' are now in common usage. Bisexuality and alternative sexual practices are talked about in ways that would have been unthinkable two decades ago. Nevertheless, many people, including many health professionals, find them embarrassing or distasteful and have difficulty in raising them or discussing them in a calm and objective way.

Language can be even more of an obstacle in more conservative communities. In most South Asian languages, for example, there are no socially acceptable words for parts of the body between the waist and knees, and no appropriate words other than offensive slang for different sexual identities and sexual activities. Where such words have not become at least partially accepted, it can be very difficult to discuss intimate personal and sexual matters.

In communities where homosexuality is strongly disapproved of, lack of vocabulary may not be the only problem. Men who have sexual relationships with men may simply not identify with words such as gay, homosexual or bisexual (see earlier). It is important to think in terms of behaviour rather than categories, and to talk, for example, about 'men who have sex with men'.

Interpreters

Great care is needed in selecting an interpreter for discussions about HIV/AIDS and related issues (see Chapter 27 *Training, supporting and managing interpreters*). Interpreters should be trained in the skills of non-directive counselling and must have had opportunities to deal with their own attitudes and feelings about HIV/AIDS and the issues surrounding it. Some people may feel unable to talk freely through an interpreter who is significantly older or younger than they or who is unmarried, or through someone of the opposite sex. Particular care may be needed in selecting an interpreter for asylum seekers (see Chapter 35 *Interpreters*).

Confidentiality is vital. It is inappropriate, for example, to use a spouse or partner, as it may be their behaviour that is in question. It is also inappropriate to use a relative or friend and it is clearly never acceptable to use a child (see also Chapter 28 *Children*). It is almost always preferable to use a professional interpreter, though some people may worry if the professional interpreter is a member of their own community.

Testing for HIV

Tests for HIV should not be carried out without the patient's explicit consent. Doctors therefore have to decide, on the basis of clinical indications and known risk factors, whether to broach the subject of testing with each individual patient. This raises particular issues with patients of black and minority ethnic groups. For example, some health professionals may assume that certain people are at risk of HIV/AIDS (and a risk to others) simply because of their skin colour or origins.

Some other people are assumed not to be at risk because they belong to a community with a strict code of conduct with regard to sexual behaviour. Health professionals may decide on this basis not to discuss HIV/AIDS with them and not to offer them testing. But assumptions are dangerous. Individuals in any community, however conservative, may be at risk from their own behaviour or from that of others.

'I am a Muslim woman who is a representative of a growing number of Muslim women throughout the world who is a recipient of HIV. I was never a drug user and was in a long-term monogamous relationship for 18 years. I thought I would never get this virus, because not only do these things happen to other people, but I am a Muslim and I believed that Muslims didn't get HIV.' (Rahman 1994)

Raising the issue of HIV/AIDS is never easy. Most people see AIDS as a remote issue that has nothing to do with them. Few people, even those who know they are at risk, find it easy to discuss their own or their partner's sex lives or to face the possibility that they might be infected. People who experience frequent discrimination may be reluctant to disclose information that might reinforce prejudice. Asylum seekers and refugees may fear that infection or the possibility of infection could be used as a reason to deport them. People in communities with a strict code of sexual behaviour may not consider AIDS testing relevant. Some may feel offended and upset that their conduct or that of their partner is being questioned.

'It is important to strike a balance between, on the one hand, adding to prejudice, racism and stereotyping, and, on the other, ignoring the issue of HIV and AIDS, which is a form of inverse racism. By colluding with taboos within a community we are jeopardising people's health. It is important to recognise and work with people's fears and to give clear information so that they can make informed choices.'
South Asian AIDS worker

Everyone who is tested for HIV should receive pre- and post-test counselling and support that takes possible cultural and religious factors into account and is in a language that they understand well. Current practice, however, seems to be patchy. One survey found that African women were less likely than others to receive post-test counselling. Women who had become infected through drug use were only half as likely to receive post-test counselling as those who had become infected through heterosexual intercourse (Positively Women 1994). In terms of education, everyone needs to know about maintaining sexual health and protecting themselves against HIV/AIDS and other sexually transmitted diseases.

Practical care

For information about confidentiality, patient care, the place of care and the needs of carers, see Part Two.

People with HIV/AIDS often need help and support from many different statutory and voluntary agencies. Those who are unfamiliar with the normal practice and routines of Western health and social support systems – for example, recently arrived refugees and asylum seekers – may feel rejected and abandoned if they are referred on to other agencies. Some people find the complexities of the system too overwhelming; they find it too difficult to contact new agencies or keep multiple appointments and so miss out on care. Such people may benefit from having a personal advocate who can steer them through the complexities of the system and ensure that they receive appropriate care and advice, not just from the health service but also from housing departments, benefits offices, legal services and voluntary groups.

Care around the time of death

In some cultures and religions it is considered to be very important for certain ceremonies to be performed when someone is dying or has just died (see Parts Two and Five for details). Great distress can be caused to relatives if these are not performed, especially when people believe that the ceremonies are essential to ensure the release of the spirit or to aid a smooth transition from this world to the next. Whenever possible, the family should be contacted and informed when a patient is likely to die. However, consent must always be obtained for this, especially if the patient may have become estranged from their family.

Consideration must also be given to gay partners, who may not share the patient's religion and who may be excluded by the family.

'Because society conditions its members to feel apprehensive towards those who lead alternative lifestyles, it is more difficult for gay men and women to receive support while they mourn their loss.' (Siegal and Hoefer 1981)

Conversely, problems can occur when a gay partner, who may not share the patient's cultural or religious roots, makes all the arrangements without consulting the family.

When someone has died

Concerns about infection risks have led many units to implement special infection control measures in relation to the bodies of people who had HIV/AIDS. Some of these have been irrational.

'In the '80s, I discovered that, in one London hospital, after a man died of AIDS the nurses were expected to tie a ligature around his penis. I asked them what they did for female patients. After that the practice was stopped.'
NHS researcher

Other measures, such as the routine use of body bags, may appear rational on the surface, but are usually unnecessary. They can cause immense distress to family members and religious communities who are unnecessarily prevented from carrying out normal religious and cultural practices after a death (see Chapter 20 *Infection control issues*).

HIV/AIDS is classified as presenting a medium risk to those who handle the body after death. Embalming is contraindicated (Healing, Hoffman and Young 1995). However, unless the person died of a high-risk opportunistic infection, there is no reason why a body bag should be used or why the relatives or the religious community should not carry out their normal rituals after a death, provided they observe routine hygiene precautions.

The Cause of Death certificate

Many families wish to prevent other people knowing that a family member has died of AIDS. This is particularly important in communities where the stigma of AIDS is often very strong. In such cases, it may be tactful to record the specific infection of which the person died rather than the underlying cause.

'My parents were very anxious that no one should know why my brother died. We had kept the secret all the time he was ill and though there were some suspicions no one actually knew. Our family doctor understood and he wrote pneumonia on the certificate. It was a very kind thing. Our whole family would have been destroyed if the truth had come out.'
Gujarati woman

Bereavement

Repeated loss is a major issue for many gay men and for people from parts of the world where AIDS affects large numbers of the population and whole families. The cumulative experience of repeated loss is likely to be especially devastating. Distress and desperation are often compounded when young adults die, leaving children and older people unsupported and impoverished. Every effort should be made to offer comfort to people in this situation, especially if they are additionally isolated because of ethnic and cultural differences.

Useful addresses

AVERT (Aids Education and Research Trust)
11 Denne Place,
Horsham,
West Sussex RH12 1JD.

Publishes educational leaflets on many aspects of HIV/AIDS.

Blackliners
49 Effra Road,
London SW2 1BZ

Run by black people for black people.

Jewish AIDS Trust
HIV/AIDS Education Unit,
Colindale Hospital,
Colindale Avenue,
London NW9 5HG.

Education, counselling and support.

The NAZ Project
Pallingswick House,
241 King Street,
London W6 9LP

HIV/AIDS and sexual health service for the South Asian, Middle Eastern and North African communities.

Positively Women
5 Sebastian Street,
London EC1V 0HE

A self-help group run by and for women living with HIV/AIDS.

35 Refugees and asylum seekers

Refugees and asylum seekers (see *Definitions* at the end of this chapter) form a particularly vulnerable group and may have special needs in terms of health care. They often present with multiple medical problems and can have difficulty in gaining access to the services they need.

Refugees and asylum seekers in Britain

Current British legislation on the treatment of asylum seekers is extremely restrictive and probably cannot be tightened any further without contravening international law. In 1997, less than 5 per cent of people who sought asylum in Britain were given refugee status. A slightly higher percentage were given Exceptional Leave to Remain (ELR) (*Economist* 1998, Runnymede Trust 1994). The vast majority of people seeking asylum in Britain are eventually refused permission to remain. Britain has a smaller proportion of people seeking asylum in relation to its population size than most comparable European countries (CRE 1997).

Despite their shared legal status, their forced exile and the difficulties they face, the asylum seekers and refugees in Britain are not a homogeneous group. They come from many different countries, cultures and religions. Most refugees are young adults, some are children (sometimes unaccompanied), a few are elderly. Some come from urban areas, some from very isolated rural areas, some are political activists, some are intellectuals, some simply belong to a religious or ethnic group that is being targeted for persecution, murder or 'ethnic cleansing'.

In the last decade most of the people applying for asylum in Britain have come from Somalia, former Yugoslavia, the former USSR, China, Sri Lanka, Pakistan, Nigeria, Turkey (mainly Kurdish people), Colombia, India, Kenya, Iran, Iraq, Ghana, Palestine, Ethiopia, Eritrea, Afghanistan, Zaire, Sudan, Uganda, Rumania, Togo and the Ivory Coast (Refugee Council 1998). Most newly arrived refugees settle in London and other major cities, because this is where they are most likely to find other people of their own community and where most refugee advice and support services are situated.

There are also many **longer-settled refugees**. Although most no longer face the immediate problems of being forced to leave their homes and make a new life in difficult circumstances, for many their refugee experience is still vivid and may give rise to additional fears and insecurities at times of illness, dependency or family crisis.

- During the first half of the twentieth century, many refugees to Britain were Jews fleeing pogroms in Russia and the rest of Eastern Europe, and later fleeing genocide in Germany and German-occupied territories before and during the Second World War.
- After the War, the destruction of much of Europe and the Soviet occupation of eastern Europe created millions of refugees. About 200,000 Poles and 50,000 other East European refugees came to Britain to help with the recovery and reconstruction of industry and the economy.
- Other groups of refugees have been allowed to settle as political crises have arisen in their home countries. These included about 15,000 Hungarians in 1956, about 5,000 Czechoslovakians in 1968, about 30,000 Ugandan Asians (many with British passports) in 1972, and about 3,000 Chileans in 1973. In the 1970s and '80s about 19,000 refugees from Vietnam, about 20,000 Iranians and about 1,500 Poles were allowed to settle (Finlay and Reynolds 1987).

Understanding the experiences of asylum seekers and refugees

Before a refugee leaves their own country, their main aim is normally to get themselves, and often their family, out of danger and into a place of safety. There may have been little time to think, or to express the feelings that arise when people are under severe threat. The shock, terror and grief that are often suppressed while people are fighting for their survival may emerge once they are physically safe, but may also be chronically delayed until a new crisis arises. Many refugees have experienced or witnessed intimidation, violence, torture and rape, and have been emotionally if not physically scarred by the events that led to their flight. Many feel bereaved by the loss of the lives they have known. They mourn their forcible separation from friends and close family and the loss of familiar surroundings. Many worry about what may be happening to the people they left behind.

Arriving in the UK often brings initial relief and a feeling of safety to asylum seekers. But these can soon be undermined by practical difficulties: anxiety about the asylum application, difficulties with accommodation, shortage of money, starting life again in an unfamiliar and very different place and in a cold climate, sorting out urgent practical issues such as health care and schools, coping with loneliness or trying to give emotional support to bewildered children and other family members, trying to learn English, trying to find work. Under the 1996 Asylum and Immigration Act, benefits for new asylum seekers were severely cut, causing additional severe hardship and even homelessness for many. Those people without regular food, shelter and money are likely to experience a decline in their health due to a poor diet, unhygienic living conditions, the cold, exposure to disease and increased risk of physical injury. Refugees and asylum seekers are often afraid to ask for the benefits to which they are entitled or to complain about difficulties in case they make their situation worse. Most live in deprived areas where health and social services facilities are already over-stretched. Of all immigrants, refugees and asylum seekers generally have the least family or community support (Goodburn 1994, BHAN 1991).

Asylum seekers waiting for a decision on whether they can stay, or people granted ELR (see above) whose situation is reviewed at set intervals, live with complete uncertainty about their future and how long they can stay. They cannot plan ahead, make commitments or put down roots. Many feel frightened, intimidated and disempowered. Uncertainty and anxiety, the well-known effects of culture shock, and the experience of racial violence and hostility add to the strain under which people live.

Research indicates that social stressors in the place of exile are a stronger predictor of depression in refugees who have been tortured than the severity of the trauma they have experienced. Depression and anxiety are common among asylum seekers and refugees in Britain, though they may not always be expressed in those terms (Gorst-Unsworth and Goldenberg 1998, Monteith 1994).

' ... people coming here had the problem of a civil war at home; people had been traumatised and lost everything; moved from their home without warning; lost friends; lost environment; lost loved ones. Those who were lucky enough to come here, when they knew they were coming to the UK, were full of hope. They thought they would forget all problems behind. But when they came here in fact the more problems started ... the promised land is not here, it is not there! ... They ended up in the inner city ... yesterday's refugee is tomorrow's ghetto dweller. This is all very sad because you don't see any way to run away from the situation ... they are on their way to this situation!'
Somali refugee (Amidu 1994)

Family reunion

Social support, especially from family members, is extremely important in reducing psychological morbidity in people who have experienced torture and exile (Gorst-Unsworth and Goldenberg 1998). Many refugees feel unable to begin the steps of creating a new life until their family members have joined them. Unfortunately, British legislation and administration have often delayed family reunion.

A person who is granted **refugee status** (see *Definitions*, later) can apply to bring in their family immediately, though the process may then take a very long time. The family is defined as spouse and dependent children (sons under 18, daughters under 21) and does not include adult children, parents and other people whom many refugees regard as their close family. During the long waits, some dependent children become too old to be brought in. When refugees are admitted under international quota agreements – for example, some people from Vietnam, Somalia and former Yugoslavia – family reunions may take place sooner. A person who has been granted Exceptional Leave to Remain may apply to bring in their family after four years but must sign an undertaking that they can support and accommodate their family 'without recourse to public funds'. An **asylum seeker** cannot bring their family over (Refugee Council 1992).

Suspicion and disbelief

The hostility shown towards asylum seekers and refugees by the British authorities and media and a general belief among many members of the public that most refugees and asylum seekers are 'cheating the system' increase people's fear and insecurity.

> 'Legal advisers [working with asylum seekers] say that a "culture of disbelief" prevails at the Home Office. Applicants are presumed to have no case, or to be fabricating a case. They are being put in the position of having to disprove negative interpretations of their case. Disproportionate emphasis is being placed early on in the process on watertight, documented evidence, which is often extremely difficult to obtain from countries of origin. A claim which is not fully supported can be abruptly refused.' (Refugee Council 1994)

While it is no doubt true that there is some abuse of the asylum system, as there is of any system, the vast majority of asylum applicants and refugees are genuine. In relation to patient care, it is important for health professionals to convey trust and respect, and to try to avoid asking questions that might be taken as implying hostility or suspicion. Many refugees and asylum seekers fear contact with people who have authority or power, including health professionals. They may fear that health professionals have links with the Home Office or the police. Some patients may be afraid to discuss problems or to be open about the past in case this somehow jeopardises their situation.

Access to health care

All asylum seekers, people granted ELR and refugees are entitled to statutory health services, including free medical treatment under the NHS and registration with a GP. Gaining access to services can, however, be difficult because of language problems and unfamiliarity with the British system. One survey found that nearly 40 per cent of refugees had difficulty registering with a GP (Goodburn 1994). People placed in temporary bed and breakfast hotels may be unable to register with a GP, because some practices refuse such patients. They may also not know how to change GPs if, as is common, they are moved on every few weeks or months. Some people use services inappropriately and may need guidance. For example, those who do not understand the role of the GP may go straight to an accident and emergency department for minor or chronic problems. Even when accessible care is offered, some patients may be distrustful, defensive and secretive towards people in authority.

Asylum seekers and recently arrived refugees also have to cope with the practicalities of normal daily life in an unfamiliar place and often on very little money. Many face a language barrier. Illness makes everything more difficult. Patients and their families may need help to find out about and use the different services and facilities available, and ensure that they are getting the benefits to which they are entitled. They may also need advice on practical matters such as school registration and eating well on a very low budget.

When someone is ill

In most cases, the practical needs of asylum seekers and refugees who are ill will be no different from those of other patients. However, illness, bereavement or the threat of new loss may dramatically affect some people's ability to cope. For some asylum seekers and refugees who have managed to survive everything else, this new event may simply be too much. Patients and families in this situation are likely to need a lot of understanding and support. It is, as always, important to take possible cultural and religious differences into account and to find out from each individual how best to meet their needs.

Place of care

Asylum seekers and refugees are particularly likely to be in temporary accommodation with inadequate and overcrowded washing, cooking and storage facilities, and to lack space at home to care for a seriously ill or dying person; they also risk being moved at very short notice (Schott and Henley 1996). Home care may therefore be impossible unless better long-term accommodation can be negotiated with the local authority.

People who have experienced torture or physical abuse

Patients who have been physically or sexually abused in any way may have particular fears and reactions in relation to medical examination and treatment. In some countries doctors are involved in carrying out torture. Normally benign medical instruments are often misused: a syringe, an oxygen mask or simple electrical equipment may reawaken terrifying memories. People who have been tortured may become extremely anxious during physical examinations, especially if they have to undress or lie on an examination couch. Many are nervous of being touched, of sudden movements or sounds, or of movements behind them or out of their sight. Some people find themselves unable to co-operate with certain medical and nursing procedures, others suffer severe panic attacks, and some hyperventilate (Bower 1994). Even people who were tortured or physically abused many years or even decades ago and who have spent most of their lives in Britain may have memories and fears re-evoked by medical and nursing procedures as well as by increasing dependency and vulnerability.

Health professionals can be most supportive by demonstrating that they are there to help, by being extremely gentle and by trying to build a relationship of mutual trust. Continuity of care is important. It may help if new health professionals are introduced by someone with whom the patient already has a good relationship. All physical treatments and interventions must be carefully explained and the patient's full consent obtained before proceeding. If the patient shows signs of anxiety or distress, it may be necessary to stop.

Long-term effects People react differently to traumatic experiences and this may affect their responses to other people and the way they react to serious illness, even many years after the event. Some people experience depression, anxiety, irritability and restlessness, and suffer insomnia and nightmares. As they grow older, they may become preoccupied with memories and with people and places that are lost. Some are left with a permanent feeling of helplessness, apathy, social isolation, fatalism and dependence. Others feel a lasting suspicion and mistrust towards other people, which may express itself quietly in bitterness or, occasionally, more aggressively (Chodoff 1970).

Some people who have been tortured feel that their health has been permanently damaged. Some feel permanently tired and ill. They may worry a good deal about physical symptoms (see also Chapter 13 *Different expectations and concerns*). They may very much want detailed and thorough examinations and investigations to rule out serious illness. It is important to recognise the real fear and inner devastation that may underlie repeated requests for investigation and reassurance, and to try to identify the concerns and worries of each patient.

HIV/AIDS

Refugees and asylum seekers who come from areas of internal or international conflict where there are high levels of HIV/AIDS and who have experienced social and family dislocation, lack of health care, possible transfusion with contaminated blood, and in some cases rape and other sexual violence, are at increased risk of infection with the HIV virus (see also Chapter 34).

Talking about the past

Some patients and family members may find it helpful to talk about their experiences before they came to Britain. In general all that is required is to listen (see also Chapter 23 *Listening with complete respect*). However, if you feel out of your depth, you may wish to get advice and support from a specialist organisation (see *Useful addresses*, below).

> 'You have to receive from people the horror of their story. It lessens the madness for them, their sense of a mad world. After a while you gain strength from listening to their stories, a strength to share them.'
> Director, Medical Foundation for the Care of Victims of Torture

Some people do not find it helpful to talk. There is no evidence that those who choose to talk about their torture do any better than those who choose not to. People's preferences are partly influenced by their culture; in some cultures, especially Western and North American cultures, there is a strong belief that people who have gone though terrible experiences or losses should help the process of emotional healing by talking about what has happened. In other cultures, talking may not be regarded as therapeutic (Bower 1994) (see Chapter 21 *The experience and expression of grief*). For many refugees, their most urgent need is to pick up the practical aspects of their lives as far as possible so as to rebuild their self-esteem, and to regain their trust and confidence in other people through positive relationships. Sympathetic and sensitive help and advice with practical problems can be very useful.

Interpreters

Where there is a language barrier a professional interpreter will be required (see also Chapter 27). There may be particular issues of suitability, confidentiality and security when selecting an interpreter for an asylum seeker or a refugee. Some communities are divided by fierce political or ethnic conflict mirroring that in their home countries. Some regimes operate intelligence services in Britain with the aim of seeking out and harming their opponents. It is very important to check that the patient and family are confident that the interpreter will not place them in any danger.

Definitions

Under the Geneva Convention (United Nations 1951), a refugee is defined as a person who has fled their home country or cannot go back to it, because of a well-founded fear of persecution for reasons of race, religion, nationality, membership of a particular social group or political opinion. In the UK:

- a **refugee** is legally defined as a person who has been granted refugee status by the Home Office;
- an **asylum seeker** is someone who has come to Britain and applied for refugee status and who is waiting for a Home Office decision. This can take many months and even years;
- some asylum seekers who are refused refugee status are granted **Exceptional Leave to Remain** (ELR) which must be reapplied for at set intervals.

Useful addresses

The Refugee Council
3 Bondway
London SW18 1SJ

The Refugees Advisers' Support Unit offers advice and information, bulletins, translated leaflets on women's health and other issues. The Community Development Team provides information on locally based refugee consortia, local refugee-geared health material and initiatives.

Medical Foundation for the Care of Victims of Torture
96–98 Grafton Road
London NW5 3EJ

A range of professional services, including consultation, counselling for people who have been tortured and training for professionals; uses in-house trained interpreters.

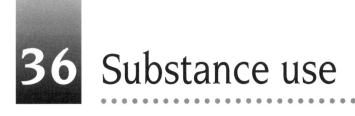

36 Substance use

In every culture some people use substances that may affect their health and well-being. The effects of substances that are widely used within the general UK population, such as tobacco and alcohol, as well as common illegal drugs, are well documented elsewhere. This chapter focuses on substances likely to be used by some people of certain cultural or religious minority groups. It is, however, important not to make any assumptions about individuals' use of substances on the basis of their group or community.

Attitudes to substance use

Most health professionals consider it risky to take any unnecessary drugs or substances that are either illegal or that have not been subjected to scientific evaluation. People who use illegal substances are often stigmatised and marginalised. People of black and minority ethnic groups may face additional problems of stereotyping, discrimination and racism. These may deter them from discussing substance use or from accepting health care.

When substance use is an accepted part of a culture, people may be unaware of any risk or may see no reason to change their habits. Giving up something that is familiar and widely accepted within one's own community can be especially hard when living in another culture. There may be little motivation to give it up if the pressure to do so comes from outsiders who may be thought ill-informed or prejudiced.

Whatever personal feelings and beliefs health professionals have about substance use, it is important not to alienate patients who use substances and to maintain good relationships. Sensitivity and a supportive approach are especially important if the health professional has good grounds for believing that substance use is harming a patient.

Cannabis

Cannabis is derived from *Cannabis sativa*, a plant that is widely grown throughout the world. It is most commonly smoked but can also be eaten or drunk. There are several forms of cannabis. The more familiar include marijuana and hashish and the Indian forms, charas and bang (Johnson 1990). World-wide there are over 100 different names for cannabis (Reynolds 1993). Cannabis use is illegal in many countries, though it is widely used as a relaxant and stimulant. It is generally believed to be beneficial and certainly to do far less harm than alcohol. The use of ganja, a form of cannabis, is part of Rastafarian religious practice (Cashmore 1992).

There is currently a good deal of debate about the possible legalisation of cannabis and its potential therapeutic use. Cannabis is believed to alleviate symptoms such as muscle spasms, tremor, ataxia and bladder dysfunction that are common following spinal cord injury and in multiple sclerosis. There is also evidence that cannabis is useful in the treatment of chemotherapy-induced nausea and vomiting (Doyle and Spence 1995).

Cannabis produces a range of effects including euphoria, dysphoria, sedation and incoordination. In high doses it produces drowsiness, bradycardia, hypotension and hypothermia. In schizophrenics, cannabis can trigger an acute psychotic reaction. Smoking cannabis can cause bronchitis and bronchial tumours (Doyle and Spence 1995, Johnson 1990). Despite these side effects, people who believe that cannabis is beneficial or who gain pleasure or relief from it, and those for whom it has religious significance, are unlikely to give it up.

Khat/Qat

Khat (also spelled qat) is the leaf of the shrub *Catha edulis*, which is found and used mainly in East Africa and in the Arab peninsula. The main active constituent of khat is cathinone, an amphetamine-like substance which is usually ingested by chewing. Although cathinone is controlled in the UK by the Misuse of Drugs Act 1971, there is no legal prohibition against the import or use of khat.

Chewing khat is generally accepted as a social activity for men in the Somali community, similar to having a smoke or a drink together in Western cultures. The use of khat by women is less common. A study of Somalis in the UK found that some people saw the use of khat as one way of maintaining Somali identity in an alien culture. It was considered preferable to alcohol or tobacco (Griffiths, Gossop et al 1997). However, not all Somalis approve of khat chewing, especially as it is expensive and a drain on already limited finances (Kahin 1997).

The normal recreational use of khat does not seem to be harmful. However, overuse seems to depress the appetite, leading to listlessness and malnourishment. Long-term overuse can result in gastric disturbances, male sub-fertility and impotence. It has also been associated with dental and oral problems, including oral cancer, and can affect the cardiovascular system (Griffiths, Gossop et al 1997, Pantelis, Hindler and Taylor 1989).

Overuse of khat is more likely to occur when people are removed from their usual social and cultural constraints (Griffiths, Gossop et al 1997, Pantelis, Hindler and Taylor 1989). Chewing khat is one of the few familiar social activities that people who have been uprooted and traumatised by civil war can maintain. In the UK, overuse is mainly a problem among Somali men, many of whom are unemployed and living in poor quality, temporary accommodation (see also Chapter 40). Some are also living under the stress of waiting for their application for asylum to be decided (see Chapter 35). Khat chewing may then become a way of alleviating distress rather than a social activity.

Pan

Pan is commonly chewed by both men and women in many parts of the Indian sub-continent and south-east Asia. It is often chewed after meals in the same way that Westerners might drink coffee or smoke. Pan is a green leaf, mixed with betel nuts and limestone to which other substances, including nuts, grains and tobacco leaves, may be added (HEA 1994). Pan turns bright red when chewed and stains the saliva, the mouth, tongue and lips. It is customary for pan chewers to use a spittoon. In hospital, people who chew pan may require a sputum pot to spit into.

There are no legal restrictions on pan or its constituents. However, there are various health risks associated with pan chewing. These include tobacco addiction, mouth ulcers and oral cancers. The betel nut contains addictive substances and can cause dizziness and sweating. It also contains high levels of copper (Trivedy, Baldwin et al 1997).

References

Adamson F (undated) *Female Genital Mutilation: A counselling guide for professionals.* FORWARD, London (See Chapter 32 *Useful address.*)

Ahmad WIU (1992) The maligned healer: the 'hakim' and Western medicine. *New Community* **18** (40): 521–6

Amidu E (1994) *Somali Refugees in London's East End: An investigation into livelihood* (unpublished MSc dissertation). University of London, London

Anionwu E (1994) Women and sickle cell disorders. In M Wilson (ed) *Healthy and Wise: The essential health handbook for black women.* Virago, London

Anionwu E (1993) Sickle cell and thalassaemia: community experiences and official response. In WIU Ahmad (ed) *'Race' and Health in Contemporary Britain.* Open University Press, Buckingham

Anionwu E (1983) *Pain in Sickle Cell Disease.* Sickle Cell Society, London

Aston J (1993) *The Construction of Pregnant Women and HIV* (unpublished MA thesis). University of London, London

Atherton DJ (1994) Towards the safer use of traditional remedies. *British Medical Journal* **308**: 673–4

BHAN (1991) *AIDS and the Black Communities.* Black HIV/AIDS Network, London

Bower H (1994) Healing the scars of torture. *Hospital Doctor* 27 Oct: 26–7

Brookoff D, Polomano R (1992) Treating sickle cell pain like cancer pain. *Annals of Internal Medicine* **116**: 364–8

Cashmore E (1992) *The Rastafarians.* Minority Rights Group, London

Chodoff P (1970) The German concentration camp as a psychological stress. *Archives of General Psychiatry* **22**: 78–87

CRE (1997) *Refugees and Asylum Seekers.* Commission for Racial Equality, London

Davies S (1986) Comprehensive care for sickle cell disease. *THS Health Summary* **3** (12): 7

Davies S, Oni L (1997) Management of patients with sickle cell disease. *British Medical Journal* 315: 656–60

Department of Health (1994) *Guidelines for Offering Voluntary Named HIV Antibody Testing to Women Receiving Antenatal Care.* Department of Health, London

Department of Health (1993) *Report of a Working Party of the Standing Medical Advisory Committee on Sickle Cell, Thalassaemia and Other Haemoglobinopathies.* Stationery Office, London

Department of Health (1992) *Department of Health Guidance PL/CO(92)5, Appendix 2.* Department of Health, London

Dorkenoo E, Elworthy S (1994) *Female Genital Mutilation: Proposals for change.* Minority Rights Group, 379 Brixton Road, London SW9 7DE

Dorkenoo E, Elworthy S (1993) *First Study Conference of Genital Mutilation of Girls in Europe.* FORWARD, London (See Chapter 32 *Useful address*)

Doyle E, Spence A (1995) Cannabis as a medicine? *British Journal of Anaesthesia* 74 (4): 359–60

Eboh W, Van den Akker O (1994) Antenatal care of women with sickle cell disease. *British Journal of Midwifery* 2 (1): 6–11

Economist (1998) A dishonourable mess. *The Economist* 14 Feb: 37–8

Finlay R, Reynolds J (1987) *Social Work and Refugees: A handbook on working with people in exile in the UK.* National Extension College, Cambridge

Goodburn A (1994) A place of greater safety. *Nursing Times* 90 (28): 46–8

Gorst-Unsworth C, Goldenberg E (1998) Psychological sequelae of torture and organised violence suffered by refugees from Iraq. *British Journal of Psychiatry* 172: 90–4

Graham-Brown R (1992) Toxicity of Chinese herbal remedies. *Lancet* 340: 673

Griffiths P, Gossop M, Wickenden S, Dunworth J, Harris K, Lloyd C (1997) A transcultural pattern of drug use: qat (khat) in the UK. *British Journal of Psychiatry* 170: 281–4

HEA (1994) *Black and Minority Ethnic Groups in England: Health and lifestyles.* Health Education Authority, London

Healing TD, Hoffman PN, Young SEJ (1995) The infection hazards of human cadavers. *Communicable Diseases Report* 5 (5): R61–7

Healy MA, Aslam M (1989) *The Asian Community – Medicines and traditions.* Silver Link Publishing, Nottingham

Hedley R, Dorkenoo E (1992) *Child Protection and Female Genital Mutilation: Advice for health, education and social work professionals.* FORWARD, London (See Chapter 32 *Useful addresses*)

Hosken FP (1994) *Genital/Sexual Mutilation of Females,* 4th edn. Women's International Network, Lexington MA

Hussein L (1995) *Report on the Ottawa Consultations on Female Genital Mutilation.* Department of Justice, Ottawa

Johnson BA (1990) Psychopharmacological effects of cannabis. *British Journal of Hospital Medicine* **43**: 114–22

Jordan J (1994) Female genital mutilation (female circumcision). *British Journal of Obstetrics and Gynaecology* **101**: 94–5

Kahin M (1997) *Educating Somali Children in Britain.* Trentham Books, Stoke-on-Trent

Khan S (1994) *Contexts: Race, culture and sexuality, an assessment of our communities.* The NAZ Project, London (See Chapter 34 *Useful addresses*)

Ladjali M, Rattray T, Walder R (1993) Female genital mutilation. *British Medical Journal* **307**: 460

Levine C, Dubler N (1990) HIV and childbearing. I. Uncertain risks and bitter realities: the reproductive choices of HIV-infected women. *Millbank Quarterly* **68** (3): 321–51

McConville B (1998) A bloody tradition. *Nursing Times* **94** (3): 34–6

Monteith C (1994) Counselling and therapy for refugees – the Refugee Support Centre. *SHARE Newsletter.* King's Fund Centre, London

NHS Management Executive (1994) *Asian Women and Maternity Services.* Department of Health/Stationery Office, London

Oni L, Bent S (1998) Sickle cell disease. *Nursing Times* **94** (37): 50–3

Panos Institute (1992) *The Hidden Cost of AIDS: The challenge of HIV to development.* Panos Institute, London

Pantelis C, Hindler C, Taylor J (1989) Use and abuse of khat (*Catha edulis*): a review of the distribution, pharmacology, side effects and a description of psychosis attributed to khat chewing. *Psychological Medicine* **19**: 657–68

Penharic L, Walton R, Murray VS (1992) Toxicity of Chinese herbal remedies. *Lancet* **340**: 674

Positively Women (1994) *Women Like Us: A survey on the needs and experiences of HIV-positive women.* Positively Women, London (See Chapter 34 *Useful addresses*)

Prohibition of Female Circumcision Act 1985. HMSO, London

Rahman TA (1994) *AIDS and the Muslim Communities.* The NAZ Project, London (See Chapter 34 *Useful addresses*)

RCN (1994) *Female Genital Mutilation: The unspoken issue.* Royal College of Nursing, London

Refugee Council (1998) *Statistical Analysis.* Refugee Council, London

Refugee Council (1994) *Increase in Refusals since the Asylum Act.* Refugee Council, London

Refugee Council (1992) *UK Asylum Statistics 1982–92.* Refugee Council, London

Reynolds J (ed) (1993) *Martindale: The extra pharmacopoeia,* 30th edn. Pharmaceutical Press, London

Runnymede Trust (1994) Refugees: Home Office research. *Runnymede Bulletin* July/Aug: 8

Schott J, Henley A (1996) *Culture, Religion and Childbearing in a Multiracial Society.* Butterworth Heinemann, Oxford

Sickle Cell Society (undated) *A Handbook on Sickle Cell Disease: A guide for families.* Sickle Cell Society, London

Siegal RL, Hoefer DD (1981) Bereavement counselling for gay individuals *American Journal of Psychotherapy* **34** (4 Oct): 518

Streetly A, Maxwell K, Mejia A (1997) *Sickle Cell Disorders in Greater London: A needs assessment of screening and care services.* Department of Public Health Medicine, United Medical and Dental Schools, St Thomas' Hospital, London

Trivedy C, Baldwin D, Warnakulasuriya S, Johnson N, Peters T (1997) Copper content in *Areca catechu* (betel nut) products and oral submucous fibrosis. *Lancet* **349**: 1447

UK Thalassaemia Society (1995) *Awareness of Thalassaemia in Asians.* UK Thalassaemia Society, London (See Chapter 33 *Useful addresses*)

UK Thalassaemia Society (1998) *Parliamentary Launch, Asian Awareness Campaign.* UK Thalassaemia Society, London (See Chapter 33 *Useful addresses*)

UNAIDS (1997) *Refugees and AIDS.* UNAIDS, Geneva

United Nations (1951) *Convention Relating to the Status of Refugees (the Geneva Convention).* United Nations, Geneva

Vallerand A (1994) Street addicts and patients with pain: similarities and differences. *Clinical Nurse Specialist* **8** (1): 11–15

Weissman DE, Haddox JD (1989) Opioid pseudo-addiction – an iatrogenic syndrome. *Pain* **36**: 363–6

PART FIVE

Specific Cultures
and Religions

Introduction

This part of the book looks at five cultures and seven religions in relation to daily living and care during illness and around the time of death. The information it contains may be relevant, in varying degrees, to individual patients and their families who identify themselves as belonging to one of these cultures and/or religions. It is important to remember that everybody is primarily an individual and that needs and beliefs vary from person to person. Never make assumptions on the basis of someone's ethnic group or religion.

Most of the content of the following chapters is based on what we, the authors, have learnt during our meetings with people of different cultural and religious groups. Christianity is included among the religions because it is as inappropriate to assume that all health professionals know about Christianity as it is to assume that they all know about Hinduism or Judaism. Five traditional cultures have been chosen on the basis of the numbers of people who may be influenced by them in the UK, or because they cover specific issues relevant to patient care. Traditional South Asian culture is discussed in some detail, both because people of South Asian heritage make up the largest minority ethnic group in the UK and because in many ways traditional South Asian culture illustrates very clearly some of the greatest contrasts with current Western European culture, values and lifestyles.

Most of the chapters in Part Five include a few paragraphs on the history of the community. It may be important, especially when caring for older people, to have some understanding of their history and heritage in order to develop a relationship based on appreciation and respect.

To save space, the information in each chapter is as specific as possible. For example, in the chapters on the different religions, washing is mentioned only when there are specific religious requirements regarding washing. For general discussion of the issues that may be important to any patient in relation to washing or to other aspects of practical care, see Part Two.

How to use this Part

We have had serious reservations about including this Part, because writing anything about the beliefs, practices and needs of different 'groups' is like walking a tightrope. We are only too aware that there is a fine balance between what may be considered 'useful information' and damaging generalisations. We are conscious of the ever-present danger of reinforcing myths, prejudices and stereotypes. On the other hand, we have found that our own thinking and our understanding of the way that culture and religion work in people's lives, as well as our ideas about practical ways of improving care, have been enhanced by learning more about other cultures and religions and about how they seem from the inside. **But this process must be combined with a greater awareness of our own personal, cultural and religious beliefs, values and practices. Reflecting on these enables us to respond more respectfully and flexibly to those of other people.** This Part will be valuable or valid only if it is read in this light and with this purpose.

So, if you have turned to this Part without first reading the rest of the book and, in particular, Parts One and Two, **it is very important that you turn back to the beginning and read the earlier Parts first.** You will also find that Parts One and Two deal in more detail with many of the themes that are, to avoid duplication, only summarised below.

Culture, religion and individuals

In some cases ethnic identity and religious identity overlap: most, though not all, people of Pakistani heritage are Muslims. In other cases there may be differences in the lifestyle and perspectives of people who share the same religion but have different cultures. For example, although Roman Catholics from Nigeria, Palestine, England and Brazil have their religion in common, they are likely to have very different cultural needs. Within every religion there are also many differences in belief and practice. It is therefore no more useful to generalise about Hindus, Jews or Jehovah's Witnesses than to generalise about Christians.

Cultures that outsiders often assume to be unified and similar are in fact extremely diverse. Particular beliefs, practices, values and traditions are more important to some people than to others. When people migrate they maintain certain aspects of their culture but may change or lose others. The children, grandchildren and great-grandchildren of immigrants may feel very strongly about certain aspects of their heritage and may reject others or find them irrelevant. In any community, each person will have their own individual cultural needs. It is extremely important not to categorise people, not to make assumptions or to generalise. **Culture is a framework, not a straitjacket** (see Chapter 1).

This Part discusses Judaism, not Jews, and traditional Chinese culture, not Chinese people. Not every Jew or Chinese person will identify with what is written here, but each chapter offers a framework for understanding things that may be important to some Jewish or Chinese patients and their families. We make no apology for including frequent reminders that the only way to provide high quality care is to find out from each person about their own needs and wishes.

37 African-Caribbean communities: history and traditional culture

Terminology

The term African-Caribbean is used in this book to mean people whose families are of mainly African descent and came to Britain from the West Indies in the Caribbean. Some people use the historical term West Indian. Others may refer to themselves as Black, Black British, Black West Indian or Afro-Caribbean, depending partly on whom they are talking to and the context (Modood, Beishon and Virdee 1994). Some, especially those of the migrant generation, may refer to their country of origin, for example, Jamaican, Trinidadian or Guyanese.

Well over half of all African-Caribbeans in Britain are British born (OPCS 1993). Most of those who were originally immigrants have been here for 40 years or more.

Certain aspects of traditional African-Caribbean culture may be important to many people. Because it is not possible to predict what will be important and to whom, the only way to find out is by listening sensitively to each individual and asking when appropriate.

The West Indies

The West Indies consists of several countries, mainly islands or groups of islands, which stretch over a 2,000 mile curve from Jamaica, near the southern tip of Florida, to Guyana on the mainland of South America, a distance equivalent to that from London to Moscow. Each country has a rich mixture of heritages. Most people are descended from the 24 million West Africans who were removed by force from their homes in the seventeenth and eighteenth centuries and transported to work as slaves on

Caribbean sugar plantations. Sugar was a source of great wealth for the white plantation owners and the European nations. During the eighteenth and nineteenth centuries, people from southern China and southern India and some other areas were brought over as indentured labourers, especially to Trinidad and Guyana (Hiro 1991). The Caribbean countries are therefore as different as those of Western Europe; each has its own history, culture, traditions and way of life.

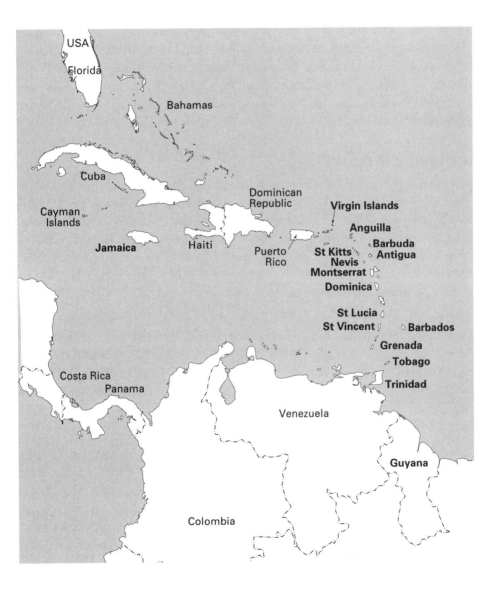

Figure 37.1 The Caribbean, showing (in bold) the main areas of emigration to the UK

The economies of the British West Indies were originally tied to that of Britain and were based on British needs. This structural dependence changed little when the West Indian countries became independent in the 1960s and '70s. Their systems of government, schools, police and judiciary were modelled on British systems; educational curricula focused on British history and literature (Edwards 1986). Most people were brought up to think of Britain as the mother country, prestigious and civilised, responsible and welcoming towards her subjects of all races. Most West Indians who migrated to Britain believed that they were coming home, equal citizens in the family of Commonwealth nations (Hiro 1991).

> 'We didn't feel strangers to England. We had been taught all about British history, the Queen, and that we 'belonged'. When I got here it was shock. A shock to discover people knew nothing about us ... I felt that Jamaica was part of England. The shock was to find I was a stranger.'
> Jamaican man (Foner 1979)

Immigration to the UK

The Caribbean has a long tradition of men and women moving abroad to work, especially to the USA. Following US immigration restrictions in the 1950s, Britain, with its strong historical ties and booming post-war economy, became an obvious focus. As British citizens, West Indians had the unrestricted right to come here to settle and work. However, relatively few came to Britain compared with the numbers that went to the USA (Blakemore and Boneham 1994, Edwards 1986).

African-Caribbean people came to Britain from several different countries, including Jamaica (the largest number), Barbados, Guyana on the South American mainland, and Trinidad and Tobago (see Figure 37.1). Most people came from rural island communities, a few from urban areas. Under British rule, island distinctions were very important; people from different Caribbean countries tended to settle and socialise separately in Britain (Hiro 1991).

The main period of African-Caribbean migration to Britain was in the 1950s and early '60s. Most immigrants were young adults, some were middle-aged, and some brought children. Some had fought for the Allies in the Second World War or worked in the war industries here and stayed on. Many were recruited through special programmes in the West Indies run by London Transport, the British Hotels and Restaurants Association and other employers (Peach 1968). In the early 1960s, the National Health Service recruited West Indian nurses and midwives.

Unlike most other immigrant groups, many African-Caribbean women came on their own to find work, sometimes leaving children in the care of relatives until they returned home or were able to send for them. About 200,000 West Indians arrived in Britain between 1955 and 1961, after which the first immigration controls on Commonwealth citizens were imposed (Edwards 1986) (see also Chapter 41 *Immigration restrictions*).

'Looking for somewhere to live was hard. I telephoned in response to adverts and arranged to visit. When I arrived I could see the shock. I have an English surname and they didn't expect a black man. They always told me the room was taken.'
Older Jamaican man

Like other immigrants, African-Caribbeans took the jobs that local people avoided because they were poorly paid, required unsocial hours or involved hard, dirty or unpleasant physical labour. Most planned to stay for only a short time, earn enough money to improve their situation at home, and then to leave. But low pay and the high fixed costs of living made it difficult to save; under new immigration laws people who left for a while could never come back; and continuing poverty and lack of employment 'back home' made return increasingly unrealistic. Once children were brought up in Britain it became even harder to leave.

Languages

In the West Indies most people speak patois (pronounced patwa) – a complete language that contains features of the vocabularies, grammar and intonation of West African languages and, depending on the island, of English, French or Spanish. There is a good deal of variation in the patois of different islands. For most older African-Caribbeans, patois is their first language and the language they feel most comfortable in.

'I am retired now and here at last I can be myself, eat my own food, talk without having to watch what I say, speak my own language and be understood.'
Older African-Caribbean woman at a day centre

Until recently in the West Indies, patois was frowned upon as the language of the 'less educated'. Many parents discouraged their children from speaking it, fearing that it would prejudice their chances of doing well in life. Some older people still feel uncomfortable about the use of patois in public. The official written language of most West Indian countries is English.

Most British African-Caribbeans are bilingual, speaking patois at home and with African-Caribbean friends and standard English at work or with other people. For many, patois is important as a mark of identity and pride (Modood, Beishon and Virdee 1994). Because patois is rarely written, it is flexible and open to new influences. Patois as spoken by younger British African-Caribbeans has special features that mark it out from a traditional West Indian patois and is sometimes referred to as Black English (Sutcliffe 1982). With older patients and relatives who are not bilingual, it may be necessary to have an interpreter (see Chapter 27).

Religions

Many African-Caribbeans, especially older people, are Christians. The main denominations represented are Anglicans, Baptists, Methodists, Pentecostalists, Seventh Day Adventists and Roman Catholics. In the Caribbean, churches serve very much as social and community as well as religious centres (Green and Green 1992). (See also Chapter 42.)

Some African-Caribbean Christians of other denominations have joined black-led Pentecostalist churches, often because they experienced racism in 'white' churches (Modood, Beishon and Virdee 1994). Some also found the style of worship conservative and dull. Members may address each other as Brother and Sister.

A study in Birmingham found that two-thirds of older African-Caribbeans go to church regularly (Blakemore and Boneham 1994). Many African-Caribbean churches provide fellowship and warmth, spiritual assurance, and practical aid such as help with getting to services and visiting when someone is ill. Some run day centres and luncheon clubs.

Some African-Caribbeans are Jehovah's Witnesses. A small but increasing number, especially of young people, are Rastafarians, or are influenced by Rastafarism. Some are Muslims, some are Hindus. (See the chapters on these religions, later.) Some are spiritualists, often influenced by traditional West African religions.

Traditional family structures and relationships

There is a wide range of family patterns in the Caribbean, influenced by factors such as class, family heritage, economic circumstances and religion. There is historically a high proportion of lone-parent families and of families where the parents live together but are not married. This pattern can be traced back to the systematic and active destruction of African families by white slave owners over a period of 200 years. Husbands were forcibly separated from their wives, and siblings from each other. Slaves were not allowed to marry and were treated as property. Children could be removed from their mothers at any time. African slaves were also used for the sexual satisfaction of white people and as breeding stock. It was believed that a slave woman would produce better children if they were fathered by different men (Hiro 1991, Fuller and Toon 1988).

When slavery was abolished in the early nineteenth century, most ex-slaves were turned out of their 'homes' and were without work or any source of income. Once the huge amount of 'free' labour on which the sugar plantations depended was no longer available, the economy of the islands collapsed, causing widespread poverty and hardship. Many men had to emigrate to find work. Women could not rely on men for security or financial support. All this had further profound effects on families and society.

Although marriage and the two-parent family were traditionally respected and regarded as ideal, especially for the security of children, poverty, insecurity, the need to travel to find work and other difficulties meant that formal marriage was often reserved for better-off or middle-class families, or for people with a long-standing relationship who already had children. Christian, Hindu and Muslim families were more likely to believe that a couple should be married before they had children.

When pregnancy occurred outside marriage, it was normal for each child to take the father's surname and for the father to support his own children. It was not considered necessary for the parents to live together, nor was it usually regarded as wrong if they did not. In many cases West Indian mothers, grandmothers and aunts took the main responsibility for children within a wider extended family. Girls were brought up to be independent and self-reliant.

West Indian families have a tradition of strong mutual support, shared responsibility, pride and independence in the face of injustice and difficulty. Families were generally expected to keep any problems to themselves. Children were expected to show respect for and obey their parents and all older people. The oldest child traditionally took on most responsibility for older parents, and for the care and guidance of younger siblings (Gopaul-McNicol 1993).

In Britain

Many African-Caribbean families came under pressure on arrival in the UK, where there was little understanding of the variety of family patterns or of the strengths of black families (see also Chapter 9 *Families, relationships and roles*). Households that did not conform to the current British norm were often regarded as immoral and irresponsible. Children in such families were expected to develop problems. In addition, the constant experience of racial discrimination and hostility, as well as, in many cases, poverty, poor housing and unemployment, placed a major strain on many families and individuals (Ahmed, Cheetham and Small 1986, Brown 1984).

Most African-Caribbean migrants had to take jobs of a lower status than they had the skills and training for. Women were sometimes able to get better jobs, while men, who generally experienced more discrimination, were more likely to be in lower-paid work or unemployed (see also Chapter 5 *The effects of racism*). As in the wider population, the resulting financial and other tensions sometimes caused relationship problems (Fuller and Toon 1988). Nevertheless, for many British African-Caribbeans, marriage or a committed permanent partnership remain the ideals, providing security and status for women and a stable environment for the raising of children. In the African-Caribbean communities there is also a strong sense of family closeness and a concern that children should be brought up with love, discipline, a clear code of good behaviour including respect for their elders, pride and independence (Beishon, Modood and Virdee 1998).

Older African-Caribbean people

At the time of the 1996 Labour Force Survey, only 17 per cent of African-Caribbeans were aged over 55, compared with 26 per cent of the white population (Church 1997). Most African-Caribbeans who are now getting old have been here since the 1950s and early '60s. Relatively few have arrived more recently as 'elderly dependants' (see Chapter 4 *Poverty*).

Older African-Caribbeans in Britain have experienced major geographical, cultural and personal changes, many of which have been very difficult. Coping successfully with these changes has demanded resilience and stoicism. Many older people feel great pride in what they have achieved, realising, however, that it is generally unrecognised and unvalued by the majority of the population. Most older African-Caribbeans never expected to spend their old age in Britain. For many, returning home is still a dream, though for most it is a dream that they know will never be fulfilled (Fenton 1987).

> 'Still, we are here in Britain now, and I think you are categorically mistaken if you now want to go back. You can't go to a country that can do nothing for you. You must stay in the country where you have done something for the country, so that it may do back for you. If you make a mistake, you can't make it right by making another mistake.'
> Older Jamaican man (Age Exchange 1984)

Finances A history of low wages and high unemployment means that many African-Caribbeans are dependent on means-tested benefits (Amin 1992). Most also sent regular contributions back to their families in the Caribbean and so have been unable to save for their retirement. Many feel a strong sense of self-reliance and pride and will not 'take charity'.

Family support In the small island communities of the Caribbean, older people were generally respected and cared for by their families, though this was combined with a strong tradition of independence. People with no close kin were often looked after by neighbours. Older women, in particular, gave advice and help and played important roles as grandmothers (Blakemore and Boneham 1994).

In Britain, African-Caribbean families share the pressures that affect other families. A high proportion of working women means that there is often no one to care for family members who are ill or frail. Small houses and flats may make it difficult or impossible to take in older people. Nevertheless, older African-Caribbeans with a strong family structure who have children nearby are likely to have considerable contact and to be supported and cared for, particularly in times of crisis (Barker 1984).

As in other communities, some older people worry that young African-Caribbeans have lost their respect for old age, and do not wish to care for older family members. Many worry about the discontent and bitterness that they often see in young African-Caribbeans, not just because such anger is unsettling in itself but because it raises questions about the value of the sacrifices they themselves made, largely for their children, and about what black people have been able to achieve in British society (Blakemore and Boneham 1994).

'I arrived in Britain here with only a small suitcase. Every morning I got up early and went to work, I worked hard all day, came home late, supported my family, educated my children. I've had it tough here and I've earned every penny of what I have. But what I really want is respect from this country, for myself and my family, and that I will never get.'
African-Caribbean man

Isolation A significant number of older African-Caribbean people do not have relatives nearby. A study in the 1980s found that 33 per cent of African-Caribbeans over the age of 60 lived alone (Fenton 1987). Some have never been part of a close family or have always lived alone. Others have adult children here, but they have moved away to find work. Because of the traditionally female-focused nature of African-Caribbean families, older men are particularly likely to be alone and isolated (Blakemore and

Boneham 1994). Many older African-Caribbeans are reluctant to leave their homes for fear of racial harassment and violence; this increases their isolation (South Glamorgan Race Equality Council 1994).

In some cases, adult children in the Caribbean or elsewhere try to come to Britain to care for ageing relatives. However, the ban on New Commonwealth immigration, increasingly strict control of visitors from the Caribbean, and immigration officials' suspicion that any African-Caribbean person visiting close relations in the UK will wish to stay, mean that they are often refused permission to come or are turned back at the airport when they arrive in the UK (Divided Families Campaign 1990, Divided Families Campaign, undated).

Caribbean foods and diets

Good food and a balanced, healthy diet are very important in traditional African-Caribbean culture. Eating well is often regarded as a sign of emotional well-being and physical health. Sharing food brings families together. Most African-Caribbeans in Britain eat traditional foods at least some of the time. Traditional foods may be especially important for older people (Douglas 1989).

'I couldn't sleep with worry when my mother was no longer eating properly.'
African-Caribbean woman

Fresh food is regarded as best, and in the Caribbean most people have plots of land where they can grow much of what they need. Older people, in particular, may be suspicious of processed and packaged foods and of additives (Age Exchange 1991). Because African-Caribbean food is often more expensive in Britain than indigenous food, it can take up a large proportion of household income.

Cooking methods and flavours vary a good deal between different islands and communities, influenced by the diets of West Africa, western Europe, North and Latin America, China and India. Important starches include yams, sweet potatoes, rice, potatoes, plantains, breadfruit, green bananas, corn meal and wheat flour. The main pulses used are kidney beans, black-eyed peas, gunga peas and split peas. Many traditional dishes are baked or stewed. One-pot dishes are popular (Shukla 1991). Fish is traditionally widely eaten. Food is often highly spiced, and hot sauces and hot peppers are used as flavourings. Fish, red meat and chicken are often marinated ('seasoned') with herbs and spices before cooking. Many African-Caribbeans, especially older people, find the food in English hospitals and residential care unappetising, bland and heavy. Some people avoid more spicy foods and red meat when they are ill and prefer light foods such as home-made clear soup.

Some African-Caribbeans follow religious food restrictions (see Chapter 11 *Religious aspects of food*, and the chapters on religions, later).

Practical care

Modesty

Physical modesty and self-respect are very important in traditional African-Caribbean culture. Older people, in particular, may not wish to be examined, washed or nursed by members of the opposite sex. Mixed-sex wards are likely to be unacceptable for many. It is very important to try to preserve people's modesty and dignity in all situations (see also Chapter 12 *Modesty*).

Washing and cleanliness

Physical cleanliness, grooming and dressing well are traditionally a matter of pride in African-Caribbean culture. Most people are used to showering and changing their clothes two, or even three, times a day. It is traditional in the West Indies to add an antiseptic to the bath water.

African-Caribbean patients often find hospital washing facilities inadequate and feel that they cannot keep themselves as clean as they would wish. People who need bed baths may want to be washed all over with lots of soap and hot water. Some may prefer to be wheeled to the bathroom rather than be washed in bed. Many people oil their skin after washing (see also Chapter 12 *Skin care*).

Hair care

'The saddest thing for a woman is to have matted hair'.
African-Caribbean woman

Good hair care is important for comfort and self-esteem. Black hair requires specific care (see Chapter 12 *Hair care*). Some older African-Caribbean women may wear a head scarf in bed.

When someone is ill or dying

Attitudes to the health service

The individual and collective experience of African-Caribbeans does not lead most people to expect equal or fair treatment from British institutions or from white health professionals. Thorogood (1989) suggests that some may therefore feel less constrained than many white people about admitting their dissatisfaction. When people do not get courteous and good health care, instead of blaming themselves or regarding it as exceptional, they may be more likely to take action. A study of African-Caribbean women found that changing GPs because of dissatisfaction was relatively common, even though it was difficult. Women seemed more likely to admit discontent than their white peers; several had confronted their GPs with accusations of poor care. Most did not feel the respect and subservience towards doctors that are common in many older English patients. Some African-Caribbeans prefer to pay for private GP consultations because they believe they will be taken more seriously (Thorogood 1989)

Many older African-Caribbeans, especially women, have also worked in the NHS, in nursing homes or in similar places (Modood, Berthoud et al 1997). They have an insider's understanding of the workings and limitations of health care institutions. They may be very much aware of pressured staff and stretched resources. They will also have had direct experience of personal and institutionalised racism in the NHS (see also Chapters 5 and 6).

Traditional remedies

Herbal and dietary remedies, some of which have been found in research to be effective, are often used for common conditions (Douglas 1989). Herbal teas, or bush teas, made from Caribbean plants, are widely used. Herbal treatment may also be administered in the form of baths, poultices and steam inhalations. Older African-Caribbean people may prefer to try herbal remedies before consulting a doctor, or may take them at the same time as pharmaceutical preparations. Some people may be reluctant to admit that they are using herbal remedies in case health professionals disapprove (Age Exchange 1991) (see also Chapter 31).

Medication

Some patients, perhaps especially older people, may prefer to be aware of and express their pain and may reject opiates. Some may be anxious about loss of control and awareness (Baxter 1989). Others may feel that illness and pain are part of God's plan and should be accepted with dignity (see Chapter 14 *Pain and pain relief*).

Family responsibilities

It is traditionally important for family and community members to visit sick people. Some patients may have large numbers of visitors, a few of these at unusual times having arrived from abroad (see also Chapter 17 *Visitors from far away*).

When a person is known to be dying, family members may wish to visit and sit with them all the time and to be present at the death. They may want to pray and sing hymns or other religious songs with the patient. In traditional African-Caribbean culture, people generally express their feelings openly and loudly. When possible, it may be helpful to move the patient and their visitors to a side room.

'West Indians are naturally demonstrative. Quite often the more reserved European staff may feel threatened, or at least feel that this behaviour is bizarre.'
Residential care manager

Organ donation

Some older people may believe that a whole body is necessary to pass into the next life, and may refuse organ donation (Green and Green 1992) (see also Chapter 19 *Organ donation*).

After the death

Last offices

Last offices may in most cases be carried out as usual. It is most important that last offices are carried out well, because the family may wish later to wash and dress the body themselves before the funeral, or to keep the coffin open until the funeral. The hair should be tidied in the style that the person normally wore. (See also Chapter 20 *Immediately after the death and last offices*.)

Embalming is common because the coffin is traditionally kept open at the funeral and because funerals are often delayed while family members gather.

Post mortems

Many people of African-Caribbean heritage dislike the idea of a post mortem, on religious or personal grounds. (See also the chapters on religions.) Some may believe strongly in the sanctity of the body and may refuse. If a post mortem is legally required, sensitive explanation must be given and care taken with repair of the body (see Chapter 20 *Post mortems*).

The funeral

Traditionally, the funeral is held shortly after the death. However, in Britain it may be delayed to allow relatives time to gather, sometimes from all over the world. In many communities it is traditional to hold a wake each night until the funeral. Relatives and friends gather to sit with close family members. Prayers may be said and memories shared. Some families keep the body at home until the funeral so that everyone, including children, can pay their last respects. Others keep the body at the funeral director's until shortly before the funeral, when it is brought home. In other cases the cortege may pass by the dead person's house on the way to the funeral. Some families may wish to fly the body to their country of origin for burial (see Chapter 20 *Repatriating the body*).

Traditionally, burial is preferred to cremation. Rituals vary a great deal, especially between different religious groups. In most Christian communities, funerals are traditionally large and emotional events with as many members of the family and community as possible attending. The funeral service may be long, with flowers, hymns, music and tributes to the dead person (Green and Green 1992).

> 'I think it's more healthy to cry and let go. Surely that's what funerals are for. For me the saddest and loneliest thing is the stiff-upper-lip behaviour at English funerals. I cannot believe how short the funerals are and how they get through the whole thing showing so little emotion.'
> Middle-aged African-Caribbean woman

Family and community support are also traditionally very important after the funeral. Homes may remain open for people to call, pray with the family and talk about the person who has died.

38 Chinese communities: history and traditional culture

According to the 1991 Census, there are about 160,000 Chinese people in Britain, almost a third of whom were born here (OPCS 1993). The origins and educational and occupational backgrounds of Chinese people in Britain vary widely.

Despite the considerable diversity of the Chinese communities in Britain, there are aspects of Chinese culture that transcend differences of background and experience and which may still be important for some people, particularly those who came to Britain as adults. Some of them may also matter to British-born Chinese people. **Because it is never possible to predict to whom they will and will not be important, the only way to find out is by listening sensitively to each individual and asking when appropriate.**

The Chinese communities in Britain

China has a strong and long-standing tradition of people emigrating to work overseas and there are Chinese communities in most of the countries of the world. There have been Chinese people in some areas of Britain, particularly the ports, since the early nineteenth century. However, the main period of Chinese immigration occurred in the 1950s and '60s. At this time there was an economic boom in Britain, a collapse in traditional agriculture and fishing in Hong Kong and in the New Territories attached to the former British colony of Hong Kong, and political uncertainty in China (Au and Au 1992, Li 1992).

Many of the first group of Chinese immigrants set up laundries, restaurants or lodging houses in the major ports, initially serving mainly Chinese seamen. As more households got their own washing machines, and eating out became more popular, many Chinese people moved into the restaurant trade. Under British law, immigration vouchers were granted chiefly to employers wishing to bring in named individuals to work in specific jobs. Most Chinese people of the immigrant generation therefore worked (and often still work) in the restaurant or retail trades. In general, men came first to find work and save. Their wives and families usually followed later. Most families were reunited in the 1960s and '70s. Some have since brought older dependent relatives to join them. There are also a number of older single men who have lived and worked in Britain for many years (Au and Au 1992).

Most people who arrived in the 1950s and '60s came from conservative farming areas and had little or no formal education. In Britain they went into unskilled or semi-skilled work, often with long, unsocial hours. Some Chinese people came from urban, Westernised backgrounds in Hong Kong and elsewhere, often as professionals – for example, nurses, doctors, accountants and engineers, and businessmen and women.

The families of about 80 per cent of Chinese people in Britain originated in the former British colony of Hong Kong (including the New Territories – see above). In addition, there are a small number of Chinese people from Malaysia and Singapore who came to Britain originally to study or to work in the health service, as well as Chinese families from other areas of the Far East, including the People's Republic of China, Taiwan, Vietnam (see below) and Indonesia (see Figure 38.1), and a few from Mauritius, the South Pacific islands and the Caribbean (Li 1992).

Although there are now sizeable Chinese communities in a few British cities, many Chinese families are fairly isolated, running perhaps the only Chinese restaurant or take-away in a small town. As a result, their existence and health care needs may not be noticed or taken seriously by service providers (Au and Au 1992).

Vietnamese refugees By the 1970s the people of Vietnam had suffered over 30 years of national and civil war. During the late 1970s and in the 1980s about 20,000 Vietnamese people came to Britain as refugees. A small number arrived later. Although only about 2 per cent of the population of Vietnam was ethnic Chinese, about 80 per cent of those who fled were Chinese. Chinese people were particularly vulnerable in North Vietnam because they were suspected of being loyal to China; in South Vietnam many were part of the merchant class to which the new Communist government was opposed. About two-thirds of the Vietnamese people in Britain came from rural areas of North Vietnam and had had little opportunity for education or contact with Western culture before they fled.

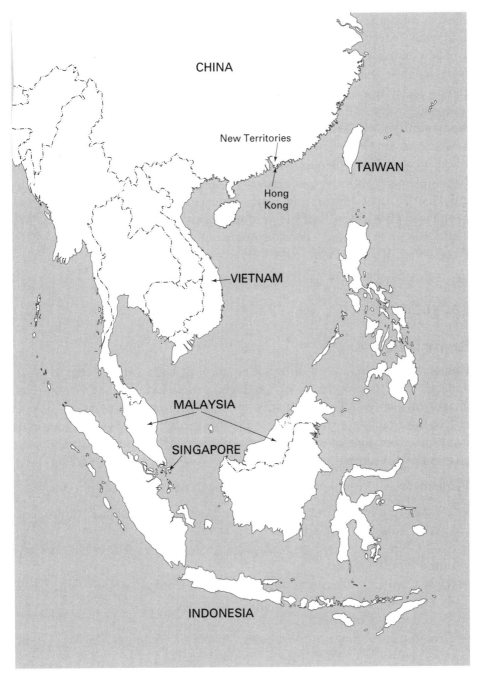

Figure 38.1 The Far East, showing the main areas of Chinese emigration to the UK

The journey of those who fled was often traumatic, and included starvation, thirst, storms, shipwrecks and attacks by pirates. Many refugees lost family members on the way. While waiting to come to Britain, many people have spent several years shut up in depressing and overcrowded 'closed camps' in Hong Kong where little meaningful activity was possible and violent gangs ruled. Most people left some close relatives behind in Vietnam; many families are further split because of the different admission policies of the receiving countries. Extended family structures and support have often broken down. People who have been through such experiences are likely to find emotional and practical adaptation to life in Britain particularly hard. Many continue to suffer serious emotional and psychological problems. They often find the complex health, Social Security and other welfare services incomprehensible and do not know where to ask for help (Tang 1994, Refugee Action 1987) (see also Chapter 35).

Languages

Spoken languages

Chinese There are over a dozen Chinese languages (often referred to as dialects) that form a family of languages rather like the Latin-based languages of Europe. The languages spoken by Chinese people in Britain reflect their families' area of origin in China, often many generations ago. Cantonese and Hakka are the most common. Most spoken Chinese languages are not mutually comprehensible.

Vietnamese is a completely different, though related, language.

- Most people from Hong Kong and the New Territories speak Cantonese, Hakka, Toi-Shan or Chiu Chao.
- Most Chinese people from Malaysia and Singapore speak Hokkien, Cantonese or Chiu Chao.
- Most Chinese people from Vietnam speak Cantonese and Vietnamese, though some speak another Chinese language.
- Most people from Taiwan speak Mandarin.
- The official language of the Chinese People's Republic is Mandarin, now called Putongwa (which means 'ordinary speech').

English All British-born Chinese people and most of those who came to Britain before they were 25 speak English. However, only about half of those aged over 45 speak English fluently or fairly well (Modood, Berthoud et al 1997). In a survey in Central London, most Chinese adults said that language problems were the main barrier to their finding out about and getting health care (Bloomsbury 1984). A more recent survey found that one-third of Chinese people who had consulted a GP in the past month had not understood the language the GP used (Nazroo 1997).

Many older Chinese people have had little or no contact with English speakers in Britain. Women with children have often led extremely isolated lives at home all day. Most men and many women have worked long hours; few people have had much real opportunity to learn English (see Chapter 25). A study of older Chinese and Vietnamese people found that only 22 per cent could speak English (South Glamorgan Race Equality Council 1994).

Written languages

Chinese has one written language. This is based on ideograms, or symbols, and was standardised over two thousand years ago. Despite the fact that each spoken language uses different words and pronunciation, they all write the same ideogram to indicate the same meaning. Consequently, everyone who reads and writes Chinese reads and writes the same language, whatever language(s) they speak.

Vietnamese is written in the Western alphabet. The tones of the words are indicated by accent marks.

Older people Older people and others with little formal education may not be able to read any language. The study of older Chinese and Vietnamese people quoted above found that 39 per cent could read only Chinese, 17 per cent could read only Vietnamese, 17 per cent could read English, and 17 per cent could not read any language.

The Chinese naming system

The Chinese naming system works differently from the British one. It is very important to check that names have been recorded correctly, to prevent dangerous mistakes and misidentification (see Chapter 30 *Recording people's names correctly*).

Traditional family structures and relationships

The extended family

The traditional Chinese family is a large unit with people of several generations all living under one roof or in close contact. The family and its extension (the clan) are traditionally the two main units of support.

Although few Chinese people in Britain live in an extended family and some live alone, many, especially of the older generation, still subscribe to its values and to the principles that have strengthened Chinese society for thousands of years. In the extended family system, the head of the family is the oldest working man. Men and women have different but mutual responsibilities. Men are regarded as chiefly responsible for the economic support and well-being of the family, and, depending on their age, are expected to make most important decisions. Marriage is considered the point at which a person takes on adult status. Traditionally, a new wife moves in with her husband's family, at least for a few years. Sons and daughters-in-law are expected to take care of older and frail members. People who are ill are traditionally expected to take on a passive role and to allow themselves to be cared for by family members. Attitudes to sexual morality are strict (see also Chapter 9 *Families, relationships and roles*).

Traditional values

Chinese people living in Britain, especially those who were educated here, are influenced by the values and norms of British society. Nevertheless, traditional values are likely to remain a powerful influence. Good manners, the love of parents for their children and of children for their parents, piety, family loyalty, kindness and social harmony are highly valued in Chinese culture. Reserve, modesty and consideration for other people's feelings are stressed. Emotions, especially negative ones, are not generally discussed, even within the family, and certainly not outside it. Disclosure of feelings may be regarded as bad manners. Chinese children are traditionally encouraged from an early age to hide personal feelings for the sake of politeness, and to avoid disputes that could disrupt social harmony. Public displays of emotion and direct confrontation are discouraged. Love and affection are traditionally demonstrated in practical ways rather than in words (Shang 1986). Work and education are highly valued; everyone is traditionally expected to study or work hard for the benefit of the family.

Respect for authority and age is very important. The views of parents and older family members should be listened to and obeyed, even if there is dis-agreement. Men have authority, at least in public, over women. Out of respect, younger people usually address their elders by titles such as Mother, Uncle, Older Sister or Grandfather, rather than by their personal name. Younger people are expected to show deference, humility and good up-bringing by listening well to older people and speaking little (Wenzhong and Grove 1991). Looking older or more senior people in the eye is generally considered disrespectful (see also Chapter 24 *Non-verbal signals*). Some Chinese people feel that questioning indicates a lack of respect; they may find it difficult to ask health professionals questions about treatments and diagnoses. Younger people may feel more able to ask questions, though probably not if older family members are present.

Reputation and honour

The reputation, honour and privacy of the family are very important and are the responsibility of all members. Sometimes this is referred to as 'face', as in 'saving face'. Families are expected to be self-reliant and to deal with their own problems. In Britain, some Chinese people may be reluctant to discuss serious illness, financial difficulties or relationship problems with health professionals or other outsiders because of the risk of bringing shame on the family (Au and Au 1992). Among small, close-knit communities gossip travels very quickly. Strict confidentiality is therefore particularly important.

Some people do not claim benefits due to them or ask for statutory assistance such as a home help because they do not wish to accept 'charity' and because of the strong belief that support should be given by the family. Others would like to claim benefits but are prevented from doing so by their lack of English.

Gratitude

It is traditional to demonstrate gratitude to people who have been very kind or who have carried out a personal service by giving gifts, including gifts of cash. Festivals (see later) are a popular time for this. Gifts should traditionally be accepted to avoid causing offence and humiliation to the giver. If grateful patients or families offer money, the refusal should be accompanied by a gentle explanation that the institution does not allow individuals to accept financial gifts. It may be appropriate to suggest that the money is given to a charitable cause.

Older Chinese people

Older people are traditionally highly respected. They are seen as at the apex of society, both because of their age and useful experience and because they represent an important link between past and present, between family ancestors and living family members. They traditionally have authority over other family members, including other adults. Their main roles are to guide and advise the family (see also Chapter 4 *Traditional expectations*).

Old age is traditionally seen as positive, bringing well-earned rewards and benefits. It is a matter of pride that an older person should be able to look after themselves. Many older Chinese people are very active, working in the family business or looking after grandchildren. Some take regular physical exercise in the form of Tai Chi. If someone becomes frail or ill, it is customary for their families to cherish and look after them.

Older Chinese people expect both to receive and to give respect. It is important for younger people, including health professionals at all levels, to behave respectfully towards them.

Approaching the end of life

It is considered fitting for Chinese people, as they get older, to reflect upon their lives and try to do good. Many people believe in rebirth (see *Buddhism*, below); living virtuously and giving to charity can have a positive influence on one's situation in the next life. For Chinese Christians and Muslims too (see Chapters 42 and 44), the idea of being rewarded or punished after death for one's behaviour in this life may be important.

In Britain

Many older Chinese people in Britain, especially men, are in poor health after a lifetime of hard physical work in unhealthy conditions and very long hours in the catering trade. Some retire early because of health problems. Many face poverty because of insufficient National Insurance contributions (see Chapter 4 *Poverty*). Some live in tied accommodation and become homeless when they lose their jobs.

A study in London found that 90 per cent of the Chinese older people interviewed had received no help from social workers, meals-on-wheels, home helps or community nurses, although there were several cases of obvious need. As well as their lack of knowledge that the services existed, some older people did not think services would be of use to them: the meals-on-wheels service would not suit a Chinese diet, and social workers would not understand the particular needs and wishes of older Chinese people. Nearly half the people interviewed found it difficult to travel alone on public transport. Most just stayed at home. Half said they felt lonely most of the time (Chiu 1989).

The same study found a high level of need for practical care such as help with bathing, dressing and going to the toilet, shopping, cooking and doing laundry. For most older people the main source of help was their family. But many received no help from family members because the latter lived too far away or worked long hours. Older people were often reluctant to ask for intimate personal care from anyone but their own daughter, who traditionally would perform this role. Many, however, had no daughter living nearby and some had no family members at all.

Most older Chinese people would rather be cared for by members of their family at home, even if they are very frail or seriously ill.

'The Vietnamese elderly [most of whom are ethnically Chinese] want to rely on and be proud of the support of their children when they are growing old. They want to stay very close to their family and feel that they should not need support from others, for example going to nursing homes or having help from social services.' (South Glamorgan Race Equality Council 1994)

Chinese philosophy and religion

Shared values

Traditional Chinese society does not contain a number of separate formal religions in the way that most Westerners find easy to understand. Instead, the Chinese philosophy and way of life are based on three main schools of philosophical and religious thought – Confucianism, Buddhism and Taoism. These have influenced each other over many centuries and form a unique philosophy and value system whose main emphasis is on people's behaviour in their daily life rather than on spiritual abstractions. For many Chinese people it is neither necessary nor possible to distinguish which of their values originated where (Küng and Ching 1993).

Formal religions In a recent survey in Britain, over half the Chinese interviewees said they had no religion (Modood, Berthoud et al 1997). However, many people with no formal religion are influenced by Confucianism, Buddhism and Taoism. They may have a shrine in the kitchen, burn incense and celebrate religious festivals. They may call on traditional spiritual beliefs and practices if someone is seriously ill or dying or after a death.

Traditional Chinese philosophy and values also remain important for many people who follow a different formal religion. Some Chinese people in Britain follow a religious form of Taoism. About a fifth (mainly older people) are Buddhist, a few are Muslim and about a quarter are Christian. Among Chinese Christians, most people are Church of England, Roman Catholic or Baptist. In Britain, there are strong Chinese churches in almost all the Christian denominations: these offer extensive social support and practical help as well as a community for worship. Some people have joined a Chinese Christian church since they came to Britain in order to reduce their isolation.

Confucianism

Confucius (K'ung Fu-tzu) was an ethical philosopher who lived in China at a time of social and moral turmoil about 2500 years ago. He taught social harmony and mutual consideration through a code of conduct that emphasises humanistic virtues such as obligations to parents and other family members, respect and obedience towards older people, loyalty, integrity, self-control, self-reliance, benevolence, respect and consideration for others. He also stressed the great importance of education and knowledge. Confucianism has strongly influenced Chinese culture and values (Küng and Ching 1993).

Taoism

Taoism is an ancient Chinese philosophy which contains the idea of a unifying force or impersonal God underlying all reality. This ultimate reality can only be perceived and understood through mystical insight. It cannot be expressed in words. Tao (pronounced dow) means The Way.

Taoism stresses the perfection and beauty of nature, and the importance of achieving purity and union with the natural world through meditation and a simple life. People are part of the natural order of the universe. They should attempt to achieve health, harmony and balance within themselves, with nature and within society by avoiding conflict and confrontation. If a course of action is blocked, Taoism stresses finding alternatives rather than persisting disharmoniously or fighting.

For some people, Taoism is a rational philosophy and an ethical guide. For others, it is a religion and has a supernatural element. Most religious Taoists believe that, by following The Way, they will be led through this transitory life to a happy eternity. Taoism is the leading religion in Taiwan.

Religious Taoism contains three classes of spirits: gods, ghosts and ancestors. There are many gods, each with different responsibilities and powers, and people pray to them for help at times of illness or difficulty. The gods are venerated at small shrines, and in special places such as the entrance to a family's home. Some people light incense sticks, offer food and other symbolic offerings in front of statues of the gods. They may also burn written prayers and requests. (Adapted from Mares 1982, by kind permission.)

An important part of Taoist tradition is the veneration of ancestors, both those who have died recently and those from previous centuries. Some Chinese homes have an ancestral shrine containing wooden or paper tablets with the names of family members who have died, and sometimes photographs of more recent generations. People may place incense and offerings of food, symbolic paper money and paper houses in front of the shrine in celebration of their ancestors' achievements and good deeds, and may pray to them for protection and help. Venerating ancestors expresses the shared community of living and dead family members and is supported by Confucius' emphasis on filial piety (Küng and Ching 1993). For some people, the knowledge that they will be remembered and venerated in this way lessens the fear of death (Huang 1989).

There is also a very strong tradition of powerful ghosts or bad spirits in Chinese culture (Huang 1989). Sometimes these are the spirits of ancestors who have been neglected and who may punish their descendants for several generations. They can cause illness and disaster to individuals and families, especially at times when people are already vulnerable, for example during illness or around a death. If the influence of ancestors or ghosts is suspected, families may organise religious services to try to appease or exorcise them. However, some people who believe in ghosts or bad spirits may be reluctant to discuss them with Western health professionals.

Buddhism

Buddhism is a world religion whose essence is a philosophy and principles rather than detailed practices, observances and rules. There is a good deal of room for differences in interpretation and expression between the different branches and schools of Buddhism. Buddhists of different heritages may have very different beliefs and follow different practices.

Buddhism was introduced to China in about CE* 65. It is based on the teachings of Siddhartha Gautama who lived in north-east India about 2,500 years ago. Gautama was horrified by the unhappiness he saw around him and sought a way to alleviate the sufferings of humankind. After many years of searching and meditation he achieved enlightenment and became The Buddha, the Enlightened One. For the rest of his life he travelled, preaching and teaching, and established a community of followers.

Teachings The Buddha taught Four Noble Truths:

- The First Noble Truth is that suffering, disappointment and impermanence are fundamental to the human condition. Nothing is secure or lasting or satisfactory in the long term. Change, loss, dissatisfaction and disappointment are inevitable.
- The Second Noble Truth is that suffering is caused by people's ignorance of the nature of reality and by their incessant wishes and desires, including their wish to hold on to things that will inevitably pass away, whether things, people, ideas, feelings or even their own life and consciousness.

---

* Common Era, used as an alternative to AD.

- The Third Noble Truth is that people can liberate themselves from suffering and disappointment by getting rid of ignorance, self-centredness and the desire to control things. When they can live without seeing everything in terms of how it affects them, they will be free of selfish needs, cravings and anxieties and of negative characteristics such as pride, jealousy, greed, fear, ignorance, selfishness and hatred. They will be reborn into a state of Nirvana where there is no more suffering.
- The Fourth Noble Truth consists of the principles that people should follow to achieve a good life and eventually reach Nirvana. These are called the Middle Way (avoiding extremes of self-indulgence and self-mortification) or the Eightfold Path. They include:
  - wisdom – understanding reality according the first three Noble Truths, combined with renunciation, detachment, overcoming greed and hatred, developing loving-kindness and compassion;
  - ethical conduct – telling the truth, avoiding gossip, slander and abusive language; living ethically, not harming others; earning one's living in a way that does not harm or exploit;
  - mental discipline or meditation – right effort so as to progress in Buddhism, being fully aware of everything and understanding its true nature, and focusing one's energies on achieving wisdom, ethical behaviour and greater awareness of the Truth (Weller 1997, Erriker 1995).

Rebirth and karma Buddhists believe in the cycle of birth, death and rebirth; every living being dies and is reborn. But in Buddhist teaching, human beings and other life forms do not have permanent, independently existing souls or identities. Each consists of a temporary combination of constantly changing forces or energies. The Buddha regarded belief in an individual eternal soul as leading to egoism and craving and thus to suffering (Erriker 1995).

> 'A simple analogy might help to clarify this process: the flame of one candle can be passed to another, and then that flame can be passed to a third candle, and so on indefinitely. The flame that passes down the line is not the same, yet neither is it different.' (Sibley 1997)

The form in which a person is reborn and what happens to them in their life are influenced by karma. Karma, a Sanskrit word, literally means 'action'. It is used in Buddhism to refer to a person's intentional acts and their ethical consequences. Through natural moral law, every act, thought or wish has karmic consequences in this life or in the next, depending on the intentions that accompanied it. Good is rewarded and bad punished. Karma also determines the form in which a person is reborn, as well as their beauty, intelligence, wealth and social status. They may be reborn as a human being, an animal, a jealous god, a proud god, a hungry ghost who can never be satisfied, or a tormented being in hell. People can improve their karma by doing good and developing loving-kindness, generosity and compassion. Each individual is therefore responsible for what happens to them.

Only human beings can achieve Nirvana, so to be born a human offers a precious opportunity. For many Buddhists, it is very important that in the time leading up to their death they should try to ensure a positive rebirth.

Boddhisattvas There were many Buddhas before Gautama and there will be more in the future. Each Buddha goes through many human and non-human lives in preparation for Buddhahood. In these lives he is known as a Boddhisattva. Boddhisattvas practise ten virtues: generosity, morality, renunciation, wisdom, energy, patience, truthfulness, determination, loving-kindness and equanimity. In the Mahayana tradition (of which Chinese Buddhism is a part), Boddhisattvas choose to delay their entry to Nirvana out of compassion to help other beings on the same path. Some Chinese Buddhists regard Boddhisattvas as permanent living deities and pray to them for help and guidance and for special causes (Goonewardene 1996, Erriker 1995).

Religious observance in hospital

Some Chinese people will wish to pray or meditate in hospital. They may wish to use a quiet room if one is available, or to have their curtains drawn. Some may wish to place incense or flowers in front of a picture or statue (see also Chapter 10 *Practical matters*). People who belong to a specific temple or church may have visits from a priest or other members of the community.

Good and bad luck

The concepts of good and bad luck have always been important in Chinese culture. Certain times, dates and numbers are considered auspicious or inauspicious, and some people take these into account when, for example, going on a journey or starting a new venture. For some people it is important to try to plan surgery and other treatments for an auspicious day when they are less vulnerable. Some days are also more auspicious for holding a funeral.

Traditionally, language, thought and reality are seen as connected. Positive thinking is emphasised and some people believe that a positive attitude and positive statements can improve the outcome of an illness. Negative thoughts and feelings and talking about illness and death may increase people's vulnerability and make bad things happen (see also *Attitudes to death and dying*, later). Some people avoid words such as death, cancer and similar words. They also avoid talking about unlucky or sad things on festivals and happy occasions. A few people may believe that their illness has been caused by someone else's ill will. Some may ask a priest to pray and to try to remove the negative energy that is harming them.

Connections between sound and meaning are important. For example, some people consider the number three lucky because in Cantonese and other languages it sounds similar to the word 'life'. Eight sounds similar to the word for 'prosperity', and nine to the word for 'eternity'. Four, on the other hand, sounds like 'death'; any number containing four, including 14, 40 and 24, may be considered unlucky or even dangerous. Some people worry about being in beds or wards with these numbers (see also Chapter 10 *Good and bad luck*).

Festivals

This section discusses specifically Chinese festivals. For those relating to Christian and Muslim Chinese patients, see also Chapters 42 and 44.

Chinese New Year *Late January/February* The most important festival in the Chinese year. The date is calculated according to the lunar calendar. Celebrations usually last 15 days, the first week being the most important. New Year is a time when people can start afresh, a time for family reunion and harmony. Many people visit grandparents and other relatives on the first day of the new year. Special 'dragon' and 'lion' dances may be performed to bring luck to the community. There are strong traditions about what people should do or avoid during this time to ensure good fortune in the coming year. A few people may prefer to stop treatment and ignore their illness at this time to avoid attracting bad luck. A death during the new year period may be perceived as particularly unlucky.

Before the festival most women clean and decorate their homes and prepare special dishes. Parents often prepare 'lucky money' in little red envelopes to give to children and grandchildren and sometimes to unmarried people. Patients in hospital over the new year may have extra visitors. It is polite to wish Chinese people a happy new year from New Year's Day onwards. Visitors to Chinese homes may be offered special cakes and sweets. (For dates of festivals see the SHAP Calendar, listed in the References.)

Lantern festival *Fifteen days later, usually February* Marks the end of New Year celebrations and welcomes the coming of spring. People may decorate their homes. They may go to the temple to get a wind chime to bring luck to their home in the new year.

Qingming (pronounced chingming) *April* Festival of souls. A solemn day when the family visits and tidies the graves of their ancestors. Buddhists may burn symbolic money in front of the graves and bring food and other symbolic offerings.

Dragon boat festival *June* Traditional to eat dumplings and hold races in dragon-shaped boats. Older members of the family are traditionally responsible for preparing the dumplings and some may worry if they are unable to do so.

Moon festival *Usually September* Fruit and round cakes called moon cakes are eaten, children carry lanterns and the lion dance may be performed.

Chung Yeung *Three weeks later, usually October* Harvest festival celebrated at the full moon. People traditionally leave their homes and spend the day in the fresh air; they may have a picnic and climb a high hill or mountain to avoid bad luck. They may visit and sweep their ancestors' graves.

The principles of Chinese medicine

(Much of this section is adapted from Mares 1982, by kind permission.) Chinese medicine is a well-organised and highly respected system of medical knowledge based on recorded observations, experiments and trials and on a rigorous body of theory. According to Chinese medical theory, illness is an impairment of balance or harmony in the body due to internal, external, physical or mental causes. The mind and the body are intimately connected and affect each other. Medical treatment involves recreating balance and harmony.

Chinese medicine has certain key concepts including ch'i, yin and yang, and five elements of matter that are believed to influence health and the functioning of the major organs. Many of these ideas arise from Taoism (see above), which places a good deal of emphasis on physical and emotional health and balance.

Ch'i (or Qi) is vital energy and gives life to all living matter. It circulates along fourteen channels or meridians, twelve of which influence or are influenced by major internal organs. The strength, flow and distribution of ch'i in the body depend on a proper balance of yin and yang. Acupuncture may be used to stimulate the flow of ch'i along the meridians of the body (Mares 1982).

Yin and yang In Western thinking and medicine, based on Aristotelian logic, opposites can never simultaneously be true. However, Chinese philosophical traditions and medicine teach that opposites can be both conflicting and complementary. All living things consist of two opposing forces or elements. Harmony and health can exist in the natural world, the human body and society, only when there is balance between the conflicting forces or energies known as yin and yang. Yin is associated with earth, night, interior, contemplation, female, cold and death; yang is associated with heaven, day, exterior, activity, male, heat and life. Although the yin and yang forces work by opposing each other, they are in fact completely interdependent and complementary, holding the universe together. Neither can exist or function without the other, and each contains the seed of the other. The interaction of yin and yang produces change, birth, growth and death. Imbalance can cause illness and even death (Chan 1995).

An excess of yin causes infections, gastric problems and great anxiety. Too much yang may cause dehydration, fever, irritability and edginess. In their daily lives people strive to achieve spiritual, emotional and physical balance. The yin and yang elements in food are extremely important, and many people place a great emphasis on maintaining and restoring harmony through their diet (see *Chinese foods and diets*, below). Different herbal and root medicines are also categorised as yin or yang and are given to counteract illness (Chan 1995).

Diagnosis and treatments Traditional Chinese medical practitioners are generally highly respected. Their aim is to correct the imbalance of the vital forces in the body. Once equilibrium is restored, the person can better overcome their illness. Diagnosis is made through visual observation, discussion, palpation and percussion, and the taking of pulses. Treatments include changes in diet, exercise, herbal treatment, acupuncture and moxibustion (a form of acupuncture which involves burning dried herbs, sometimes in a cradle on top of an acupuncture needle). There are few if any major invasive procedures; surgery is not part of traditional Chinese medicine. If part of the imbalance that caused the illness is thought to be due to immoral behaviour, for example neglecting family duties, the patient may be encouraged to do things to restore harmony with family members, both living and dead (Jang 1995).

In the 1970s the Chinese government officially encouraged the integration of the Western and Chinese medical traditions as 'New Medicine'. In Hong Kong and other countries where the two systems run side by side, people are accustomed to using both, depending on the condition and on experience. Chinese medicine is often more popular for chronic conditions and Western medicine for acute, urgent conditions. There is no sense, as there often is in the West, that people should choose one medical system and stick with it (Cheung, Lau and Wong 1984).

Chinese medicine in Britain

Many Chinese people who are familiar with the basic biomedical concepts of Western medicine also accept the principles of Chinese medicine and use the two in parallel or when Western medicine seems ineffective or too invasive. Older people and people who speak little or no English in Britain may rely entirely on Chinese medicine.

> 'Most older people here prefer traditional Chinese doctors. Some go home to Hong Kong for treatment and only use the NHS if they really have to. They don't do well in Western institutions.'
> Chinese advice worker

Many people use home remedies and tonics based on herbs and other substances, as well as self-prescribed dietary remedies. Home remedies are passed down through generations. Cold, damp, heat and wind are often perceived as causes of both common and serious illness. Some Chinese people feel that many of their health problems in Britain are due to the weather and their diet (Tang 1994).

Practical implications

Experience indicates that many Chinese medical and herbal treatments are effective. Others may not be, or may lead people to delay seeking other medical treatment, occasionally with serious consequences. A few are thought by Western pharmacologists to be harmful or to interact with Western medication (see Chapter 31).

In some cases Western and Chinese treatments clash directly. Sometimes Chinese medicine prescribes a treatment that exacerbates symptoms in order to achieve a cure. For example, where Western medicine traditionally recommends cooling a fever, Chinese medicine recommends heating the body in order to sweat the fever out and regards cooling a fever as dangerous. Some treatments contain substances that are contraindicated with the conventional Western medical treatment for a particular condition (Chan 1995).

Most Western medicines, including antibiotics, are regarded as yang, or hot. Some people are reluctant to take them or may prefer to take a reduced dose, possibly for longer. Some may take special food or drink to try to counteract the negative effects of medication. It is helpful to ask Chinese patients whether they are prepared to take Western medicines and whether they are taking Chinese medicines (Fong and Watt 1994) (see also Chapter 31).

In a few cases a patient may wish to consult a traditional Chinese medical practitioner. Some will invite a sacred healer who may chant and perform healing rituals. People's wishes and beliefs should be respected and supported as far as possible. Visits by alternative practitioners should usually be allowed in hospital and other residential care, and privacy provided. If staff are worried about any aspect of alternative treatment, they should discuss their worries sensitively and tactfully with the patient and the family.

Chinese foods and diets

There is no one Chinese diet. China is a huge country with tremendous variations in climate and agriculture, and individual diets are affected by the family's area of origin within China. Farming in many parts of China is difficult and is frequently threatened by drought, flood and other disasters. Because of a long history of food shortages and hunger, food is regarded as very precious. Nothing is wasted.

Rice is the staple food of most Chinese families in Britain, and is eaten at all main meals. However, people whose families originated in Beijing and northern China may eat mainly wheat- and corn-based dishes such as noodles, dumplings and bread. Rice is normally steamed or boiled, but can also be eaten as rice noodles or porridge. It is regarded as an essential and balanced food and as the most important part of a meal. A meal without rice may not be considered a meal at all.

To accompany the carbohydrate, people eat small quantities of other dishes including vegetables, meat (mainly pork and chicken) or seafood. Vegetables are always cooked for hygienic reasons. (Salads and raw food are not part of traditional Chinese cooking.) A few people eat a vegetarian diet for religious reasons (see below). Most eat all kinds of meat, including offal. Some do not eat pork or beef. Vegetables and meat are usually steamed, stewed or stir-fried. Onions, ginger and garlic are often used to add flavour. Soy sauce, chilli sauce and vinegar are often placed on the table rather than salt. Chinese people of Vietnamese or Thai origin may use a fish sauce instead of salt. Food is usually eaten very hot; cold food is regarded as unhealthy. English boiled vegetables and bland food can seem heavy, overcooked and tasteless to people used to a more flavoured diet.

Soup is eaten with many meals, often as part of the main course, and usually using the water in which the vegetables or meat have been cooked. Noodles, vegetables and other ingredients may be added. The soup can be spooned over the rice to moisten it, or spooned into the empty rice bowl at the end of the meal and drunk.

Milk and dairy products are not part of most Chinese diets and some people dislike the taste. However, some people drink warm milk. Some Chinese people are lactose-intolerant and cannot tolerate milk or dairy products.

Many Chinese people believe that cold unboiled water is unhealthy because it shocks the system. In many hot countries water is always boiled for hygienic reasons. Most Chinese patients prefer to have a thermos of hot water by their bed rather than a jug of water, and may prefer to take medication with warm water. Other cold drinks may also be avoided. Many people drink hot tea without milk at mealtimes.

Serving Food is normally eaten with chopsticks or a spoon (for soup) and so is chopped into bite-sized pieces before cooking. Each person usually has their own bowl of rice and helps themselves to meat and vegetables from communal dishes in the middle of the table.

Religious aspects of food

Some Buddhists and Taoists eat a vegetarian diet. Some Buddhists abstain from meat on the days of the new and full moon. A few may avoid garlic and onions, which are thought to heat the blood and make meditation more difficult. Chinese Muslims are likely to follow Muslim food restrictions (see Chapter 44 *Dietary requirements*).

Food and health

Chinese medicine (see above) places great emphasis on the role of diet in health care. Dietary remedies are often used to cure disease (Chan 1995).

Food, when metabolised, becomes ch'i or energy, either as a cold energy force (yin) or as a hot energy force (yang) (see above). When a person is ill, they should eat more yin or yang food in order to rebalance their body. Older people are believed to have a tendency to coolness (yin) and may choose more hot (yang) foods. Foods are defined by type, not temperature: alcohol, red meat, chilli, radishes, ginger, carbonated drinks, curry, wheat products, shellfish, nuts and spicy and fatty foods are generally regarded as yang. Most vegetables and fruits, milk and dairy products, water and salt are yin (Chan 1995). Different cooking methods also affect the attributes of food; for example, boiled and steamed foods are generally considered cold, and fried foods hot. Foods are also divided into five flavour categories – sour, bitter, sweet, salty and spicy-hot. Particular flavours may be considered beneficial or harmful, depending on the illness (Mares 1982). Spices, herbs and salt also affect the attributes of food. Rice is particularly valued because it is a balanced or neutral food. People who are ill may eat rice porridge, which is easier to digest.

Although some people think consciously in terms of yin and yang foods and the other dietary categories, many take them into account automatically in planning their diet or choosing food when they are ill.

Some people, especially older people, may believe that the appearance or shape of a food will cure a particular disease. For example, walnuts may be taken to cure brain disorders (because of their shape); red dates and liver for the blood; and bananas for the bowels. A person with heart disease may be given soup containing pig's heart.

Food in hospital

'The worst suffering for my father was not his illness. It was being forced to eat food he did not understand and did not like.'
Chinese woman

English cooking methods and hospital food pose major problems for people who eat a traditional Chinese diet and who are concerned about the effects of what they eat on their medical condition. Chinese people may need help in selecting a diet that is acceptable in terms both of familiar taste and texture, and of nutritional and medicinal qualities (see also Chapter 11 *Providing food in hospital and other residential care*). Even people who are used to English food may strongly prefer Chinese food when they are ill or away from home. Some people will require rice with both main meals. This must be long grain, not pudding rice, ordered specially if necessary. Food should always be served hot. Cold meat and salad, sandwiches or other cold snacks are unlikely to be seen as nourishing.

Families who can, will often bring in food for hospital patients. They are likely to bring chopsticks but the patient may also need a spoon, bowls and a plate. Family members are often very concerned if a person is not eating and may see this as a bad sign. Occasionally, relatives may try to force feed them to help them regain their strength. If a patient cannot eat, it is important to explain this sensitively.

Some visitors bring special healing teas, soups and other dishes that contain Chinese herbs and medicines. This is an important way of expressing love and concern. Soup is considered particularly nourishing, and families often make special soups with expensive medicinal ingredients, boiling them for up to six hours. They may also bring herbal teas, made from dried flowers or grasses (Chan 1995). It may be important to find out from the family – respectfully and sensitively – what special herbs or foods the patient is receiving and to check that these do not conflict with the other medication they are receiving (see also *Chinese medicine in Britain*, above, and Chapter 31).

Practical care

Modesty

Physical modesty and dignity are very important in Chinese culture. Any form of exposure in front of strangers or even other family members is extremely embarrassing for many people, especially older people. Physical contact across the sexes is generally avoided except between husband and wife. Sitting on the bed may be seen as intrusive. Close friends of the same sex sometimes hold hands or put an arm around each other's shoulders. (See also Chapter 12 *Modesty and physical examination.*)

Washing and cleanliness

Chinese culture places great emphasis on physical cleanliness. Most people wash by pouring hot water over themselves from a bowl or sponging themselves down with very hot water. Many Chinese people dislike sitting in a bath of water; some worry that it will make them ill.

Draughts, chills and cold air are often thought to cause serious health problems. In Britain many Chinese people, especially older people, worry a lot about catching chills and other illnesses. They may want to keep very warm and wrap up well, especially when they are ill and their resistance is low. Some people do not wash their hair when they are ill. Lying in a bed near an open window or in a possible draught between two doors will worry some people.

Gaining consent

Chinese culture traditionally emphasises courtesy and the maintenance of social harmony. Behaviour that causes disharmony – for example, assertive questioning and publicly standing up for one's rights – is traditionally avoided. The expression of anger may be regarded as unacceptable, indicating disrespect and undermining the dignity of everyone involved (Wenzhong and Grove 1991). Because of the importance of maintaining harmony, and because of ideas about the respect due to doctors and other professionals, many Chinese people feel unable to question medical decisions or to complain about inadequate or inconsiderate treatment. This does not necessarily mean that they are happy or satisfied. It is particularly important to be sensitive to non-verbal signs of distress, agitation or anger and to be careful to obtain informed consent for all procedures (see also Chapter 15 *Informed consent*).

Home visits

People in the catering trade often work late and so sleep till noon the next day. Visits should, wherever possible, be arranged between two and four in the afternoon or on a day off (Au and Au 1992).

Certain chairs in a home are sometimes reserved for particular members of the family, especially older people. It is polite always to check before sitting anywhere.

Most Chinese people take pride in how their home is kept. Some may be distressed and embarrassed if they cannot keep it clean and tidy. Some families always remove their shoes when entering their home. If you see a pile of shoes, it is polite also to remove yours.

It is customary to offer food and drink to all visitors. Visitors should try always to accept at least some of what is offered because total refusal can cause serious offence.

When someone is ill or dying

Family responsibilities

> 'It is very important to involve the relatives as well as the patient. Practical care should be a joint thing.'
> Chinese advice worker

The family is generally the most important source of health care advice and treatment. Much illness is treated by family members, often with no outside help being sought. Even when outside help is sought, decisions about treatment are usually made either by the patient and family together or by other family members without the patient. The family has the patient's best interests at heart and the patient usually trusts them to make the right decision. Family members may therefore expect to be responsible for all decisions. This contrasts strongly with current Western ideas of patient autonomy and confidentiality (Tong and Spicer 1994) (see also *Discussing the diagnosis*, below, and Chapter 15 *Maintaining patient confidentiality*).

Some Chinese people, particularly older members, do not see emotional issues or family problems as a matter for discussion with health professionals. They may consider practical help with treatment and medication, with caring for a patient at home, or with finances, more acceptable (Boston 1993) (see also Chapter 9 *Different families*).

Attitudes to death and dying

In traditional Chinese culture, death and illness are often regarded as dangerous and frightening subjects. Because language, thought and reality are seen as connected, open discussion of dying and death before they happen may be considered dangerous and unlucky. People who are ill or dying and the bodies of dead people are considered to be surrounded by a negative energy that could affect others. Some Chinese people therefore strongly prefer to avoid admission to hospital at all costs, however ill they are.

People traditionally cleanse themselves physically and spiritually after touching a dying person. Many modern Chinese customs and rituals surrounding death and funerals reflect these beliefs. For example, some families may strongly wish a relative to die in hospital, because a death at home may bring ill-fortune to those still living there. Some families may feel that the approaching death should be kept a secret from outsiders. Children and pregnant women may avoid a dying or dead person in case contact brings bad luck. Some patients and their families may refuse to accept that death is approaching and may want curative treatment continued even when there is little or no point.

At the same time, many Chinese people have a pragmatic attitude to death. Everyone is destined to die at a certain time and there is nothing they can do about it. Many people, especially older people and those with a formal religious faith, believe that there is a better life after death to look forward to. In the meantime it is important to get on with practical matters and to finish things well. This ties in with the Buddhist belief that each person has a purpose to fulfil in their life. By completing things properly a person can have a positive influence on their next life. People who know they are dying may wish to put their practical affairs in order, pay any debts, make provision for their children, decide on a burial plot and a coffin and choose the clothes they will be laid out in. In contrast to current Western thinking, however, there may be little emphasis on discussing feelings and dealing with emotional issues.

'Try to understand what we do, and don't look down on us because we do things differently. Much of what we do is in order to have a good life when we are reincarnated.'
Chinese midwife

Discussing the diagnosis

Traditionally, it is important to spare a patient worry and distress, to help them to be calm and hopeful, and to allow them quiet and privacy for reflection. The patient's task is to let go and let others take over and look after them. Some Chinese people may consider talking about death with a seriously ill patient, especially an older person, very bad practice. They may feel that it is like wishing death on them. Some feel that explicit discussions about poor prognoses, treatments, resuscitation and so on should be held with other family members (see above).

Although the seriousness of the illness and impending death may not be spoken of, Chinese patients are usually perfectly aware of their condition and of what is happening. **Many things can be understood without being spelt out in words.** Patients observe their physical symptoms, the treatments they are given or not given, and the behaviour of the people looking after them. They realise that the pattern of visits has changed, that people are coming from further afield or even from abroad to see them. A relative or friend may stay at their bedside as death approaches. Realising that they have not got long to live, they may make a will, allocate their personal possessions and even plan for the funeral. It is simply that open explicit discussion is often regarded as unnecessary and distressing, even as destructive (Tong and Spicer 1994).

Culture-based assumptions about the benefits of speaking out and 'facing the reality of death', and insensitive encouragement of open discussion can lead to discomfort, distress and frustration on both sides. However, some Chinese people, possibly those brought up in the UK, prefer more explicit and open communication, and this sometimes may lead to tension and conflict with other family members.

Medication

Most Chinese people have no objection to opiates and other methods of symptom control. At the same time, stoicism and self-control are generally highly valued and some people, particularly older people, are reluctant to ask for pain relief. Because it is important in Buddhist tradition to be aware and focused at the time of death, some Chinese Buddhist and other patients may wish to avoid any medication that could cloud their minds. Some also fear loss of control; it is important to find a dosage that balances the need to relieve pain without causing disorientation. Some people may feel that the suffering they are enduring in their last illness is the result of negative karmic effects (see *Buddhism*, above). They may prefer not to have pain-relieving or other medication so as to pay their karmic debt now, rather than in a future life (Sibley 1997).

Visitors

It is extremely important that family members and close friends visit a person who is seriously ill or dying. Relatives and friends who work long hours may not be able to visit at conventional times. Visitors from abroad may arrive from the airport at unusual hours and should be allowed to visit. Sometimes several people will wish to stay by the bedside of someone who is seriously ill or dying and this too should be accommodated wherever possible (see also Chapter 17). Visitors do not traditionally bring flowers, which may be considered unlucky.

Chinese visitors often talk to the patient even if he or she is unconscious, telling them who is present and who is expected, and offering reassurance and support. By tradition, older Chinese people are expected to pronounce 'last words of wisdom' to the younger generation when they realise that death is near (Tong and Spicer 1994). If close family members are not present and a patient suddenly deteriorates it may be very important to call them. Wherever possible, the family should be asked beforehand what they would like done.

Buddhist patients

Buddhism recognises that death, which represents an annihilation of our identity, is the ultimate fear or barrier for most people. Many Buddhists believe that the state of mind of a person who is dying will influence the form in which he or she is reborn or even liberate them from rebirth altogether. In general it is believed that a state of conscious and focused peace is best as a preparation for death. Some Buddhists may wish to have peace and quiet for meditation. Some may wish to chant quietly. Some may wish to have Buddhist scriptures read to them by relatives or by a monk (Erriker 1995).

Organ donation

Traditionally it is important that the body is buried whole. Some Chinese people may therefore be reluctant to donate organs or tissues.

After the death

Last offices

It is traditional for the body to be left undisturbed for some time to allow the soul to depart. In Buddhist tradition it is generally believed that consciousness remains with the body for up to three days after the death. Although most Chinese families in Britain have no objection to a body being removed from the room quickly it is always important to check. The open expression of grief at a death is regarded as normal and encouraged. Some people grieve and wail loudly. People who do not express their grief may be thought to have had a bad relationship with the person who has died. Whenever possible, a side room should be provided for bereaved family members.

Most Chinese families have no objection to hospital staff washing and wrapping the body. However, it is always important to check first. People are often buried with the things they had about them in their daily life such as a watch, a wedding ring, a comb, spectacles and a walking stick. Some families therefore wish nothing to be removed. Unless the dead person is a Christian, a non-denominational shroud should be used. Some families bring their own special shroud. Some put a coin in the dead person's mouth to symbolise helping the soul to cross into the next life. (See also Chapter 20 *Immediately after the death and last offices*.)

Patient's property

Some families may be reluctant to take property home with them. If this seems to be the case, ask sensitively whether they would like the hospital to dispose of any property for them (see also Chapter 20 *The patient's property*).

Post mortems

There is no religious prohibition against post mortems unless the patient is a Muslim (see Chapter 44 *Post mortems*) but many people find the idea distressing. It may be important to reassure families that the body will be complete and repaired before burial or cremation.

The funeral

Some Chinese families prefer to prepare the body for burial themselves, usually at the funeral parlour. The dead person is usually dressed in new clothes, with the things that they carried with them every day. Sometimes they have chosen their own burial outfit beforehand. Bundles of symbolic paper money may be put in the coffin to express good wishes for the person's next life.

Burial is generally preferred but rising costs mean that some families now choose cremation. Providing a lavish funeral is traditionally a sign of respect and may also be seen as ensuring good luck for the remaining family members. Some families wish to fly the body 'back home' for burial (see

Chapter 20 *Repatriating the body*). It is very important that all family members and friends attend the funeral. People who are older than the person who has died may, however, sometimes stay away. Close relatives traditionally wear white and other people black. Bright colours are not worn at a funeral, as they are considered disrespectful.

At the funeral the coffin is often kept open so that people can pay their last respects. A photograph of the dead person is often placed on a stand beside the coffin. Later this will be taken home, to be put in a place of honour and incense burned in front of it.

Some families may want the burial to be conducted by a traditional Chinese priest who specialises in burials, but this can be difficult to organise in Britain. Buddhist, Christian and Muslim families are likely to follow their own religious practices (see *Buddhism*, earlier, and Chapters 42 and 44). People may send flowers to the funeral, because they are not considered unlucky after a death (as they are before a death). Some people give money to the family. Incense and symbolic paper money may be burnt.

After the funeral the family normally provides a comforting meal for the mourners. Each person may also receive a small white packet with a red stripe containing items to bring them good luck. Most people change their clothes when they get home. Some throw away the clothes they wore at the funeral.

Mourning rituals

A wake may be held for several days, though this is becoming less common. Some people consider it important to grieve loudly, believing that the louder the crying the sooner the gods will hear.

In Chinese tradition, association and contact with death and misfortune are considered unlucky (see *Good and bad luck*, above). Some Chinese people, especially those from conservative rural areas, avoid a family in which a death has recently occurred. The relatives of a person who has died may stay away from festivals and weddings for some time in order not to bring bad luck.

Some families ask a Buddhist priest to chant for several days, for the soul of the person who has died. On the 49th day families usually hold a memorial ceremony. Paper money and other symbolic things such as a cardboard house may be burnt to express the family's wish that the person will be happy and prosperous in their next life.

39 Nigerian communities: history and traditional culture

●●

The continent of Africa covers an area of nearly 12 million square miles and contains over 600 million people. Within its boundaries there is a huge variety of climates and terrains. There are over 50 different countries, each with its own customs, languages and religions, many of which are further subdivided into separate very different regions. It is therefore as impossible to write anything general about the culture, values and needs of 'African people' as it is to write anything useful about the culture, values and needs of 'European people' (even though Europe is only about one-third the size of Africa). We have therefore chosen to focus on people from two countries, Nigeria on the west coast of Africa, and Somalia (see Chapter 40) on the east coast.

Nigeria

Nigeria is situated on the Gulf of Guinea on the Atlantic Ocean (see Figure 39.2). It is bordered by Benin to the west, Niger to the north, Chad to the north-east and Cameroon to the east. The area now called Nigeria originally consisted of a very large number of separate states and kingdoms. At the end of the nineteenth century these came increasingly under the control of Britain and other European countries that were dividing Africa up between them during the 'scramble for Africa' (Pakenham 1991). In the early 1900s, Britain claimed the territory covered by Nigeria as a British colony.

In 1960 Nigeria became an independent nation in the British Commonwealth. Since independence, ethnic conflicts and religious and political differences have led to friction, unrest, violent changes in government and periods of civil war.

Nigeria is traditionally agricultural, though it also has large oil reserves. However, long-standing civil and political unrest and the drop in oil prices

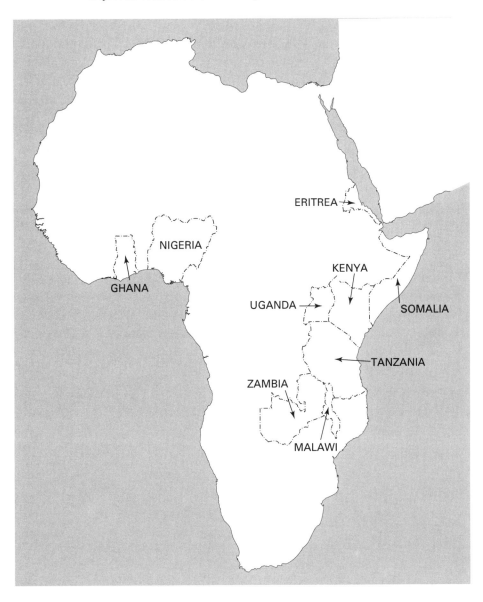

Figure 39.1 Africa, showing the main countries from which people have come to the UK

in the 1980s have led to substantial foreign debts. As a consequence, Nigeria is ranked by the World Bank as a low-income country.

Nigeria has the largest population of any African country – about 112 million people. It contains more than 250 ethnic groups, each with its own history, culture, traditions and language or dialect. The largest ethnic groups are the Hausa (21 per cent of the population) and the Fulani (9 per cent) from the north, the Yoruba (20 per cent) from south-west, and the Ibo from south-east (17 per cent) (*Encarta World Atlas* 1998). The other ethnic groups make up rest of the population and include the Edo, the Ijaw and the Ibibio from the south, the Nupe and the Tiv from central Nigeria, and the Kanji from the north-east. Each ethnic group also contains several sub-groups. Although people often mix socially, most marry within their own ethnic, linguistic and religious group. The majority of Nigerians in the UK are Yoruba or Ibo, and we focus mainly on these two groups in this chapter. There are also some Hausa and Fulani people.

The Nigerian communities in Britain

People from Nigeria came to the UK from the 1940s onwards to study at universities and for professional qualifications. Most were members of the educated elite from the cities, principally Lagos (the capital at the time).

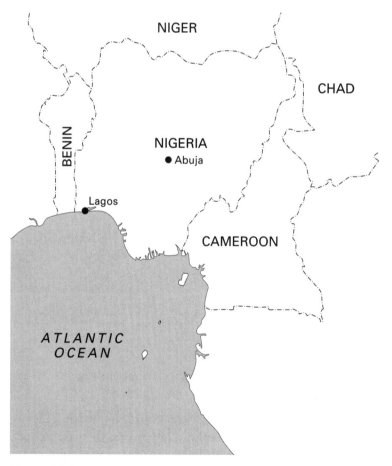

Figure 39.2 Nigeria

Although most people went back to Nigeria, some stayed on, working in the professions – for example as accountants, engineers, quantity surveyors, nurses, midwives and doctors. Later on a small number of business people came to Britain. (As British subjects, all Nigerians had the unrestricted right to come to Britain to live and work at that time. The first pieces of legislation restricting the entry of immigrants from the New Commonwealth were enacted in 1962 and 1971 (Commonwealth Immigrants Act and Immigration Act). As political and economic instability in Nigeria increased, many Nigerians working in the UK decided to settle here permanently. Once people had families here, it became still harder to return. A few Nigerians have come to Britain more recently, seeking political asylum (see Chapter 35).

Many Nigerians have lived in the UK for much of their adult lives. Some of these people are now reaching retirement age. Most younger people of Nigerian heritage were born here.

Certain aspects of their traditional culture may be important to many Nigerian people. For some, religious beliefs will also be very important. Because it is not possible to predict what will be important to whom, the only way to find out is by listening sensitively to each individual and asking when appropriate.

Languages

Nigeria is a multilingual country with over 450 different spoken languages. English is the official language and is used in both primary and secondary schools. After English, Hausa is the most widely spoken language, followed by Yoruba, Ibo, Fulani, Kanuri and Tiv. Although each of these is a different language, most educated Nigerians are fluent in several languages. There is a strong oral tradition, and it is very common to use proverbs, adages and metaphors in conversation to make a point or express meaning.

The English spoken by most Nigerians in Nigeria is known by linguists as West African Coastal English (WACE) and differs in certain respects from standard British English. The key differences are: different syllables may be stressed in a long word; extra words or changes in word order which are used instead of stress to indicate emphasis; and intonation (see also Chapter 24 *Paralinguistic features*). Most Nigerians in Britain have adapted their English so that it is understood more easily by British English speakers. Older people may retain more features of Nigerian English. People of Nigerian heritage under stress or in the grip of strong emotion may also unconsciously use more Nigerian English forms.

Naming systems

The Yoruba and Ibo naming systems are similar to the British one: each person has one or more personal names followed by a shared family name. Some personal names, however, indicate a person's role or status in the family, and are very common. There are also differences in the way that names are used, and it is easy to cause unwitting offence. (For more information on recording and using Nigerian names correctly, see Chapter 30 *Other naming systems*.)

'Never make the mistake of being too familiar by calling a Nigerian adult by their first name. They will feel offended. Always ask or wait until you are invited to use the first name.'
Nigerian nurse

In traditional Nigerian culture greetings are very important: failing to greet a person is a sign of disrespect. It is particularly important to greet and address older people respectfully. In Nigeria people often drop a small curtsey or bow when greeting an older person.

Religion

Most Nigerians believe in a divine higher power. The Hausa, Fulani and Kanuri peoples in northern Nigeria are predominately Muslim (see Chapter 44). The Ibo and Yoruba people of the south are mainly Christian (see Chapter 42). They include Roman Catholics, Methodists, Anglicans, Brethren of the Church of Nigeria, Lutherans, Baptists, Seventh Day Adventists and Pentecostalists. There are also some Muslim Yorubas and Ibos. Traditional African religions are also practised, especially in rural areas throughout the country. Some Nigerians believe in witchcraft, though this is often disapproved of by more educated people.

Traditional family structure and relationships

The concept of the nuclear family does not exist in Yoruba and Ibo cultures. All relatives are regarded as 'the family'. Children may be cared for by grandmothers, aunts and other family members as well as by their parents. The father is regarded as the head of the family and is traditionally the main provider. As in Britain, traditional male and female roles are shifting in Nigeria, and more women are in paid employment so there is more joint decision-making.

Both in Nigeria and in the UK there are now an increasing number of single-parent families headed by women. Children in these families generally retain their father's family name.

Marriage

Men and women are traditionally expected to marry and have children. Unmarried women may be considered very unfortunate, disapproved of and socially isolated. Polygamy is accepted among Nigerian Muslims and also occurs among Christians and followers of traditional African religions (see also Chapter 9 *Men and women* and Chapter 44). Divorce is becoming more common.

Before a marriage is agreed, each family traditionally investigates the other to find out if there are any psychiatric illnesses, hereditary diseases, beliefs or practices that they might not agree with. Many families then have an engagement ceremony when they gather to meet each other.

Family and community

The family is very important in traditional Yoruba and Ibo cultures, and family loyalties and responsibilities are taken extremely seriously. Personal self-respect and dignity, and family pride are central to Yoruba and Ibo cultures. There are important family ceremonies to mark all major life events such as birth, marriage, naming a baby and death. Children are not seen as only the responsibility of their parents: childcare and discipline are shared among the adults of the family. Everyone is expected to keep an eye on and look after older or ill family members and pregnant and newly delivered women, and to rally round during a crisis or when someone dies. Community networks are also very important: everyone knows everyone else, and people support each other.

'Nigeria has a very rich culture and we are a warm, generous and expressive people. I love the discipline instilled in our children and the healthy reverence and respect we have for our elders.'
Nigerian nurse

Education is highly valued. Great emphasis is often placed on academic achievement and qualifications.

Older people

In the UK, Nigerian families tend to be more scattered, and younger members are involved with their own work and lives. This can be especially hard for retired and older people. They may become isolated and miss the traditional community network and the companionship and support it offered. Many older people would prefer to return to Nigeria but financial constraints and the social and political instability in Nigeria often make this frightening or impossible.

It is very important to show respect and deference towards anyone older and especially to parents (see *Addressing people*, above). Younger people traditionally kneel or prostrate themselves before older people.

Nigerian foods

Food is very important in Yoruba and Ibo cultures. It is impolite not to offer visitors food and drink. However, most people will not be offended if they are refused politely.

Each region has its own style of food preparation and people will not necessarily like food from another region. Some people follow religious restrictions on diet (see Chapters 42–48).

The staple carbohydrates of Yoruba people are cassava pottage (which is thick enough to eat with the fingers), rice and pounded yam. Meat and fish are eaten, and food is hot and spicy. Meals are often accompanied by a hot pepper sauce. Ibo food tends to be less spicy. Staple carbohydrates include yam, cassava, corn and sweet potato.

Some meals, especially those that include pottage, are eaten with the fingers. Most Nigerians in the West use cutlery when they are out, but many prefer to use their hands when they are at home. Some, especially older people, may be unaccustomed to using cutlery.

British food is generally considered bland and unappetising as well as less nutritious. Newcomers often find it difficult to eat. Many Nigerian patients in hospital and other residential care prefer to have home-cooked food brought in to them if possible. Because the range of local fruit and vegetables is far more restricted in the UK, and imported foods are more expensive, some people of Nigerian heritage, especially the elderly, may be deficient in vitamin C and folate.

Food when ill

Light and nourishing flavoured gruels and custards are traditionally prepared for people who are ill. Herbs may be given to promote healing (see Chapter 31). Some people give herb teas or hot peppery foods to people with colds, flu or a fever in order to encourage sweating and to reduce their temperature. Relatives may want to bring special food for someone in hospital.

Practical care

Prayer

Some Muslim patients will want to pray five times a day and to wash before doing so (see Chapter 44 *Worship*).

Modesty

Modesty and privacy for washing and examination are likely to be very important, especially to older people. Some people may strongly prefer to discuss intimate matters with a professional of the same sex (see Chapter 13 *Codes of modesty*). Interpreters should, whenever possible, be of the same sex as the patient (see Chapter 27).

Washing and cleanliness

For many people of Nigerian heritage it is very important to have a bath at least once a day. Many people consider it unhygienic to immerse themselves in a bath full of the water in which they have washed. Instead, they sit in the bath with a large bowl or bucket of water and pour the water over themselves with a small bowl. Nowadays many people take showers.

Patients who are no longer able to wash themselves may prefer to take a shower, or to sit in a bath and have water poured over them, rather than have a bed bath. If a dependent person needs to be immersed in water, they are likely to appreciate having clean water poured over them before they are taken out and dried (see also Chapter 12 *Practical care*).

Most people use paper after using the lavatory. Some more traditional people prefer to wash themselves with soap and running water. Muslim patients may need to wash before prayer (see Chapter 44).

Clothing

Most Nigerians in the UK wear Western clothes, though some women prefer traditional dress. This consists of a blouse, a full-length wrap-around skirt and a head tie, all in a matching fabric. Some women wear a sarong-type wrap wound round the waist and draped over one shoulder. Muslim women may keep their heads and bodies covered at all times (see Chapter 44).

Traditional Yoruba dress for men consists of loose trousers over which is worn a long loose gown, sometimes with a shawl round the shoulders and a small round brimless hat. A long, full and flowing robe may be worn over the top. Ibo men sometimes wear a full-length wrap round the waist instead of loose trousers. Most men in the UK wear traditional dress only for special occasions.

Many people wear Western-style nightwear, though some women prefer full-length loose gowns for reasons of modesty. Some women wear a headscarf at night to keep their hair neat. Some men wear a wrap, similar to a sarong.

Tribal marks

Some people have tribal marks, usually on the cheeks but sometimes on other parts of the body. These may indicate family or tribal allegiance, or may have been done as part of traditional medicine rituals or to protect a small child. Small children are considered especially vulnerable to evil sprits. Tribal marking is still practised in some rural regions of Nigeria and tribal marks are a matter of pride to many people. However the practice is generally declining and some people with marks may be sensitive about them.

Jewellery and religious items

It is customary for women in Nigeria to wear wedding rings, and becoming more common for men to do so too. Some Hausa women paint their nails and decorate their feet and palms with henna. Once applied, henna cannot be removed but fades and grows out with time. Patients for whom elective surgery is planned should be asked to let the henna grow out so that they can be properly observed during and after surgery (see Chapter 13 *Recognising clinical signs in skin*).

Some people may wear or keep with them special items given them by traditional healers. (See also Chapters 42 and 44.)

Female circumcision – female genital mutilation

Some Nigerian women are circumcised, though attempts are being made in Nigeria to abolish this practice (see Chapter 32).

When someone is ill or dying

Traditional medicine

Western medicine is generally highly regarded. However, this regard may co-exist with strong belief in traditional ways. Some people may also consult a traditional healer or diviner, who may prescribe herbs or potions or advise sacrifices (see also Chapter 31).

Confidentiality

Traditionally, people are often reticent about illness because it can adversely affect the social standing and potential marriage prospects both of the individual and of the family. The immediate family may close ranks to ensure that others do not know that someone is ill. This is particularly likely if the person requires surgery or a blood transfusion, or has cancer, a hereditary condition or an infectious disease. It is therefore especially important to be scrupulous about confidentiality. In some cases a patient may not want their spouse to know what is wrong with them or what treatment they need (see also Chapter 15 *Maintaining patient confidentiality*).

Some people, especially older people, may believe that their illness is the result of the 'evil eye' and is caused by someone wishing them ill or casting a spell on them. They may also believe that illness makes them more vulnerable to the ill will of others. This increases the need for discretion.

Some people may not seek medical help until their illness is acute or well advanced. This may be due to a reluctance to acknowledge or talk about illness, to reliance on the power of prayer or to the belief that what happens is God's will and must be accepted.

Physical examinations

Privacy and modesty are important for most Nigerians, and especially for women. Some women may prefer to have a female doctor. Some, especially older people, may be reticent about discussing intimate matters and symptoms. They may also be offended if they are asked their age.

Medication and surgery

Many people believe that injections are more effective than tablets because the medication 'goes straight into the bloodstream'. Some more conservative patients who are prescribed oral medication may feel dissatisfied and worry that their illness is not being taken seriously.

Fear of surgery, and of anaesthesia in particular, is quite common. Some patients may refuse surgical intervention unless it is the only option (see also *Confidentiality*, above). For some this is simply due to fear of the unknown. Others know of people who have died during surgery in Nigeria where perioperative mortality rates were high. A few people may believe that surgery makes them especially vulnerable to evil spirits. Patients who are anxious need support and careful explanations about what will happen and how they will be cared for. Religious patients may feel reassured if a religious leader or family members pray with them before-hand. Some may want to take religious items into theatre to protect them.

Telling the truth

It is traditionally unacceptable to tell a person that they are going to die. Some people may regard revealing a poor prognosis to a patient as tanta-mount to putting a curse on them. A person who predicts a death may be believed to be responsible for it.

As in many communities, some relatives may want to know the likely prognosis but might object to the patient being told (see Chapter 15 *Telling patients the truth*).

Families and illness

It is still the norm in Nigeria for sick or dependent people to be cared for at home by their relatives. This is one advantage of large, extended families. In the UK, however, care at home may be impossible: families are often scattered, there may be no supportive community network, and most women – who traditionally do the caring – go out to work. Older dependent people who cannot be cared for at home may particularly lament the loss of the old traditions and may feel abandoned and rejected. They can be very distressed by the prospect of going into hospital or other residential accommodation.

Visiting a person who is ill is a strong social obligation. Anyone who does not visit is likely to cause lasting offence. Some patients may have large numbers of visitors (see Chapter 17).

Beliefs about death and dying

Many Nigerians, including some Christians and Muslims, have some belief in rebirth (see also Chapters 42 and 44). Some people believe that the spirit of a dead person can come back to the family in a newborn baby. Such a person is particularly loved. Some Nigerians believe that the spirits or souls of people who have died can haunt the living.

Dying at a ripe old age is traditionally considered a good death. Dying young, or dying as a result of an accident, suicide or violence or of certain stigmatised diseases, is considered a bad death. Many patients would want every treatment possible to delay death.

When a person is dying

In many families it is very important for close relatives to be present when someone dies so that they can say goodbye and hear any last wishes, advice or instructions that the dying person may want to give them. Great distress and lasting pain can be caused to relatives who are not able to be present. Visitors may express their grief openly, both physically and verbally. A person who does not do so may be considered odd and uncaring or even responsible for the death.

Last offices

The adult children of a person who has died may want to wash and dress the body themselves. When carrying out last offices, it is important to remember that the coffin will be kept open before burial so that people can pay their last respects (see Chapter 20 *Immediately after the death and last offices*).

Traditionally, the parents of a person who dies are not involved after the death and do not attend the funeral. Other family members will make all the arrangements on their behalf.

Organ donation

This is a matter of personal choice. More conservative people may find the idea of organ donation offensive but there is a growing awareness of its importance. It is always worth asking the family.

Post mortems

Attitudes to post mortems vary from person to person.

Funerals

A funeral in Nigeria is very much a community affair. Large numbers of people attend and emotions are expressed openly. Burial is customary: many people find the idea of cremation distasteful. Some people place certain items such as a Bible in the coffin. The coffin is kept open and is carried by male family members. It is customary to take photographs and, these days, to make videos of the ceremony so that people can remember it in detail.

The funeral of a young person is generally quieter; relatives who are older than the person who has died, including the parents, traditionally do not attend.

Suicide is generally considered an abomination, and people who have committed suicide are usually buried swiftly and without ceremony.

Repatriating the body

Many people would like to repatriate the body for burial but this is often impossible because of the cost. Sometimes the community will club together and offer financial help to a family who want repatriate the body (see also Chapter 20 *Repatriating the body*).

The funeral and afterwards

After the funeral of an older person it is customary to celebrate their long life. There is usually a large wake at which food and drink are served. There is music and dancing, and people wear bright clothes. Wakes in Nigeria often last for several days and nights. In the UK they are usually more modest and may last for only the day of the funeral.

If the person who has died was young, or has parents who are still living, the wake is much more subdued and people wear dark clothes.

After a death, close relatives are traditionally never left alone. Family and community members gather to offer comfort, to bring food and to celebrate the life of the person who has died. Some widows stay at home and dress in black for 40 days after the burial. Ibo women may shave their hair as a sign of grief.

A year after the death it is traditional to remember the person who has died by holding a remembrance service and party. Similar ceremonies may be held on later anniversaries.

40 | Somali communities: history and traditional culture

● ●

This chapter outlines aspects of traditional Somali culture that **may** be important to some people of Somali origin in Britain. Most Somalis are Muslims and follow Muslim practices in their daily lives (see Chapter 44). **Because it is never possible to predict what will and will not be important to an individual, the only way to find out is by listening sensitively and asking when appropriate.**

Somalia

Somalia lies above the Equator on the east coast of Africa, with a long V-shaped coastline forming what is known as the Horn of Africa (see Figure 40.1, below, and Figure 39.1). To the east, Somalia faces the Indian Ocean. To the north it faces the Gulf of Aden, the other side of which is the Arabian peninsula. For centuries there has been strong commercial, cultural and religious contact between the people of Somalia and the people of the Arabian Peninsula.

Somalia became independent in 1960. Before that it was divided into two colonial territories: British Somaliland (in the north) and Italian Somaliland (along the east coast). In recent times Somalia has been severely affected by drought, armed political conflict and a brutal civil war that began in 1988. By 1993 roughly three-quarters of the Somali population of about 8 million had been displaced by the civil war (Lem 1994). Most of those who left Somalia fled to neighbouring countries such as Ethiopia and Kenya. A small number have gone to the Gulf States, to Europe and to North America.

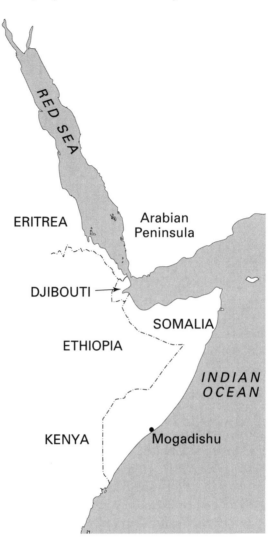

Figure 40.1 Somalia

The Somali communities in Britain

There have been small Somali communities in the UK since the end of the nineteenth century, mainly in east London, Cardiff, Hull and Sheffield. These consisted largely of merchant seamen and, after the two World Wars, demobilised servicemen who had fought for Britain. During the 1950s, a small number of ex-seamen settled in industrial centres such as Sheffield and Manchester and in London's East End. Some were joined by their wives and children in the 1960s (Kahin 1997).

However, most Somalis in Britain have come more recently as refugees from the deteriorating political situation in the 1980s and the civil war. Initially, many were professionals from urban areas. However, as the violence increased, more and more people, some from rural areas, were forced to flee. It is estimated that there are about 60,000 Somalis in Britain. Most of the refugees live in east, north-east and west London, Sheffield, Cardiff and Brighton (Kahin 1997, Refugee Council 1994).

Languages

Spoken languages

The official language of Somalia is Somali. There are several different dialects but most people understand the Northern dialect. Members of some Somali minority clans speak a different first language. Somalia has a very strong oral tradition of history, poetry and story-telling. In general, oral communication is very highly valued.

Since the beginning of the civil war, normal life in Somalia, including education, has more or less come to an end. Most people have had little schooling. English is not taught in Somali schools, so even Somalis who have been to school are unlikely to speak English when they arrive. People who have had secondary education in Somalia usually speak Arabic. A few speak Italian, English or French.

Written languages

Lack of resources and the civil war have seriously affected schooling in Somalia. It is estimated that literacy in Somalia is about 24 per cent, and in the refugee Somali communities in Britain about 65 per cent (Kahin 1997). Women may be less likely to read or write. Somali is written in the Roman alphabet. Some people read Arabic, English or Italian.

The Somali naming system

The Somali naming system is different from the British system; there is traditionally no shared family last name (see Chapter 30 *Recording people's names correctly*). The need to have a consistently written name for records causes particular problems for people who cannot read or write and therefore do not fill out or check their own details on forms. Because many Somalis in Britain are refugees, their initial documentation is often filled out by immigration officials who may not understand the Somali naming system. Any errors they make are perpetuated or compounded in health service and other records.

The celebration of birthdays is not part of Somali culture, so most people do not know their date of birth. Many simply give a year and January 1st. Since many Somalis live in temporary accommodation and are moved frequently, addresses are also inadequate for precise identification. It is not uncommon for Somali patients to have several sets of notes under different names.

Religion

Islam has been the main religion of Somalia since before the twelfth century CE*. Somalia is an Islamic state. Almost all Somali people are Muslims and adhere carefully to the beliefs and practices of Islam (see Chapter 44). Because they are newly arrived and poor, few Somali communities have been able to set up their own mosques and meeting places. Most Somalis worship in mosques attended by other communities. Although the prayers are in Arabic, the sermons, teaching and discussions are usually in a language they do not understand.

Traditional Somali society

Much of this section is adapted from Kahin (1997), by kind permission.

There is a complex network of clan (or tribe) and sub-clan loyalties in Somalia, stretching back hundreds of years. People within each clan and sub-clan have shared loyalties, rights and obligations, and are expected to support each other in times of difficulty and crisis. The main unit of practical support, however, is the extended family (see below).

Over two-thirds of Somalis belong to one of the four or five main 'noble clans', which are divided into a number of sub-clans (reer). The members of the 'noble clans' are believed to have a common ancestry and each traditionally inhabits a certain area of Somalia. Their traditional occupation is tending sheep and camels. Many are nomadic or semi-nomadic, used to moving around with their animals through a fairly hostile terrain in a hot climate. The 'noble clans' have traditionally dominated Somali society.

There are a number of minority clans and sub-clans with lower-status occupations such as fishermen, craftsmen and agricultural farmers. Most live in

---

* Common Era, used as an alternative to AD.

relatively small, distinct communities in southern Somalia and often speak a local dialect. One of these is the Bravanese, from the coastal city of Brava. They speak a dialect of the East African language Swahili and have historical connections with East Africa. Some fled to Kenya before coming to Britain.

There is also a small number of minority, clans traditionally labelled 'low caste', who work as, for example, barbers, shoemakers, blacksmiths, street sweepers and peddlers. Most of them come from northern Somalia where they lived among other Somalis. They speak Somali (Kahin 1997).

The 'noble' majority clans and sub-clans do not usually socialise with those of the minority or intermarry with them. The minority clans have always experienced varying amounts of discrimination (though some have higher status than others).

The civil war Different clans and sub-clans in the complex Somali social system have often taken opposite sides during the recent period of turmoil and conflict. People at all levels of Somali society and in all the different communities have suffered appallingly. However, many of the more recent Somali refugees come from the minority clans, which have experienced extreme violence, looting and intimidation from the armed militias. Many of the minority clans used to live on valuable farmland or in potentially wealthy port areas and so became targets in the battle for resources. They were not protected by the leaders of the more powerful 'noble' clans and sub-clans, were unarmed and had no political allies. The divisions and conflicts that have occurred between the different majority and minority clans and sub-clans in recent years are likely to affect relationships between Somalis in Britain.

Traditional family structure and relationships

The Somali family system is traditionally patriarchal. Family membership, property and lineage are transmitted though the father. Many people know their lineage through the paternal line back through 20 or 25 generations. Such things are not written down but are part of a strong oral tradition and culture. Children belong to their father's clan and women retain their allegiance to their own father's family when they marry. In nomadic life and where there are few other sources of support, the clan and the family provide crucial practical and emotional support and protection. Many Somalis feel a very strong sense of family and clan loyalty and responsibility. Members of the same sub-clan may, for example, visit a patient in hospital even if they have never met.

The most common family unit in Somalia is extended; usually three generations live together or very close to each other. Marriages are traditionally arranged by the families, though the young people make the final decision themselves. Marriage between cousins is common (as it is in some other Muslim communities) and is seen as having many advantages for both the families and the couple. In rural areas it is traditional for a wife to live with her husband's family. In the cities, couples who can afford it may live on their own but near both sets of parents. Relationships with other members of the extended family are usually close and very important.

Somali people traditionally give unquestioning support and loyalty to their family and sub-clan and put these first, especially in times of crisis. The bonds of love and obedience between parent and child are expected to last into old age. Parents are normally more involved in the lives of their adult children than is at present customary in the West. The reputation of the family is extremely important. Immoral or unacceptable behaviour by one person brings shame on the whole family and on all its members. Because the reputation of female family members is particularly important for the whole family and the sub-clan, close limits may be set on their freedom.

Men Somali men are traditionally the head of the family and are responsible for providing for the whole family, making decisions, maintaining authority and discipline and ensuring the unity, honour and social standing of the family, and protecting female family members, particularly outside the home (Kahin 1997).

Women The traditional responsibility of most Somali women is to care for the home and the children. Within the family Somali women often have a good deal of power, especially as they grow older, though they are expected to behave self-effacingly and modestly in public. Women are not generally expected to work outside the home. Unlike women in some other Muslim communities in Britain, Somali women do not traditionally observe purdah (see Chapter 44 *Physical separation*).

Differences in the roles of men and women are generally more marked in families from rural areas and among people who have had little formal education. People socialise mainly within their extended family – men and women usually separately – and often out of doors. Non-family members do not usually visit each other's homes.

In Britain Most Somali refugee families in Britain have lost members and many are divided, possibly permanently (see also Chapter 35). Few extended families are able to live together. Many Somali women in Britain are widowed. Others arrived in Britain alone with their children because their husbands had disappeared or were unable to flee with them. Some families have now been reunited but many of these marriages then break up because of the pressures on the men (see below), and because many women, who have been used to running their own lives for several years, are unwilling to return to a more traditional female role. Although there is a strong tradition of mutual family and sub-clan support in Somalia, this is often very difficult to sustain in Britain where most people are themselves only just surviving.

'Most Somali women feel extremely lonely, so bear with us if three or four of us come with a woman to support or interpret for her.'
Somali woman

Unemployment among Somali men in Britain is extremely high, owing to a combination of factors including language barriers (see *Languages*, above) and disorientation, lack of marketable skills and knowledge of employment opportunities, limited opportunities for training and employment, and racism (Kahin 1997). Unemployed men are particularly vulnerable to depression, and there are increasing reports of mental illness and suicide among younger Somalis (Silveira and Ebrahim 1995) (see also Chapter 36 *Khat/Qat*). Almost all the Somali people in Britain are very poor and rely on Income Support. Many are in temporary accommodation and may be moved frequently. Most families are divided (see above).

'An inquiry into the daily lives of Somali refugees in Tower Hamlets found a high level of poverty and disillusionment. Few people were receiving the benefits to which they were entitled. There were extreme difficulties in getting health care and very few interpreters to help. Of a random sample of 360 people, 88 per cent lived three to a bedroom in flats which were generally damp and infested with vermin. Somalis were also frequently victims of racist attacks and racial abuse and many feared going out. Unemployment was the norm and, despite strong attempts at community organisation by self-help groups, "there is an atmosphere of despair and a pervasive sense of communal depression".'
(Refugee Council 1994)

Older Somali people

Older people are traditionally highly respected and powerful in Somali society. The older people of each clan and sub-clan have public authority. During the past turbulent decades in Somalia, clan elders have played a major part in trying to restore peace (Kahin 1997). However, many older Somali people in Britain are extremely isolated. Those, mainly ex-seaman, who have been here for many years are often cut off from more recent arrivals and have little in common with them. Their English may be poor and may be limited to the language they needed on board ship. Many never brought their families to Britain to join them and live entirely alone.

Older people who arrived more recently as refugees are more likely to have family members here. Nevertheless, most find the adjustment to life in Britain extremely difficult. They are unlikely to speak English and often lack people of their own age to talk to. They are very often reluctant to go out and become completely house-bound.

Somali foods

Most Somalis follow Muslim food restrictions strictly and also fast during the month of Ramadan (see Chapter 44 *Dietary requirements*).

The main sources of carbohydrate in the Somali diet are sabayad (a fried unleavened bread made of wheat flour), pasta and rice. In Britain many Somalis also eat UK-style bread and pitta bread. The main meats are lamb, beef and chicken. Somalis also traditionally eat some fish, especially tuna. Onions and tomatoes are used in many dishes and salads are popular. Cheese is not generally popular, though many people drink warm milk and yoghurt mixed with water (Northwick Park and St Marks NHS Trust 1994).

The main meal is traditionally eaten at midday and usually consists of meat or chicken cooked with vegetables, sabayad, rice or pasta, and salad. This is often followed by the cooking liquid from the main dish (eaten as a soup), and then by fruit. Many people like their food hotly spiced with chillis, though they may avoid chillis when ill (Northwick Park and St Marks NHS Trust 1994). At home most people eat with their fingers, but they may prefer to use cutlery in public. Some may prefer a spoon if they are not used to using a knife and fork.

Practical care

Prayer

Most Somalis will want to pray five times a day. It is important to wash before praying (see Chapter 44 *Worship*).

Modesty

Modesty is extremely important. Most Somalis will wish to follow the Islamic code of modest behaviour and should be given every help in doing so. Somali women are likely to want to keep their bodies covered as much as possible during examinations and treatment. Unnecessary exposure of any part of a woman's body, including her legs, is likely to cause extreme anxiety and distress (see *Clothing*, below, and in Chapter 12). Somali men are likely to want to keep their bodies covered from the waist to the knees.

Most Somali women and some men strongly prefer to be examined and cared for by someone of the same sex. Some people may feel unable to discuss intimate matters with a professional of the opposite sex (see Chapter 13 *Codes of modesty*). Interpreters should, whenever possible, be of the same sex as the patient (see Chapter 27 *Training, supporting and managing interpreters*).

Washing and cleanliness

Like many people from hot countries, most Somalis prefer a shower to a bath, and are accustomed to washing frequently. For Muslims it is important to wash after using the lavatory and before the five daily prayers (see Chapter 44 *Worship*).

Traditionally the right hand is honoured above the left, as in many Muslim societies. The right hand is used for all honourable purposes and the left for actions that are necessary but considered unclean. Somalis are brought up never to use their left hand for giving things, pointing or shaking hands. Some may be shocked and embarrassed if they are given things with the left hand and may feel unable to take them (Kahin 1997) (see also Chapter 12 *Practical care*).

Clothing

Somali women, especially those from urban areas, traditionally wear a diric (pronounced diri). This is a full-length, long-sleeved loose cotton garment. They may also wear a head scarf, a shoulder wrap and, under the diric, a waist slip. These clothes are also worn in bed (see Chapter 12 *Clothing*).

Men, when relaxing or in bed, may wear traditional dress, a sarong, which is wrapped round the waist and reaches the knees.

Jewellery

Somali women are unlikely to wear jewellery with special religious or other significance. Some women wear earrings but are usually prepared to remove them if necessary.

Make-up

Many Somali women wear henna (a brownish-yellow vegetable dye) on their finger and toe nails. They may also henna their hands and feet. Once applied, henna cannot be removed but fades and grows out with time.

Patients for whom elective surgery is planned should be asked to let the henna grow out so that they can be properly observed during and after surgery (see Chapter 13 *Recognising clinical signs in skin*).

When someone is ill or dying

'What I notice is that Somalis feel more satisfied if they are examined by the doctor. They need lots of reassurance. Time, courtesy and listening is what they need. They don't necessarily want a prescription.'
Somali health advocate

Many Somali people, especially those from rural areas, find the British health care system unfamiliar and worrying, though most have great faith in Western medicine. Many are cut off by language barriers. Some, especially refugees, worry about confidentiality.

Families and illness

Family members and members of the same sub-clan are under a strong obligation to visit anyone who is ill and to bring them food and presents. Not to visit can cause lasting shame and resentment. Somali patients may therefore have a lot of visitors. If this distresses the patient or other people, restrictions should be imposed as tactfully as possible and with an understanding of the obligation to visit (see also Chapter 17).

Physical examinations and treatments

Somalis who have experienced torture or physical violence may become extremely frightened and distressed during physical examinations and treatments (see also Chapter 35 *People who have experienced torture or physical abuse*). These patients need special care and understanding. Whenever possible, procedures should be carried out in such a way as to minimise fear and to avoid anything that reminds them of their experiences. People who have experienced torture and injustice may find it very hard to trust or to be open with anyone in authority, including health professionals.

Women who have undergone female genital mutilation may be anxious about any procedure or treatment that involves their genital area. They too are likely to need sensitive help and support (see Chapter 32 *Physical examination*).

When someone is dying

It is most important for the family to be with a dying person. Family members may want to read the Qur'an or to invite a religious leader, a sheikh, to read it. When the person has died, the family may want to close the eyes and kiss their forehead.

Last offices

See Chapters 44 and 20 *Immediately after the death and last offices.*

Organ donation

See Chapter 19 *Organ donation and transplantation.*

Post mortems

See Chapter 20 *Post mortems* and Chapter 44.

The funeral and afterwards

Following a death, relatives and community members traditionally visit the family at home. They may bring money or offer other practical support to the immediate family. The funeral is normally held as soon as possible (see Chapter 44 *Timing*). Traditionally, women do not attend the burial, but may attend the ceremony at the mosque beforehand. There is often a full reading of the Qur'an, ending on the seventh day when people gather to pray for forgiveness for the dead person and to share a special meal.

41 South Asian communities: history and traditional culture

· ·

Terminology

The term 'South Asian' is used here to refer to people whose families originated in the Indian subcontinent: India, Pakistan, Bangladesh and Sri Lanka. It does not include people whose families originated in other Asian countries such as China, Hong Kong, Vietnam, the Philippines and Singapore (for information about traditional Chinese culture, see Chapter 38).

The terms 'South Asian' and, more commonly, 'Asian' are widely used in the health service and elsewhere. Although they can be useful, they are in fact artificial, coined by outsiders to designate a 'racial group' whose families originated in the Indian subcontinent, a huge area as diverse as Europe. (Gujarat and Bangladesh for example, are over 2,000 kilometres apart, the same distance as London from Athens.) 'South Asian' and 'Asian' mask tremendous diversity in terms of national and regional origins, cultures and religions. Few people in Britain identify with either label in a meaningful way, any more than most English people, when asked what group they belong to, reply European (Modood, Beishon and Virdee 1994, Bowler 1993). Nevertheless, in the face of continued discrimination and racism, 'Asian' has become a unifying political label for many British people whose families originated in the Indian subcontinent.

Most people prefer to define themselves in terms of the region or country from which they or their family emigrated – for example, Indian, Pakistani, Gujarati, Punjabi, Mirpuri, and/or the religious community to which they belong. Nevertheless, because certain cultural traditions occur throughout the Indian subcontinent, the term South Asian has its uses. This chapter discusses those aspects of traditional South Asian culture that may be important in providing culturally sensitive care. (It does not cover religious beliefs and practices. For these see the chapters on religions, later.) Older people may be more likely to feel strongly about traditional aspects of South Asian culture than people brought up in Britain, but individual views vary a good deal. **Because it is never possible to predict what will be important to whom, the only way to find out is by asking each patient and listening sensitively.**

Diverse communities The South Asian communities in Britain include people of different occupational and educational levels and lifestyles. They include people whose families originated in several different areas of the Indian subcontinent (see Figure 41.1) as well as from East Africa; from towns and cities as well as from more conservative farming areas; Hindus, Jains, Sikhs, Muslims, Christians, Zoroastrians and Buddhists, and people with no religious affiliation. In addition, the experiences and circumstances of each of the South Asian communities in Britain have been very different (see Chapter 5 *The effects of racism*).

Almost half the South Asians in Britain were born and brought up here and are the children and grandchildren of immigrants (OPCS 1993). Among the immigrant generation, most people arrived in the 1950s, '60s and '70s. A few have arrived more recently, in particular women and children from Bangladesh joining their husbands, a very small number of 'elderly dependants' and refugees from Sri Lanka.

Where people came from

The Indian subcontinent – migration for work

A small group of men, mainly Muslims, came to Britain in the 1930s and '40s as sailors and cooks on British Merchant Navy ships. They often settled around the ports. Later some brought their families. There were also a few other people from British India, mainly professionals and students.

The main period of immigration from the Indian subcontinent was after the Second World War when British industry and government were recruiting workers to fill chronic labour shortages. Most people came from a few small areas of north-western India, Pakistan and Bangladesh that already had strong links with Britain, often through the British Indian Army or the Merchant Navy (see Figure 41.1). In general, the families who emigrated were somewhere in the middle of their society, neither very wealthy, because the wealthy have little incentive to migrate, nor very poor, because the poor are unlikely to be able to afford, or to have the mental and physical energy, to embark on such a huge step (Anwar 1979, Rose 1969). A number of professionals, mainly doctors and nurses, came to Britain from all over the Indian subcontinent (Vadgama 1982).

In most cases, men came first. Most assumed that they would stay for only a short time, to save enough money to improve their family's lifestyle at home or to get a better education. But saving proved hard. What had seemed like high wages from afar, turned out to be very low in relation to rent and basic living expenses. Moreover, most people found themselves, whatever their experience and qualifications, limited to the poorly paid and unattractive jobs that local people did not want (Barker 1984).

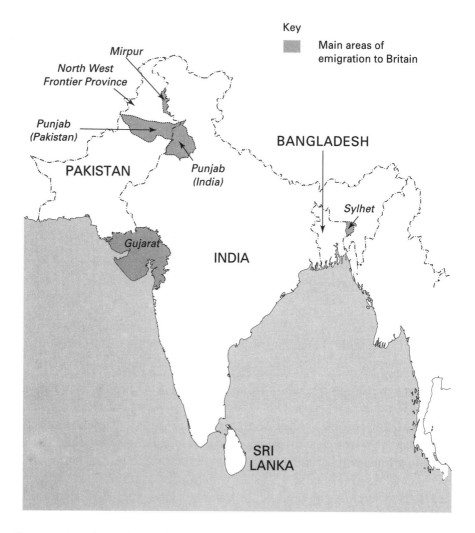

Figure 41.1 The Indian subcontinent, showing the main areas of emigration to Britain

Wives and children After several years, when they realised that their return was not imminent, most men brought their wives and children, or fiancées, to Britain. A few brought their dependent parents. Family reunions were often delayed many years while people waited for the British authorities to process their applications (Gordon and Klug 1985).

'I remember I came off my shift at the bakery and I heard the news. I had been here about five years then. Somebody said, "There's an Indian woman in the High Street!" We were all amazed. None of us had seen an Indian woman since we left home. After that a few more came and then it became quite common and there were families here and everything changed.'
Sikh man in Southall

Most men in the Hindu and Sikh communities brought their families over in the late 1950s and the 1960s. Muslim men, mainly from Pakistan and Bangladesh, often delayed, feeling that their wives and children would be happier and safer at home with their families. Most Pakistani women joined their husbands in the 1960s and '70s; many Bangladeshi women came in the 1980s and '90s. Some men, mainly Muslims, never brought their families and see them only on visits home. There are quite a lot of single or unaccompanied middle-aged and older men, especially in the Bangladeshi community (Blakemore and Boneham 1995).

Immigration restrictions Until 1962, all citizens of the British Empire and the Commonwealth could come to Britain to work and to live, and could travel in and out at will. After 1962, Commonwealth citizens had to have a voucher to fill a specific vacancy or to be joining the head of their family (Rose 1969). In 1971 the Immigration Act was introduced to end immigration from the New Commonwealth. Since then most immigration to Britain from the Indian subcontinent has been of the wives and children under 16 of men already living here.

East Africa – refugees

In the 1960s, several of the African countries of the old British Empire became independent. During the previous decades a large number of South Asians (mainly from Gujarat and Punjab – see Figure 41.1) had settled in British East Africa (Kenya, Tanzania, Malawi, Zambia and Uganda – see Figure 39.1). They were encouraged by the British government to form a commercial and professional middle layer between the white colonisers and the African majority. As independence approached, the African communities increasingly saw the South Asians as allied with the unpopular colonial authorities and unwelcome.

Recognising their vulnerability, the British government gave all South Asians in East Africa the right to keep their British citizenship at independence. It guaranteed them passports and the right to come to Britain at any time. However, in 1968, in response to media and public pressure in Britain, the government withdrew this right. From then on, East African Asians with British passports had to apply for entry vouchers to Britain. Because it is illegal under international law for any state to refuse entry to its own citizens and following international pressure, the British government allowed a quota of 1,500 British East African Asian families to enter the country every year. Nevertheless, thousands of British Asians were stranded in East Africa, many forbidden to work, with no source of income and with nowhere to go except the UK (Tandon and Raphael 1978).

In 1972, all the remaining South Asians in Uganda were forcibly expelled; most were allowed to come to the UK. Most Asians with British citizenship also had to leave the other East African countries. The British government eventually removed the quota system and most British East African Asians were allowed into the UK by 1980.

Because East African Asian refugees came as whole families, they spanned the entire age range from infants to people in their 60s, 70s and 80s. Many people from long-established East African families had never been to the Indian subcontinent (Blakemore and Boneham 1995) (see also Chapter 35).

Sri Lanka – refugees

Since the mid 1980s a number of Tamil people from Sri Lanka have come to the UK as refugees from the civil war. These are mainly unaccompanied young men; a few have brought their families (see also Chapter 35).

South Asian naming systems

In general, each religious community has its own naming system. Because some of these differ from the British system on which records are based, all names must be recorded carefully to prevent dangerous confusion (see Chapter 30 *Recording people's names correctly*).

Most older South Asian people prefer to be addressed formally except by members of their family and close friends. It is not always correct to use 'Mr' or 'Mrs' with the last name; in some naming systems the last name is a title or a personal name. Ask each person how they would like to be addressed.

In some communities, personal names are rarely used. Respectful titles such as Mother, Auntie, Uncle, Grandfather, Brother and Sister are used instead, especially with older people. An older woman may be called Mother or Auntie by all the younger women she knows.

Languages

English Everyone born in the UK speaks English, as do most people who came here as children or young people. In general, people who came to Britain as adults, especially women, have had less opportunity to learn and use English (see Chapter 25 *Who speaks English?*).

South Asian languages Although many South Asians in Britain speak English as their first language, there are also speakers of Punjabi (including the Mirpuri dialect), Urdu, Hindi, Tamil, Gujarati (including the Kutchi dialect), Pashto, Bengali (including the Sylheti dialect), Marathi or one of the other over 800 languages and dialects of the Indian subcontinent. Table 41.1 shows the main South Asian languages spoken in the UK. Many people speak several South Asian languages. South Asians from East Africa may also speak Swahili (an African language). Some people brought up in the UK may not speak any South Asian language.

Table 41.1 The main South Asian languages spoken in the UK

India
- People from Punjab State speak **Punjabi**
- People from Gujarat State speak **Gujarati**
- People from the northern part of Gujarat State speak a dialect of Gujarati called **Kutchi**
- The language of higher education in Northern India is **Hindi**

Pakistan
- People from Punjab Province speak **Punjabi**
- People from Mirpur speak **Mirpuri**, a dialect of Punjabi
- People from the North-West Frontier Province State speak **Pashto**
- The language of education in Pakistan is **Urdu**

Bangladesh
- People from Sylhet speak **Sylheti**, a dialect of Bengali
- The language of education in Bangladesh is **Bengali**

Sri Lanka
- Tamil people from Sri Lanka speak **Tamil**

Dialects Because they do not expect outsiders to be well informed about dialects, many Sylheti speakers say they speak Bengali, Mirpuri speakers say they speak Punjabi, and Kutchi speakers say they speak Gujarati. It may be necessary to check when choosing an interpreter that they can really understand each other (see Chapter 27 *Working well with a professional interpreter*). Table 41.2 shows how much people who speak one language are likely to understand other languages.

Table 41.2 How much speakers of one South Asian language are likely to understand of another language

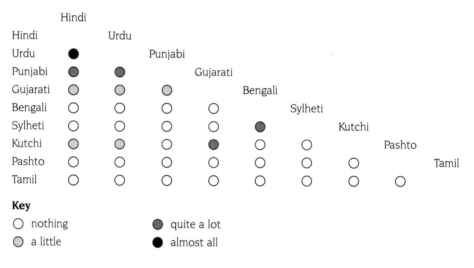

	Hindi	Urdu	Punjabi	Gujarati	Bengali	Sylheti	Kutchi	Pashto	Tamil
Urdu	●								
Punjabi	◐	◐							
Gujarati	◐	◐	◐						
Bengali	○	○	○	○					
Sylheti	○	○	○	○	◕				
Kutchi	◐	◐	○	◕	○	○			
Pashto	○	○	○	○	○	○	○		
Tamil	○	○	○	○	○	○	○	○	

Key

○ nothing ◕ quite a lot

◐ a little ● almost all

Traditional family structures and relationships

Although there is now a general trend towards more Western-style nuclear families and responsibilities, both in the Indian subcontinent and in Britain, many people still hold on to traditional South Asian family values. Each family and each individual will differ in what is important to them. In some cases there may be tensions between family members with different values and experiences. In general, families of East African Asian and Indian heritage in Britain are less conservative than families of Bangladeshi and Pakistani origin (Beishon, Modood and Virdee 1998).

The traditional South Asian family

In the farming communities from which the families of many South Asian people originated, the male head of the family and his wife, their sons and wives, and their grandsons, their wives and children, usually lived in one household and ran the family farm. Daughters, when they married, went to live with their husband's family, bringing up their children and growing old there. This large, multi-generational or extended family provided all financial, social, physical and emotional support for older, frail or ill members.

In Britain, few families are all able to live together under one roof. A recent study found that only about a fifth of South Asian couples lived with other family members, usually the husband's parents. Pakistani and Bangladeshi couples are most likely to live with older people or with other in-laws. Families of South Asian and Indian heritage are less likely to want to live as an extended household but still maintain close, often daily, contact and a strong sense of responsibility for family members who are ill, old or frail (Modood, Beishon and Virdee 1994).

Authority and decision making

Traditionally, there is a formal hierarchy in which the male head of the household has overall authority. Beneath him, older adults have authority over younger adults, and men over women, at least in public matters. A husband may be seen as the guardian of his wife, responsible for her well-being and for taking decisions in her best interests. Respect, obedience and gratitude are due to parents and other older relatives because of their age, experience and wisdom; they are seen as still contributing to the family. Older people often expect to be fully informed about important family matters, to make decisions, and to be consulted and deferred to by younger members. Expectations about who will be involved in and make decisions may be significant when discussing tests, treatments and other issues (see also Chapter 15 *Informed consent*).

Many South Asian families maintain strong links with family members 'back home'. The views, advice and judgements of these family members, who are often more conservative and have very different experiences, may sometimes affect decisions taken here.

Marriage

In South Asian tradition, marriage brings together not just two individuals forming a new independent unit but all the members of the two extended families. The bride's relationships with her husband's family members, especially the women, are often as important as her relationship with her husband. The marital relationship is traditionally less exclusive and in many ways less pressured. People are not totally dependent on their husband or wife but have other sources of support and companionship.

In the Indian subcontinent, marriages are traditionally arranged by parents and other older relatives. The members of the family who guide or make the choice are responsible for supporting and advising the young couple after marriage. Marriage is regarded as a life-time commitment. The wise guidance of older members is generally seen as a far more reliable basis for long-term success than Western 'romantic love'. The bride and groom are expected to come to know and love each other after marriage, rather than before it. Because the woman is generally regarded as responsible for ensuring the success of a marriage, she is often seen as having a particular duty to fit in and make it work (Aitchison 1994, D'Alessio 1993).

Most South Asian parents in Britain guide rather than arrange their children's marriages; some allow a completely free choice. Young people usually accept their family's concern and advice. Some, however, feel unable to accept their family's choice of partner and refuse. This may lead to a breakdown in relationships, often with disastrous consequences for the young person. They may have to survive alone in a racist society that will never completely accept them.

Men and women – traditional roles and responsibilities

In traditional South Asian families the roles of men and women may be very different. In conservative communities, marked differences in gender roles are generally unquestioned and regarded as normal and natural. Men are expected to be the breadwinners, and to support and protect the whole family, including the old and the sick. The eldest son has a special duty to support his parents. In conservative communities men are also expected to take charge of all matters outside the home, and of all contacts with non-family members.

In most communities in the Indian subcontinent it is traditional for a woman to leave her own home when she marries and to live with her husband's family. She becomes responsible, with the other women in the household, for running the home and all day-to-day domestic matters, and for the practical and emotional care of children, the sick and the old. As she grows older her position becomes important and powerful. In many communities, women's social life traditionally revolves around family and religious celebrations and visits to other women in their own homes.

The oldest son's wife is traditionally responsible for the physical and emotional care of her in-laws as they grow older. In some communities it may be regarded as shameful if a married woman has to support and care for her own parents. That responsibility belongs to her brothers and their wives.

The relationships and responsibilities of South Asian men and women in Britain vary a good deal. In some families, relationships are much like those in the average English family. In others they are more traditional. For example, in some South Asian Muslim communities it is considered to be one of the marks of a caring husband to protect his wife from the risks and gazes of the outside world and to enable her to remain in the safety of her home. Women, particularly once they are married and have children, do not work outside the home. Many husbands do the shopping and other errands. Women who lead secluded lives may have had little or no experience of British society or institutions and may find it particularly hard to take decisions or to organise the care they or their families need in times of crisis. They are also less likely to speak or read English.

In contrast, in many families of East African Asian and Indian origin, it is regarded as desirable for women to work outside the home provided this does not have a negative impact on the children. Gender roles are less clearly differentiated, though it is still common for women to carry out most of the domestic duties (Beishon, Modood and Virdee 1998). Decisions are often shared, though ultimate authority may still lie with the husband or the oldest man.

Family responsibilities

In traditional South Asian culture, each person is seen and sees themselves primarily as a member of their family rather than as separate and autonomous. The needs and interests of the family and of the individual are often assumed to be the same; the independence and self-assertion so valued in the West may be seen as immoral, selfish and irresponsible. Each person has duties, responsibilities and expectations, depending on their position in the family, their age, sex and marital status. Although these are not rigid, and individual personalities always play a part, most people accept them. People are more likely to be admired for the way they carry out their family responsibilities than for developing their individual potential (Stopes-Roe and Cochrane 1990) (see also Chapter 9 *Families, relationships and roles*).

Mutual dependence and support are traditionally regarded as desirable and healthy. People have a duty to be concerned about other family members and to become involved in their lives and difficulties. Children belong to the whole family, not just to their parents. In conservative families no one is expected to live alone; large and small possessions are often shared; loans may be given within families rather than by strangers; younger people are expected to accept advice and support from older people, and siblings to take responsibility for each other throughout their lives; older people may take decisions for younger family members. People are not expected to separate from their family when they become adult; unmarried adult children are expected to live with their parents. If the wishes of the family and those of the individual conflict, most people accept the need to find a compromise. Many people accept the restrictions that are bound to accompany close family involvement and dependence, preferring these to the loneliness and self-centredness that they see in Western societies.

A person's reputation and honour are traditionally a family rather than an individual matter. The achievements of any member enhance the whole family's reputation. Conversely, unacceptable behaviour or a failure of duty may damage everyone's reputation. As in many societies, women are traditionally expected to set higher moral standards and to follow stricter codes of behaviour. They represent the honour and reputation of the family. An unmarried couple living together or a child born outside marriage are generally regarded as extremely shameful for the whole family.

Public behaviour

In some communities there is a strict code of behaviour between the sexes to preserve mutual respect and ensure morality. Men and women do not mix, and friendships across the sexes are traditionally rare. In an extended family household where there may be several married and unmarried adults, the women and children traditionally spend their days in separate rooms from the men. Men and women may prefer to remain physically separate in public. In conservative communities it is considered improper for a married couple to touch each other in front of other people, even their own children.

'My parents had an excellent marriage and we were a very happy family, but I never once saw my parents kiss or hug each other. That was something private.'
British Asian doctor

In conservative communities men and women may visit an ill relative at different times of the day. A female patient may be chaperoned by a female family member. For reasons of modesty, some patients may prefer to draw their curtains at visiting time (see also Chapter 12 *Modesty*). Personal matters to do with intimate physical care or bodily functions are unlikely to be discussed between men and women or, in conservative communities, between husbands and wives. This can be important if family members are asked to interpret (see Chapter 28 *Using friends and relatives to interpret*).

Older South Asian people

Old age in the farming communities from which most South Asian people in Britain originated is generally seen as a time when people give up their work and other burdensome duties, whether inside or outside the home, and become respected focal points for the family, cared for and listened to (Boneham 1989). It is the most important duty of an eldest son, as well as a matter of pride and honour, to care for his parents. Not to do so is a matter of family shame.

Although the number of older South Asian people in Britain is still small, many of the pioneering generation of immigrants are now at or approaching retirement age. Many South Asian older people feel that their family is their only real source of companionship and support. They expect their families to respect, love and care for them. Many younger South Asian people, in turn, feel a great sense of responsibility for their older parents and wish to support and care for them. However, changed circumstances and lifestyles in Britain, changing values in some communities and the physical break-up of the family can make this very difficult (see also Chapter 4 *Traditional expectations*).

> 'We are torn between the two cultures and it is so often impossible here. Often the husband and wife both have to work, the children are at school or college, no one is at home all day and the old people feel very separate and lonely. Loneliness is a major cause of depression for many old people here.'
> South Asian community worker

Traditional South Asian medicine

The Indian subcontinent contains three main traditional systems of medicine, all of them over 2,000 years old. These are the Ayurvedic system, based originally on ancient Hindu texts and influenced over the years by medical knowledge from different cultures; the Unani or Hikmat system, which originated in Greece and the Middle East and is largely used in Muslim areas; and the Siddha system, used mainly by Tamils in southern India and Sri Lanka. All three work on the basis of different elements and humours which make up the body and are believed to affect people's physical, spiritual, emotional and mental well-being. Imbalances within the body cause illness and distress and must be restored through treatment. Treatment often involves changes in the person's diet and lifestyle. Medication containing herbs, minerals and other substances is also used. Traditional practitioners diagnose conditions mainly through observation, detailed discussion with the patient and taking the patient's pulses (Godagama 1997, Ahmad 1992).

These three medical systems are recognised by governments in the Indian subcontinent, where there are training colleges and systems of registration for practitioners, and are generally highly respected. Trained practitioners of traditional medicine are usually more accessible and less expensive than practitioners of Western medicine. There are also large numbers of untrained or semi-trained practitioners who are generally even cheaper. In addition, preparations based on traditional South Asian medicine are sold across the counter in pharmacies and general stores (see also Chapter 31).

South Asian foods

The staple diet of people in the Indian subcontinent varies hugely, according to local climate and agriculture. There is no such thing as an Asian diet. For example, Sylhet (see Figure 41.1, above) is one of the wettest places in the world. The climate is excellent for rice, and fish (often reared in the flooded rice fields) is plentiful. People in the fertile Punjab area (divided between India and Pakistan) eat chapattis made of wheat or maize. People in Gujarat eat both rice and chapattis as their staple carbohydrate. Most meals consist of a large amount of carbohydrate and relatively little protein.

Most of the fruit and vegetables that grow in the different climatic regions of the Indian subcontinent are different from those grown in Britain. Cooking styles also differ. Food is usually fried briefly and then stewed, with none of the cooking water thrown away. Vegetables are rarely boiled. Pulses such as lentils and chickpeas are a major source of protein, especially for vegetarians. A wide variety of spices are used, and many people used to South Asian food find English food heavy and tasteless.

Meals Rice and/or chapattis and the different accompanying dishes are normally laid out in the centre of the table and people help themselves to food during the meal as they wish. Salads (mainly of chopped up vegetables such as cucumber, onion and tomato with lemon juice squeezed over them) are served as a side dish and are not normally a meal in their own right. In some communities it is traditional for men and visitors to eat first, followed by women and children.

South Asian food is traditionally eaten with the fingers, usually of the right hand which is reserved for handling clean things, or with a spoon. It is usually served in bite-size pieces. Most people will want to wash their hands before they eat.

Religious aspects of food

In the Indian subcontinent, food has a spiritual significance that it has almost completely lost in the West. Many South Asians in Britain follow religious prohibitions on food (see Chapter 11 *Religious aspects of food* and the chapters on religions).

Food and health

Like all cultures, traditional South Asian culture contains beliefs about what people should eat and avoid to keep healthy. Certain foods are classified as 'hot' or 'cold' in terms of their effects on the body and the emotions. This has nothing to do with the physical temperature of the food, and details vary between communities. 'Hot' foods are generally salty, sour or high in animal protein. They are believed to raise the body temperature and to excite (and in excess to over-excite) the emotions rather like alcohol. 'Cold' foods are generally sweet, bitter or astringent. They are believed to cool the body temperature, calm the emotions, and make a person cheerful and strong.

Too many hot or cold foods can unbalance the body and emotions and cause ill-health. Certain illnesses are also thought to 'cool' or 'heat' the body and to require more or less of certain foods. For example, for a cold or a sore throat – both 'cold' conditions – people may avoid cold drinks, fruit juices, salads and yoghurt. After an operation some people may avoid tomatoes and citrus fruits, which are believed to delay healing. Many people, especially older people, automatically follow these principles in order to maintain a healthy diet.

Sick people also traditionally avoid foods that are very spicy, oily or rich. Many invalid-type dishes are soft: for example, very soft rice mixed with a little ghee (clarified butter), a soft mixture of rice and lentils, light lentil soups, lightly fried lightly salted potatoes, bread, dry chapattis, or a soft pudding such as tapioca. Fresh fruit is often highly regarded.

Food away from home

It is important to ensure that people have food that is both appetising and religiously and culturally acceptable. Relatives may worry if a patient is not eating properly or is not getting the right food. Some may bring in food as a way of showing their love and concern for a patient, especially if the patient follows strict religious dietary restrictions. This should be facilitated wherever possible (see also Chapter 11 *Relatives bringing in food*).

Practical care

Modesty

Physical modesty is extremely important in most South Asian communities, especially for more conservative and older people. Women traditionally cover their legs, upper body and upper arms. For a South Asian woman to uncover her legs may be as humiliating as for an English woman to have to uncover her breasts in public. Some women keep themselves completely covered at all times. Backless gowns and garments that leave the legs bare are immodest and degrading for many women, particularly in the presence of strangers. Men traditionally cover themselves from the waist to the knees. To be naked, even in the presence of other men, may be very humiliating (see also Chapter 12 *Modesty*).

At home As in many cultures, most women feel able to take on the physical care of a sick husband at home, and, in some cases, of other male relatives. It may be more difficult for a man to take on the physical care of his wife. Men may feel embarrassed or incapable. Women may feel humiliated and ashamed if they have to depend on intimate care from a man, even their husband. Nevertheless, many people are able to overcome these difficulties.

> 'I was working with a very conservative elderly Sikh couple where the wife had to have a permanent indwelling catheter. This meant that when she went home her husband would have to empty her bag for her. They both found this distressing and undignified, but the man said to me, "Tell me what I have to do and I'll do my best. After all, she has looked after me all my life."'
> British Asian doctor

Clothing

Many **women** wear traditional styles that reflect their background, culture and religion. Some South Asian women who wear Western clothes prefer to keep their legs covered with trousers or a long skirt. They may change into traditional clothes when in their own community and when relaxing.

- **Shalwar kameez** are the traditional everyday wear of most Punjabi women (in both India and Pakistan) and of most Muslim women in Gujarat. The kameez (shirt) is a long tunic with long or half sleeves. The shalwar (or salwar) are trousers. There is also a long scarf called a chuni or dupattah, which lies over the shoulders and across the breasts. Some women pull one end of the dupattah over the head as a sign of modesty and respect in front of strangers, older people or men. In some communities the width of the shalwar legs changes with fashion.

- **Sari** Most Hindu women and most Bangladeshi women traditionally wear a sari over a blouse and underskirt. Hindu women sometimes leave the midriff bare. The underskirt is full length with a drawstring waist. A sari is about five or six metres long. Like the dupattah (see above), one end may be pulled over the head as a sign of modesty and respect. Tamil Hindu women often wear Western clothing.

Most South Asian **men** wear Western-style shirt and trousers outside the home, but may relax in traditional dress. This is usually a kameez (loose shirt) and pyjama (trousers) or a dhoti (a length of cloth wrapped round the waist and drawn between the legs). Some men wear a lunghi (a cloth wrapped round the waist).

When ill Most people prefer to wear familiar clothes when they are ill or away from home. Many women wear a lighter, looser version of their sari or shalwar kameez in bed. Most men wear pyjamas or a tunic top with pyjama bottoms. (Pyjama is originally a Hindi word.) Some wear a dhoti or a lunghi (see above).

Shoes

The feet are considered dirty and, by some people, polluting. At home, most people take their shoes off when they come into the house, especially when entering a room where prayers are said. Visitors do the same as a matter of courtesy. Shoes are not put with other possessions, for example in a bag with other clothes or on a locker.

Washing and cleanliness

In traditional South Asian culture, physical cleanliness is linked to ideas about spiritual pollution and purity. Certain things, including all body fluids, pollute both the body and the soul. People try to avoid them and wash thoroughly under running water if they come into contact with them. Incontinence and suppurating wounds may cause additional distress. The degree to which South Asian people in Britain follow these beliefs varies a good deal. For some older people in all communities and for conservative Hindus they may be crucial, for others they are irrelevant or even unknown. (See also Chapter 12 *Practical care*.)

Showers Many South Asian people shower or wash at least twice a day. Some people find the idea of a bath disgusting because it involves sitting in one's own dirty water. Patients who are too weak or frail to stand in a shower may prefer a bed bath to a bath. A few people consider it unhealthy to shower when they are ill or weak.

For reasons of modesty, some people always shower in their clothes, putting on clean, dry clothes when they have finished. Jewellery with special religious significance is normally kept on while showering but it may be important to keep it dry.

Some people clean out their nasal passages and throats with water and spit out any phlegm, particularly first thing in the morning. Handkerchiefs are not traditionally used in the Indian subcontinent, and a few older people may blow their noses into the fingers of their left hand and then clean their fingers under running water. Some people may need a jug and a bowl for cleaning out their nasal passages and for gargling and spitting out phlegm.

Washing before and after meals Many South Asians wash their hands, rinse out their mouths and clean their teeth when they wake up and also before and after every meal. Offer people who cannot get out of bed a jug of water and a bowl so that they can pour water over their hands.

People with false teeth may want to rinse them after a meal. After cleaning their teeth, some people clean their tongues using a U-shaped metal tongue cleaner.

Before prayers Many South Asians always wash before praying, usually in running water. People who cannot get out of bed may need a glass or jug of water for pouring, a tooth bowl, a larger bowl and a towel. Muslims follow a special prescribed washing routine before the five formal daily prayers (see Chapter 44 *Worship*).

Lavatories Some South Asians always wash their perineal area with running water after using the lavatory. Using the lavatory and keeping clean afterwards causes extreme anxiety to many people (see also Chapter 12 *Elimination*).

'When my mum went into hospital she was more worried about the lavatories than anything. At one point she couldn't get out of bed and the nurses didn't realise how important it was to her to wash after using the bedpan. They just didn't understand. She felt so dirty and disgusting. She stopped going to the toilet altogether and became faecally impacted.'
South Asian woman

Hair care

The head is traditionally regarded as sacred and is not touched by others without good reason (see also Chapter 48 *Hair care*). Some South Asian women oil their hair with coconut oil when they brush it, to keep it healthy and shiny (see Chapter 12 *Hair care*).

Jewellery and make-up

See Chapter 12 *Jewellery and other items*.

When someone is ill or dying

Families and illness

Traditionally, all members of the extended family must visit and sit with anyone who is ill or dying. No one who is ill is ever left alone. People who do not visit may be considered callous and discourteous. Visitors may arrive in large groups or at 'unusual' times and may find standard visiting restrictions upsetting and difficult to deal with (see also Chapter 17).

> 'What I found most difficult when my father was so ill was that we could not be with him all the time. He wanted us all to be there but we were only allowed two or three at a time and we had to leave at night. There were no facilities for anyone to stay overnight with him and to just be beside him. He was so alone and we felt so bad.'
> South Indian woman

Expectations of medical care

Many South Asian people, like many other people, place great trust in the knowledge and authority of doctors. Specialists may be thought to have more expertise than general practitioners. Faced with a range of treatment options, some people may prefer the doctor to make decisions for them (see Chapter 15 *Informed consent*).

The place of death

Many South Asian people prefer to die at home in a familiar environment surrounded by their families. However, some may feel safer in hospital where they know everything possible will be done for them. Work routines and other pressures may also make it difficult for family members to look after people who are very ill at home.

> 'When I am dying I want to be at home with the people I love. I know that the doctors and nurses in the hospital are very good, but it is all so different, the surroundings, the feeling, the smells, the sounds. I want to be able to wash in my way and to taste the food that I have eaten all my life. I want everything to be familiar and comfortable. I want to hear my family moving and talking around me. No effort, no strain, just familiarity and utter contentment.'
> North Indian man

In most South Asian communities it is very important that family members are present at the time of death. This is one of the last things they can do for the dying person. Often large numbers of people will want to gather and pray (see Chapter 18 *Care when death is imminent*). After the death they may want to stay with the body for a long time, especially if they are waiting for other relatives to come and pay their respects (see Chapter 20 *Spending time with the body*).

After the death

Last offices

The rituals and practical tasks to be carried out after a death vary according to the family's religion (see Chapters 42–48). Sometimes family members will want to wash and prepare the body for the funeral themselves. This should be facilitated wherever possible. (See also Chapter 20 *Immediately after the death and last offices*.)

The funeral

It is a binding duty for members of the extended family and the community to attend a funeral. Not to attend may be considered shameful and unforgivable, so funerals are often extremely large. In many communities it is important to hold the funeral as soon as possible (see Chapter 20 *Paperwork and certificates*).

42 Christianity

●●●

The information below will apply only to certain Christian patients and their families. There are also different denominations of Christianity; people's practices and wishes may vary a good deal. Never assume. Always check everything with the person concerned.

Christian communities in Britain

Christianity is a missionary religion and, in the 2000 years since its foundation in the Middle East, has spread throughout the world, in particular to Europe, much of the old Russian Empire, Latin America, North America, the Far East, central and southern Africa, and Australasia. During this period it has divided into a large number of different churches or denominations, each with certain different views and practices.

It has been estimated that there are about 7 million practising Christians (those who attend church services, for example) in the UK, but that probably about 40 million people would categorise themselves as Christian (Weller 1997). The families of Christians in Britain originated in many parts of the world. Their practices and wishes may be influenced by their cultural heritage as well as by denominational differences.

The Christian churches in Britain

The main Christian churches in Britain are:

- the Anglican Church (the Church of England and its sister Churches in Wales, Ireland and Scotland) (see later);
- the Roman Catholic Church (see later);
- the free or non-conformist churches; for example, the Baptist Church, the Methodist Church, the Seventh Day Adventist Church (see later), the United Reformed Church, Pentecostalist Churches (see later) (including the Elim Church, the New Testament Church of God, the Church of God of Prophecy and the Assemblies of God), the Society of Friends (Quakers) and the Salvation Army;
- the Eastern Orthodox Churches, including the Greek, Russian and Serbian Orthodox Churches.

There are also a number of smaller independent churches, often local and with small congregations. Many of these have been set up to meet the needs of particular black and minority ethnic communities.

Although all these churches share a belief in God and the divinity of Christ, there are often major differences between them in terms of beliefs, practices and attitudes. Some have very strict rules governing daily behaviour and worship; others are looser and leave most decisions to the conscience of individual members. The different churches also attach different importance to congregational worship, to the sacraments and rites such as baptism and communion.

In the last 50 years there have been attempts to try to increase unity and understanding between the different denominations; these have met with some success. Inter-church relations are now generally more positive and ministers frequently co-operate, for example, in visiting and caring for people in hospital. Nevertheless, for most Christians their own particular denomination and its rituals, traditions and practices are very important.

This chapter contains a general account of Christian belief and practice and then focuses on four denominations: Anglicanism, as representing the majority of Christians in Britain; and Roman Catholicism, Seventh Day Adventism and Pentecostalism, all of which have a significant black and minority ethnic membership (Weller 1997).

Christianity – a brief description

Christians believe in a loving God who is revealed in three persons – Father, Son and Holy Spirit. They believe that everything is created and given life by God the Father. He entrusted the world to humanity but people's weakness and susceptibility to temptation led them away from Him. This story is told in the books of the Hebrew scriptures known to Christians as the Old Testament. The Old Testament is also seen as foretelling the coming of Jesus Christ, the Saviour of humankind.

Jesus Christ

Christians believe that God the Father eventually sent His son Jesus as a human being to save humankind and to show people the way back to God. Jesus was a Jew who lived in Israel at the time of the Roman Occupation about 2000 years ago. In His teachings and example, Jesus, known as the Christ (the Anointed One), summed up the whole of God's law as to love God and to love one's neighbour as oneself.

Many of Jesus' contemporaries became His followers and believed in Him as their Saviour; others saw Him as a wise teacher and kindly prophet. However, to many of the religious leaders in His society He was a threat because His followers claimed that He was the divine son of God. Jesus Himself accepted His mission as a suffering servant and anointed one (Messiah) whom the prophets had predicted would deliver the Jewish people. Accused by the religious leaders of blasphemy and high treason, He was crucified by order of the Roman governor of Jerusalem.

Christians believe that Jesus Christ rose from the dead on the third day after His crucifixion and remained on earth appearing and preaching for 40 days. He then ascended into heaven. For most Christians the resurrection of Christ is central to their faith because it shows that Christ overcame death, redeemed humankind and offered the hope of eternal life; death is therefore not the end. They believe that each person is an eternal soul who lives on after their body dies. After their death, each person will be judged by God and will be received by Him in heaven or will be sent to hell.

Some Christians believe that God will judge each person on the basis of the life they have lived and whether they have followed His commandments. Others believe that the only route to salvation is through recognising Christ as Saviour and through baptism in His name.

The founding of the Church

Before Christ died He held a meal with His closest followers, the twelve apostles. At this meal, known as the Last Supper, Christ entrusted His message to the apostles and in particular, to the apostle Peter. He blessed bread and wine and gave it to the apostles, asking them to do the same in memory of Him. This is the basis of holy communion (see below).

Christian beliefs and values

Christianity stresses the importance of living a good life in response to God's love. Much of Christ's message is summed up in His Sermon on the Mount, also known as the Beatitudes:

'Blessed are the poor in spirit, for theirs is the kingdom of heaven.
Blessed are those who mourn, for they shall be comforted.
Blessed are the meek, for they shall inherit the earth.
Blessed are those who hunger and thirst after righteousness, for they shall be satisfied.
Blessed are the merciful, for they shall obtain mercy.
Blessed are the pure in heart, for they shall see God.

Blessed are the peacemakers, for they shall be called the children of God. Blessed are those who are persecuted for righteousness' sake, for theirs is the kingdom of heaven.'

St Matthew's Gospel, 5: 3–10

For some Christians, evil is simply an absence of good and a denial of the love of God. Others believe in Satan, the devil, originally an angel who defied God's love and was cast out of heaven. They see him as an active force in the world, causing evil, suffering and despair, and trying to turn people away from God. Some of the latter believe that physical and mental illness can be caused by Satan or the forces of evil and may pray or carry out special rituals to try to destroy Satan's power. Some Christians also believe strongly in angels, beings of pure light who act as God's messengers, and support people on earth.

Most Christian churches regard marriage and family life as very important, but attitudes differ widely on issues such as divorce, premarital sex, contraception, abortion, homosexuality and so on. (For more on specific practices and beliefs of members of the Anglican, Roman Catholic, Seventh Day Adventist and Pentecostalist Churches, see below.)

Religious observance

Few of the Christian churches prescribe precise details of daily life such as daily prayer, diet and dress. These are usually regarded as personal issues. In many churches, Christians are expected to make their own decisions based on their personal beliefs and values. Although these beliefs and values are individual, they are not flexible. **It is important to find out what each patient requires and to respect their decisions.**

Worship

Prayer, both formal and informal, is a major source of support and comfort to many Christians, and may become particularly so at times of crisis. Some people pray quietly or read the Bible. Some may wish for a chaplain or another Christian to pray with them. Some may pray or sing with members of their congregation. People's privacy and need for quiet should be respected and different needs accommodated wherever possible (see also Chapter 10 *Practical matters*). The most frequently said Christian prayer is the Lord's Prayer, which was given by Jesus to His followers:

Our Father, Who art in heaven
Hallowed be thy name.

Thy kingdom come.
Thy will be done on earth as it is in heaven.
Give us this day our daily bread
And forgive us our trespasses
As we forgive those that trespass against us.
And lead us not into temptation
But deliver us from evil.
For thine is the kingdom, the power and the glory
For ever and ever. Amen.

Some Christians also derive great comfort from the saints, people who have led exemplary lives on earth and have died, who are now praying for those still on earth. Many Christians have a special devotion to Mary, the mother of Jesus (see below). Others strongly disapprove of this.

The Bible

The stories of Jesus' life and mission are recorded in the four gospels of the New Testament, the most important holy book for most Christians. Many Christians also regard the books of the Old Testament (the history of the Jewish people's relationship with God) as having unique significance. Together these are known as the Bible. Members of some churches regard every word of the Bible as the literal and sacred truth. They set detailed standards of belief, practice and behaviour for their members based on a literal reading of biblical texts. Other Christians regard the Bible as a record of how people have understood God's activity, which must be re-interpreted for each generation in the light of Christian tradition and of modern thinking and circumstances. People who are ill and those who care for them may find comfort in reading or listening to passages from the Bible.

Some people may bring religious items such as a Bible, prayer books, statues, pictures or a rosary into hospital with them. These should be treated with respect.

Sundays and church attendance

In most Christian churches (though not Seventh Day Adventists – see later) Sunday is a special day of rest and church attendance celebrating the resurrection of Christ. Services on Sunday may include communion (see below). Some patients may wish to attend church services on Sundays and other days if at all possible.

Holy communion

Holy communion is consecrated bread and wine, shared in memory of Christ's Last Supper (see above). The significance attached to holy communion varies in the different Christian churches (see also *Roman Catholicism*, later). Some patients may wish to receive communion in bed. It is normally brought by a priest, minister or lay assistant.

Ministers, priests and pastors

In most Christian churches there is a minister, priest or pastor (who may also have another title) who leads services, administers sacraments and carries out pastoral care and counselling for the community. In many churches, including the Anglican Church, the minister may be a woman. Many people who no longer attend services or follow the formal requirements of their church still regard themselves as Christian and may be grateful for the sensitive offer of a visit by a minister at times of distress and worry.

Baptism

The sacrament of baptism or christening is practised by nearly all Christians. It is seen as the beginning of an individual's relationship with God through the church and takes place only once in a person's life. In some churches baptism takes place only when the person is old enough to understand the commitment they are making. Most churches baptise infants on the basis of the faith and commitment of the parents and godparents or sponsors. The mainstream churches generally recognise the validity of each others' baptism (Green and Green 1992).

Sometimes a seriously ill person may wish to be baptised before they die. Normally a minister of the appropriate denomination should be called. In an emergency, anyone – though preferably a baptised person – may baptise. The essentials are the use of water, which may be lightly sprinkled on the forehead, and the words, 'I baptise you in the name of the Father, the Son, and the Holy Spirit.' Prayers may be said and the sign of the cross may be made over the person. A baptism should always be recorded, using the full Christian names.

Religious jewellery

Some Christians wear religious jewellery – for example, a cross, a medal of Christ or a saint, or a picture on a chain or thread around the neck. Some religious jewellery may have been blessed and may sometimes be worn specially to protect the wearer at times of illness and vulnerability. However, most people will be willing to remove religious jewellery if necessary, for example before surgery (see also Chapter 12 *Jewellery and other items*).

Religious dietary restrictions

Most Christians do not follow religious dietary restrictions. A few are vegetarian or vegan (see *Seventh Day Adventists*, later). Some fast or abstain from meat at special times. A few may fast more strictly. For example, members of the Aladura International Church (an African independent church) take no food or drink from midnight until six o'clock the next evening twice a month (Hebblethwaite 1996).

Festivals

Most Christians celebrate festivals related to the life, death and resurrection of Jesus Christ. In Britain and in most other parts of the world these have also become social celebrations. The most important religious festivals for most Christians are Easter and Christmas. The dates of these and other festivals fall later in the Orthodox churches than in the Western churches. The dates of some festivals depend on the lunar calendar. (See also the SHAP Calendar, listed in the References.)

Christmas Eve and Christmas Day *24 and 25 December in Western churches; 6 and 7 January in Orthodox churches.* Celebrates the birth of Christ and is a time of rejoicing and thanksgiving. Also a time of family reunions and visits and present-giving. Many Christians go to church and some attend a service on the evening of Christmas Eve.

Ash Wednesday *February or March* (depending on the date of Easter Sunday, see below). Marks the beginning of Lent, the 40 (in Orthodox churches 42) days before Easter Sunday. Traditionally this was a period of fasting and penance in preparation for Good Friday and Easter. Nowadays, it is generally observed less strictly in the West but many Christians give up something special, take on an extra task or say extra prayers during Lent. Some Catholics attend extra masses.

For many Orthodox Christians Lent, known as the Great Fast, is still a period of abstinence and fasting. Some eat no meat, butter or milk for the whole period; some make an extra fast in the final week, known as Holy Week. All these practices are intended as an offering to God and to enable the person in some way to share in Christ's suffering in the saving of humankind.

Easter is preceded by **Holy Week** in which the days leading up to Christ's death are remembered. It is a week of sorrow and repentance for many

Christians. On **Good Friday** *March, April or May* (see below) Christians focus on the suffering and death of Christ on the cross. Some devout Christians go to church, especially around three o'clock in the afternoon when Christ is known to have died.

Easter Sunday *March or April in Western churches; April or May in Orthodox churches.* Easter celebrates Christ's resurrection from the dead after His crucifixion and burial. It is extremely important and joyful for most Christians. Many go to church. In the Orthodox churches, Easter is a far more important festival than Christmas.

Other festivals may be important to some Christians; for example: the Ascension (Thursday, 40 days after Easter Sunday), which commemorates Christ's ascension into heaven; Pentecost or Whitsun (seven Sundays after Easter), which commemorates the gift of the Holy Spirit to Jesus' apostles after His death; and the Assumption, or Dormition (*15 August*), which commemorates the tradition of the ascension into heaven of Mary, the mother of Jesus. The latter is mainly celebrated by Roman Catholics and members of the Orthodox churches.

When a person is seriously ill or dying

Attitudes to death and dying

Many Christians regard this life as a preparation for life after death. For many, the suffering and pain of this life are only part of the picture, and are viewed as part of the wider framework of God's law and plan for humankind. This may influence the decisions that some people make when they are seriously ill or dying.

Prayers and anointing of the sick and dying

Families members may wish to pray beside the bed of a person who is sick or dying. Some people may want a minister or other members of their congregation to pray with them. In some churches this may involve a large number of people. These should be accommodated wherever possible (see also Chapter 17).

In some denominations a minister may anoint the patient with consecrated oil. The minister may also pray to God to give the person courage for whatever lies ahead of them, to forgive their sins and, according to His plan, to restore them to health or to receive their soul into heaven.

Organ donation

Most Christians have no religious objection to organ donation.

After the death

Last offices

As always, it is important to check if the relatives have any preferences about how the body is prepared. Most Christians are not particular about who touches the body after death. Normal procedures will be acceptable to most people. (See also Chapter 20 *Immediately after the death and last offices*.)

Post mortems

Most Christians have no religious objection to post mortems.

Funeral services

Funeral services are often held in church, usually led by a minister, after which the family and close relatives and friends may accompany the body to the cemetery or crematorium. Alternatively, the whole service may take place at the cemetery or crematorium. Most Christian denominations permit both burial and cremation; some require or strongly prefer burial. It is traditional in some Christian communities for people to go to the home of the family after the service to express their sympathy and to share a meal together.

ANGLICANISM

The Anglican Church includes the Church of England and its sister churches, the Church in Wales, the Episcopal Church in Scotland and the Church of Ireland. There are about 70 million Anglicans in the world, including the Indian subcontinent, Hong Kong, the Caribbean, east, west and southern Africa, North and South America, and China. Some Anglicans may describe themselves as Church of England or C of E, Church of Wales, or Episcopalian.

Anglican beliefs and values

The Anglican Church contains a very broad range of beliefs, practices and attitudes. There are few regulations binding members' daily lives. Each individual makes their own decisions on matters of personal morality based on Christian principles and their own conscience. Anglicans whose families originated in other parts of the world may also be influenced in their religious practice by different cultures and heritages. Within the Anglican Church there are also various traditions or groupings, ranging from the High Church or Anglo-Catholic tradition, which has much in common with traditional Roman Catholicism (see below), to the evangelical tradition, which is generally less formal and ritualistic and has more in common with the free or non-conformist churches. **Although most of the information in the general section on Christianity above will apply to many Anglican patients, it is always important to ask each patient and family what they would like and not to make any assumptions.**

Most hospital religious provision in Britain has evolved on the basis of traditional Anglican practices and therefore meets the basic religious needs of Anglican patients. There is an Anglican chaplain in most hospitals who offers pastoral care and comfort and administers the sacraments. He or she also offers care to members of other religious denominations and to people with no formal religious attachment if asked, and can liaise with representatives of other religious groups as necessary.

When a person is seriously ill or dying

Prayer and anointing

When a person is seriously ill or dying the patient or family may wish for a minister to come and pray with them. They may also request anointing. This involves making a sign of the cross with consecrated olive oil on the person's forehead (and sometimes chest and wrists) while offering prayers. People may also be anointed before a serious operation or at other special times (Green and Green 1992) (see also *Holy communion and Baptism* in the general section on Christianity, above).

At the time of death

A minister may say a prayer of commendation at the bedside. Prayers may also be said afterwards at the bedside or in the chapel. The soul of the person who has died is commended into God's keeping and thanks are given for their life (Green and Green 1992).

ROMAN CATHOLICISM

Roman Catholics in Britain

In the UK, Catholics make up about 13 per cent of the total population (Green and Green 1992) and are of very mixed heritages: a survey in the 1970s found that one-quarter of the Catholics in Britain were immigrants and another fifth were the children of immigrants (Hornsby-Smith 1991). In Northern Ireland, Catholics currently make up 38 per cent of the population (Northern Ireland Office, personal communication 1994). There is a small number of old English Roman Catholic families in Britain whose forebears survived the Protestant Reformation in the sixteenth century. The families of most other British Catholics originated elsewhere in Europe, including the Irish Republic (the largest number), Italy, Spain, Portugal and Poland. There are also smaller Catholic communities whose families originated in the West Indies, the Philippines, Latin America, southern India and Sri Lanka, Hong Kong, China, the Middle East, and central and southern Africa.

Roman Catholicism – a brief description

Most of the information in the general section on Christianity above also applies to most Catholic patients.

The Pope, the head of the Roman Catholic Church, is regarded by most Catholics as having God-given spiritual authority. He speaks out on moral and spiritual issues, setting out matters of faith and what the Church requires of its members.

Beginning in the 1960s there were major changes in the Catholic Church, including greater lay involvement and more open discussion. These coincided with major changes in social values and behaviour in Britain. Although official Vatican teaching has now become more conservative, there is a great variety of beliefs, attitudes and practices on many key issues in the British Catholic community. There is also a wide range of cultural influences and traditions, reflecting the many different heritages of British Roman Catholics. Some people adhere very strictly to traditional expressions of Catholic beliefs and official rulings; others make their own decisions based on Christian principles and ethics and on their own conscience. **It is very important therefore not to make any assumptions about the wishes or needs of a Catholic patient but to find out from each person and family what is important to them.**

Religious observance

Sunday mass and holy communion

Mass is the most important Catholic religious service, at which the sacrifice of Jesus Christ on the cross is remembered and bread and wine are consecrated by the priest. Catholics are required to go to mass once a week on Sunday or on Saturday evening, though not everyone does this.

Catholics believe that the consecrated bread and wine are transformed into the actual body and blood of Jesus Christ. Holy communion, when the bread (and sometimes the wine) is distributed, is therefore regarded as a miraculous gift from God and extremely sacred. Out of reverence, people do not normally eat or drink for at least an hour before taking holy communion. Some may fast for longer. If a person has committed a serious sin or has not been to holy communion for a long time they may want to go to confession (see below) before receiving holy communion.

When someone is ill Some Catholics may wish to attend mass if at all possible, especially on Sundays. If they are unable to move they may like holy communion to be brought to them. This should be arranged with the Catholic priest or chaplain. The bread and wine are treated with extreme reverence. It is important to try to ensure peace and privacy while people are preparing for and taking holy communion, as well as for a short time afterwards.

Confession

Confession (also called penance or reconciliation) is a sacrament at which people confess their sins privately to a priest, say that they are sorry and promise to try never to do wrong again. They receive forgiveness (absolution) and are usually asked to say certain prayers as a token of their sorrow. They may also receive counselling. The priest is believed to act as a representative of Jesus Christ in confession; when he forgives a person's sins, they are regarded as forgiven by God.

Some people may very much wish to make their confession before receiving holy communion or if they are seriously ill or dying. This should be arranged with the Catholic chaplain.

Additional devotions

Some Catholics have a special devotion to Mary, the mother of Jesus Christ. Mary is regarded as particularly holy and virtuous, because she dedicated her life selflessly and generously to fulfilling God's will. She is regarded as having special power to intercede with her Son. People may have pictures of Mary on their locker and may ask her to intercede with God for special causes. They may also say the rosary, a prayer of special devotion to Mary.

Catholics (and some other Christians) may also pray to saints. They are believed to have particular power to intercede with God for people on earth.

Some Catholic relatives may bring holy water, blessed by a priest, to a patient. A cross may be made on the patient's forehead or the water may be sprinkled over them (see also Chapter 10 *Holy Water*).

Families and relationships

The Catholic Church lays down clear guidelines relating to marriage and relationships. The family and marriage are regarded as extremely important, especially in relation to bringing up children. Sexual intercourse is permitted only within marriage. Divorce is normally prohibited, as are abortion and most forms of contraception. Homosexuality is forbidden. Some Catholics who have gone against these or other rulings but who still wish for religious contact and comfort may be anxious about their relationship with the church.

Dietary restrictions

Catholics are required to abstain from meat and alcohol on Ash Wednesday or on Good Friday (see Festivals, earlier). Traditionally it was also forbidden to eat meat on all Fridays, again as a symbolic sacrifice in memory of Christ's death. Some people still eat fish or vegetarian meals on Fridays and these should be available.

When a person is seriously ill or dying

Prayer and anointing

The family may call a priest to carry out the sacrament of the Anointing of the Sick (also known as last rites or extreme unction). He prays that the patient may be absolved from sin and given spiritual healing, while anointing them with holy oil on the forehead and hands. A dying person who is able may also wish to receive holy communion (see above and also *Baptism* in the general section on Christianity).

If a person has died without being anointed, a priest can anoint the body up to three hours after the death to comfort the family.

Beliefs about death

Many Catholics believe that a soul must go through a period of preparation and purification before it can enter heaven; this is known as purgatory. Many people pray for the soul of someone who has died, that they may be released as soon as possible from purgatory and go to Heaven. A mass for the soul of the dead person may be held either at the funeral or afterwards.

SEVENTH DAY ADVENTISM

The information below will apply only to certain Seventh Day Adventist patients. Never assume. Always check everything with the person concerned.

The Seventh Day Adventist Church developed from Protestant Christian roots in Europe and the USA during the nineteenth century. There are now about 8 million Seventh Day Adventists in 204 countries. In Britain there are approximately 17,000 Seventh Day Adventists, most of whom live in southern Britain. About 85 per cent of British Seventh Day Adventists are of African-Caribbean heritage and may also be influenced by aspects of African-Caribbean culture (see Chapter 37). (See also the general section on Christian beliefs and practices at the beginning of this chapter.)

Seventh Day Adventist beliefs and practices

The Seventh Day Adventist Church bases its beliefs wholly on the Old and New Testaments of the Bible and has informally developed 27 fundamental beliefs. Among these are belief in the Trinity, consisting of God the Father, God the Son and God the Holy Spirit; in the Second Coming of Jesus Christ when the righteous dead will be resurrected; and in the binding nature of the Ten Commandments.

The Seventh Day Adventist Church places great emphasis on the biblical statement that the body is the temple of the Holy Spirit and so must be respected and kept pure. This affects the way people live and the decisions they make. The church teaches the importance of chastity before marriage, monogamy, healthy family relationships and the equality of men and women. Divorce is viewed as a last resort. The church offers education and guidance to its congregants and expects them to maintain high moral standards; within this framework people take responsibility for their own choices in relation to observance and religious practice.

> 'Adventists as a whole have tremendous respect for the quality of life and this affects the decisions we make for ourselves and our families. We ask that you are sensitive to our needs and wishes.'
>
> Seventh Day Adventist pastor

As an organisation the church supports medical research and health care. It runs hospitals and health centres as well as educational and philanthropic establishments. Many Seventh Day Adventists contribute a tenth of their income towards charitable church institutions and activities. Many local churches run health education programmes for their communities.

Religious observance

The Sabbath

> 'The Sabbath, Saturday, is our rest day. How we observe it is a profoundly personal choice. It is not imposed on us by the church and we would like our individual needs and beliefs to be respected.'
>
> Health care assistant

Seventh Day Adventists observe Saturday as the Sabbath, the seventh day of the week, a day of rest and worship. The Sabbath starts on Friday night at sunset and ends at sunset on Saturday. Traditionally it is a day for prayer and meditation and for being with family and the community. Most Adventists attend church and Bible study sessions. Many prepare food beforehand in order to cut down their work on the Sabbath, so Fridays may be particularly busy. Most people do not watch television or listen to the radio on the Sabbath.

In hospital or other residential care, Seventh Day Adventist patients may appreciate peace and quiet on Friday evenings and throughout the Sabbath. They may be disturbed if there is a television on in their ward or room, especially if the sound is up. Seventh Day Adventist patients may appreciate having their beds positioned so that they are not able to see it. Other patients should be asked to use headphones. Some Adventist patients may prefer to sit in a day room if one is available.

Prayer and the Bible

Although there are no set times for prayer, most Seventh Day Adventists pray, meditate and read the Bible every day. It is important to respect and accommodate people's privacy and need for quiet at these times.

Adventists do not have formal prayer books because prayers are expected to be spontaneous. Some may wish to listen to tapes of sacred music and singing. Most people do not have other religious items or jewellery.

The pastor

Each community has a pastor who offers support and comfort as well as being a source of information and advice. Sometimes a pastor will visit to pray and read the Bible with a patient. Quiet is appreciated at this time if possible. The pastor may also bring communion of unleavened bread and grape juice. Seventh Day Adventists in hospital may appreciate the offer to ask their pastor to visit them.

Festivals

Christmas and Easter are celebrated to varying degrees by different congregations. Seventh Day Adventists recognise that the dates on which most Christians celebrate these festivals are not historically accurate.

Dietary requirements

The church teaches that a vegetarian diet is preferable; many Adventists are vegetarians. Some are vegan and do not eat cheese, eggs or milk. Others eat most food but avoid shellfish, offal and pork (considered unclean). Although each person's decisions are individual, they are firm and should be respected. It is important to ask each person about their dietary requirements, to ensure that any advice on diet takes these into account, and to check that acceptable food is available (see Chapter 11 *Providing food in hospital and other residential care*).

At baptism, Seventh Day Adventists promise to abstain from alcohol and recreational drugs including tobacco. Many Adventists do not drink tea or coffee.

Medication

There is no objection to opiates or any other medication to relieve symptoms. Most Seventh Day Adventists accept alcohol in medication if necessary. Some vegetarians may be concerned about animal products such as gelatine in capsules. Some Adventists may also wish to avoid medication containing pork products such as porcine-derived insulin or pig's heart valves.

When someone is seriously ill or dying

Beliefs about life and death

'We believe that life here is a preparation for the life beyond.'
Seventh Day Adventist minister

The Church teaches that a person is an integration of body, mind and spirit. Life is sacred and the quality of life – seen in terms of righteous living – is very important. When someone dies, the 'breath of God' is withdrawn from them. They then sleep until the Second Coming of Christ, when He will return to the earth and when all those who have died will be resurrected, each with a new physical body made in the image of God. At that time all the dead will be judged and the just will be rewarded accordingly.

A person who knows that they are dying is encouraged to make peace, seek reconciliation and ask for forgiveness, both directly of the people they have wronged and of God, through prayer. Some people may want a pastor to be present as death approaches.

After the death

Last offices

Provided the family so wishes, the normal last offices can be carried out. Some families, especially those of African-Caribbean heritage, may wish to keep the coffin open at the funeral, so it is particularly important that the dead person's face is clean and as serene as possible and the hair groomed in their usual style. (See also Chapter 20 *Immediately after the death and last offices*.)

PENTECOSTALISM

The information below will apply only to certain Pentecostalist patients. Never assume. Always check everything with the person concerned.

The Pentecostalist movement is historically rooted in Protestantism but came into prominence in the twentieth century. In Britain the main Pentecostalist Churches include the Elim Pentecostalist Church, the New Testament Church of God, the Church of God of Prophecy, the Assemblies of God and Apostolic Church. Several Pentecostalist Churches in Britain have their roots in the Caribbean and have mainly African-Caribbean members (Weller 1997). The term Pentecostalist is derived from Pentecost, seven weeks after the resurrection of Jesus Christ, when the Holy Spirit descended on a gathering of His apostles and disciples, inspiring them to go out and preach and to 'speak in tongues' (see below).

The Pentecostalist Churches stress the importance of each person's active and loving relationship with God through Jesus Christ, the Saviour of the world, and through the Holy Spirit. Faith in God, in His purpose and love for humankind, and in His power to intervene directly in people's lives, are very important. Although life can be very hard, God will help people get through the difficult times. Many members of Pentecostalist Churches follow the literal meaning of the Old and New Testaments, and believe that everything that happens is the will of God. There is, however, a great deal of variation in practices and customs. (See also the general section on Christian beliefs and practices at the beginning of this chapter.)

Religious observance

Worship

There are no formal times for prayer; people may pray privately at any time of the day or night. Some may bring a Bible into hospital with them; this should be treated with respect. It is very important to pray for other people. Communal prayer is considered particularly important and powerful. Family and other church members may gather to pray out loud and sing hymns with the patient, often in large numbers. They may prefer privacy and a separate room so that they need not worry about disturbing other people. This should be accommodated wherever possible (see Chapter 17).

Many Pentecostalists believe in physical and emotional healing through the power of prayer to God. Some may practise spiritual healing through the laying on of hands. Some may anoint the patient on the forehead with consecrated oil.

Sunday services

Sunday is traditionally a special day, set apart for congregational worship and private prayer. People often read the scriptures and spend time with their families. In some homes no television is watched on Sundays.

Congregational worship is very important and is generally participative and emotional. People may be moved to give testimony, pray out loud and, sometimes, to speak in tongues. Speaking in tongues – speaking in an ecstatic, unlearned language other than one's own – is recorded in the New Testament as a sign of the coming of the Holy Spirit, and is generally regarded as a great gift. Some churches hold services of healing. Many Pentecostalists attend several church worship meetings a week and are very involved in church activities.

Every month Pentecostalists celebrate the Lord's supper with bread and wine followed by ceremonial washing of feet. This is known as congregation or communion. A minister may come to celebrate congregation with a patient in hospital.

Festivals

Christmas, Easter and Pentecost are celebrated, and Good Friday is a solemn day when many people fast (see *Festivals* in the general section, earlier). Easter is particularly important and is a joyful festival. Some people may want to go home at Easter if at all possible. At Pentecost (seven weeks after Christ's resurrection) many churches hold a convocation, a large gathering with prayer and celebration. Again, people in hospital or residential care may wish to go home for this.

The minister

In many churches the minister, and sometimes his family, are the focus of much community activity. One of his main duties is to preach the word of God based on biblical revelation. The minister also has important pastoral duties and may visit patients in hospital.

Families and communities

Most Pentecostalist Churches stress a strong moral code of behaviour, including traditional family values and sexual morality. They also stress social responsibility and practical and emotional support for other members of the congregation, especially those who are ill, lonely or troubled.

Many churches are a focus for community self-help projects, especially in areas such as education and care for older people, where statutory provision often fails to meet the needs of black and minority ethnic members and their families.

Practical care

Many women will want to dress modestly at all times and may be anxious about physical exposure during examinations and treatments. Most are prepared to be examined by a male doctor (see also Chapters 11 *Modesty* and 12 *Modesty and physical examination*).

Fasting

Fasting is part of the Pentecostalist tradition, though individual practice varies. Sometimes a congregation sets aside special days for fasting and communal prayer, sometimes people decide to make a fast themselves. People may also fast to ask God to help and support someone who is ill or going through a bad time. The length of fasts varies. Some people may drink and eat very little for several days (see Chapter 11 *Fasting patients*).

When a person is seriously ill or dying

Worship

The family and the congregation may wish to pray and sing at the bedside (see above).

Attitudes to death and dying

Most people combine faith in prayer and in God's power to heal with acceptance of God's will. People who know that they are seriously ill or dying may wish to set things straight and seek reconciliation for things that they regret in their lives. Minister and church members often help by listening and praying with the patient for forgiveness.

It is generally very important for the family to be present when a person is dying. The minister may also be called. They may pray and sing the patient's favourite hymns.

43 Hinduism

The information below will apply to only some Hindu patients and their families. Never assume. Always check everything with the person concerned.

Hindu communities in Britain

Almost all Hindus are Indian in origin. It is estimated that there are about half a million Hindus in the UK (Weller 1997). Most of their families originated from:

- East Africa, in particular Kenya, Uganda, Tanzania, Zambia and Malawi (see Figure 39.1). A number of Hindus moved to these countries from India one or more generations ago. Most originated in Gujarat and Punjab States (see below). Most Hindu families from East Africa came to Britain in the late 1960s and the 1970s, many as refugees.
- The states of Gujarat and Punjab in north-western India (see Figure 41.1). Most Hindu families from these areas came to Britain in the 1950s and '60s.

There are also a small number of Hindu families in Britain from other areas of India, as well as from countries such as Fiji, Guyana, Trinidad and Mauritius, to which some Hindus emigrated in the nineteenth century. In addition there are a number of Tamil Hindu families from Sri Lanka, most of whom arrived in Britain more recently as refugees.

Diversity Hindus whose families originated in different parts of India may follow different religious practices and customs and celebrate different festivals. Older people are particularly likely to feel more comfortable among people who share their religious and cultural heritage and language. This chapter focuses particularly on the beliefs, practices and customs of Hindus in north-western India. (For more about the traditional culture of the Indian subcontinent, see Chapter 41.)

Languages

Most Hindus whose families originated in Gujarat speak Gujarati. Those whose families originated in Punjab speak Punjabi. Hindus from other areas of India speak the local language of that area (see Chapter 41 *Languages*).

Hindu naming systems

In general, it is most acceptable to use title plus last name, especially with older people. Names must be recorded correctly to prevent dangerous confusion in records (see Chapter 30 *Recording people's names correctly*).

Hinduism – a brief description

Hinduism is the religion of most of the people of India. It is, however, much more than what many Western people would think of as a religion. It is a social and cultural system and a way of life as well as a set of beliefs, values and religious practices.

Hinduism has no one founder, no one holy book, and no central authority or hierarchy to control or define Hindu beliefs and practices. It has developed over thousands of years in response to different ideas and circumstances in the Indian subcontinent, and is still developing. Within the overall uniting framework of Hinduism there is a great range of beliefs and customs, depending mainly on people's family, place of origin and religious tradition. Differences in belief and practice are accepted and there is no insistence on one unequivocal version of the truth (Green and Green 1992). Some people also choose to follow a living guru or spiritual guide. However, despite the great variation within Hinduism, for each individual his or her own religious beliefs and duties are clear and important.

> 'For me being a Hindu shows me the right way to lead my life, what I must do and what I must not do, how I should look after my children. It also shows me what I must teach them so that they become good people, doing their duty in life. And it provides a spiritual centre too; I pray and meditate and I read the holy books and I try to come closer to God.'
> Hindu man

Hindu beliefs and values

There are certain fundamental truths and values that almost all Hindus believe and practise, including: the existence of a Supreme Spirit (Brahman or Parabrahman); an immortal soul that exists in all living things; the cycle of birth, death and rebirth through which everyone must go; release from the cycle of rebirth as the ultimate aim of life; a clear code of dutiful and right behaviour; compassion and non-violence; and the supreme duty of seeking Truth. Care and respect for older people, obedience to parents, and hospitality to visitors are all major religious duties.

> 'And when one sees that the God in oneself is the same as the God in all things and everywhere, one does not hurt oneself by hurting others; then one attains the highest level.'
>
> Bhagavad Gita 13: 29

It is part of Hindu belief that, because human mental, emotional and intuitive powers are limited, not everyone can begin to understand the Supreme Spirit, the ultimate reality. Most people need easier ways to approach and worship It. Many Hindus therefore worship the Supreme Spirit through symbols or manifestations, often personified as gods and goddesses or as incarnations. Each god or goddess or other representation, being part of the whole divinity, has certain qualities that represent aspects of the Supreme Spirit. Some of the gods and goddesses most important in Hindu worship today are Brahma, Shakti, Vishnu, Mahadeva, Shiva and Parvati. Different gods and goddesses complement each other. Sometimes they are worshipped under different names.

Duty, karma, death and rebirth

Hindus believe that the purpose of life is to do good in order to seek the Truth; for each person this means fulfilling the duties that have been assigned to them. Different people have different duties, depending on the situation into which they were born. For everyone the cycle of birth and death continues until they have completed the purpose for which they have come here and can be finally united with the Supreme Spirit in perfection (moksha or mukti).

> 'Oh Lord, lead us from untruth to truth,
> From darkness to light,
> From mortality to immortality.'
>
> Brihadanayaka Upanishad

The idea of rebirth is linked to belief in karma, the natural moral law of reward and punishment for all thoughts and deeds. Belief in karma leads to a strong sense of personal responsibility. People are responsible for what they are now, because what they are now is a result of what they have done and thought in the past. In the same way, their actions and thoughts now will determine their future and their next life. Karma involves acceptance and responsibility but not fatalism. In other words, nothing is an accident or the simply result of fate; everything has a cause. Belief in karma may affect the way people react to illness and crises. One must do one's best in any situation, however difficult.

> 'We strongly believe in rebirth. Whatever you do in this life affects your next life. It is just the body that dies, the soul goes on and never dies.'
> Hindu woman

For Hindus, death is the end of one life and the beginning of the next. It is not the end.

> 'Just as a man leaves an old garment and puts on one that is new, the Spirit leaves its mortal body and then puts on one that is new.'
>
> Bhagavad Gita 2: 22

Devout Hindus trust that a good life and death will ensure a favourable rebirth. Some older people spend a lot of time praying and preparing, both spiritually and practically, for death. It is a very important religious duty for relatives to ensure that the correct prayers and rituals are carried out around the time of the death (see later).

Different faiths within Hinduism

There are many different Hindu branches and spiritual groups in Britain, whose members may observe different practices and customs. One such group is described below.

The Swaminarayan faith was founded by a holy teacher and reformer, Sahajanand Swami, who was accepted as Godhead by 2 million followers and known as Lord Swaminarayan. He lived in Gujarat (north-western India) at the beginning of the nineteenth century. At that time Gujarat was torn by violence, famine and despair. Lord Swaminarayan preached the worship and glorification of God through righteous living, including non-violence and vegetarianism, honesty and hard work, dutiful and chaste behaviour, and service to the family and to others. All initiated members of the Swaminarayan faith promise to adhere to five spiritual vows: not to steal, not to eat meat, not to take alcohol or any intoxicating substance, not to commit adultery and to lead a pure life. They follow a strong written code of behaviour, the Shikshapatri, written by Lord Swaminarayan. This gives clear guidance on family, social, financial, moral, managerial and spiritual matters. Since Lord Swaminarayan left this earth (took Samadhi) in 1830, the movement has been led by a succession of spiritual leaders or gurus through whom the Spirit of God is manifest on this earth (Swaminarayan Hindu Mission 1995, Williams 1984).

It is estimated that over 5 million Hindus in Gujarat follow the Swaminarayan faith (Williams 1984). Different branches, based on different views concerning the proper line of succession to the founder, tend to worship in their own temples. There are about 10,000–15,000 followers of the Swaminarayan faith in the UK. Because they do not expect health professionals to have heard of their faith they may give their religion as Hindu.

Jainism Jains may also give their religion as Hindu. However, Jainism is a separate religion – see Chapter 45.

Religious observance

(see also Chapter 10 *Practical matters*)

Worship

Many devout Hindus pray at least three times a day: at sunrise or when they wake up (usually before eating or drinking), around noon and just before sunset. Many people also pray before meals and before going to sleep. Physical and spiritual cleanliness are closely linked: it is important to be clean to pray. Most people shower or wash, put on clean clothes, and rinse out their mouths to get rid of the influence of impure acts or thoughts. Hindus traditionally pray sitting on the floor or standing. Some Hindus apply a coloured paste to their foreheads when they have completed their morning worship (see *Make-up*, later). Women do not pray formally while menstruating or for 40 days after giving birth.

Some people use a rosary or mala – a string of sandalwood beads – to help them concentrate. This is often kept in a cloth bag to protect it from dirt and pollution. Some people may set up a small shrine in front of them with pictures or statues (murti), on which to focus while praying. It is traditional to place in front of this a symbolic offering of a glass of milk or water or some fruit, a small light, oil lamp or candle, and sometimes a lighted stick of incense. People may ring a small bell to catch the attention of the gods when they begin their prayers.

People who cannot get out of bed or do not have enough floor space may pray sitting cross-legged on the bed. Some may cover their heads with a scarf or cloth. They may wish to have their curtains drawn for privacy while praying and should not normally be disturbed.

Washing before prayer A patient who cannot get out of bed may need a bowl of water, a cup and a flannel so that, at the very least, they can make a symbolic wash. This involves wiping the face, rinsing out the mouth, pouring running water over the hands and sprinkling water over the head. Many Hindus always wash their perineum with water after using the toilet so that they are clean for prayer. An incontinent patient may need help in ensuring that they are clean before praying (see also Chapter 12 *Practical care*).

Holy articles and books

The most popular Hindu holy book is the Bhagavad Gita (often simply called the Gita). Other important books are the Ramayana, the Hanuman Chalisa and books of devotional poems. The two most important Swaminarayan holy books are Vachnamrut and Shikshapatri. All holy books and other items used for worship are kept clean and safe. They are often wrapped in cloth for protection. They are not put on the floor or near the feet or near shoes, leather articles or dirty clothes; nothing is put on top of them. People usually wash their hands before they touch a holy book or other holy items.

Holy water and prasad

Religious pilgrimages to holy places are highly valued. Some people may make a pilgrimage for special blessings for themselves or for someone who is ill. People who have been to the Hindu sacred river, the Ganges (Ganga), may bring home a bottle of holy water for a patient. This is believed to purify a person and remove sins (see also Chapter 10 *Holy water*).

Family members may sometimes bring a patient a small amount of prasad, food that has been blessed at the temple. Discuss with the family how to dispose of any uneaten prasad, because it is customary not to throw it away.

Prayer at home and a family shrine

Hindus believe that God is everywhere; worship in the home, where people feel comfortable and at ease, is particularly important. Many Hindu homes contain a small shrine with statues and pictures of the gods where people can worship. This may be in a corner on a shelf, in a wood or glass-fronted cabinet, or, if there is space, a separate room. Sometimes the shrine is in the kitchen, which is often regarded as the purest and cleanest room and as a consecrated space because food is prepared there.

The room containing the shrine is kept pure and is not entered without an invitation. People take off their shoes at the door and should be modestly dressed. Women visitors may be asked to cover their heads. No one touches anything on a shrine unless specifically invited.

The temple and the pandit

Community members may go to the temple (mandir) to pray, to sing devotional songs in front of statues of the gods and goddesses, to hold classes, and to celebrate special religious occasions and festivals. A temple is usually run by a managing committee with a president and a secretary. In Britain, Hindu groups originating from different areas tend to have different traditions and practices as well as speaking different languages; each community may have its own temple.

Most temples have a resident priest, a pandit or pujari, who performs sacred ceremonies and tends the holy shrines. He may sometimes be asked for guidance on religious matters. Many pandits are from India, and are here only temporarily. Their English may therefore be limited and people who want to make contact with the temple may sometimes do better to contact the secretary or the president (Weller 1997).

The pandit does not traditionally have a pastoral role, though this is changing in some communities in Britain. Relatives and other community members usually undertake such duties as visiting and praying with the sick and comforting the bereaved. If a person in hospital requires a pandit, he should, wherever possible, be of the same community and religious tradition and speak the same language.

Astrology and good and bad events

Astrology has been studied in India for thousands of years and many Hindus believe that people's lives are influenced by the movements of the planets. Some may regard certain days as more propitious for operations and treatments, and may prefer to arrange non-urgent procedures on these days. It may be important for them to avoid operations at the time of the new or full moon, at eclipses of the moon, or during certain festivals if possible. In some families the exact timing of a funeral and other mourning rituals is traditionally decided by a pandit. This is often impossible in Britain where families have to fit in with crematorium and other arrangements (Laungani 1997).

Some people believe that illness and other problems can be caused by a poor astrological constellation, past misdeeds or failure to act correctly, or by other people's jealousy or ill-will. They may consult an astrologer or a pandit, who may advise special ceremonies and prayers to alleviate the situation.

Festivals

There are many Hindu festivals celebrated by different communities and in different parts of India. Most are dedicated to particular gods and goddesses. Some people fast during or before certain festivals (see *Fasting*, below). The dates of Hindu festivals vary slightly each year, depending on the date of the full moon. (See also the SHAP Calendar, listed in the References.) The major Hindu festivals celebrated in Britain are:

Holi *February/March full moon* A spring festival celebrated in northern and central India. Celebrates an ancient legend in which Good triumphs over Evil. Bonfires are lit and coloured water and dyes thrown at participants.

Raksha bandhan *August full moon* Celebration of the strong bond between brothers and sisters, with the exchange of gifts.

Navratri *September/October* Festival of the nine nights dedicated to the goddesses Lakshmi, Durga and Sarasvati. Especially celebrated in Gujarat.

Divali (or **Deepavali**) *October/November*. Five-day celebration of the victory of Good over Evil, as told in the Ramayana (see above). Also the festival of the goddess Lakshmi. Candles and lamps are lit. Family celebration. Marks the end of the Hindu year.

Other festivals may also be important to certain communities – for example, the birthdays of Lord Rama and Lord Krishna, and of Lord Swaminarayan and other holy Swaminarayan leaders. It is helpful to ease any visiting restrictions over a festival (see also Chapter 10 *Religious festivals*).

Families and relationships

The family is central to Hindu life, and supporting the family is an important religious duty. In India, the family traditionally consists of three generations with several adult couples and their children (see Chapter 41 *Traditional family structures and relationships*). Even when families no longer live together, or live on different continents, their mutual responsibilities and commitments may remain strong. Family bonds are particularly likely to matter to older people, who may also expect to have authority in the family. Extended families are less common in certain Hindu communities, for example among Tamils in Sri Lanka.

Marriage

Hinduism stresses the sanctity of marriage. Hindus are expected to marry and have children, with both men and women taking an active part in bringing up the children. Parents remain responsible for their children all their lives. It is part of the traditional duty of Hindu parents, grandparents, aunts and uncles to arrange the marriages of younger family members. Children are expected to repay the care of their parents and older relatives by obedience, by marrying and bringing up their own family well, and by supporting and caring for them when they are ill or old. Brothers have particular responsibility for their sisters. Showing respect for and caring for one's elders are religious duties.

In most traditional Hindu families men and women share decisions, although men are considered to have ultimate public authority. One of the religious duties of a Hindu woman is to honour and obey her husband. In turn, a husband must treat his wife with kindness and respect. Women are traditionally considered responsible for the upbringing and religious and moral education of their children, the practical care, comfort and well-being of their families, and the atmosphere and conduct of the home. They are particularly honoured and respected as mothers. A married woman is often regarded as bringing good luck to religious ceremonies.

Divorce is generally strongly disapproved of. Divorced people, especially women, may be socially isolated.

The caste system

Hindu society is traditionally divided into four castes and many hundreds of interdependent sub-castes, based on social and occupational status and on geography. The caste system goes back many thousands of years. Some historians say that originally people could improve their caste position as they became spiritually more enlightened. However, over time the system became rigid and inflexible. The caste and sub-caste into which a person was born defined their social and spiritual status, occupation, social contacts, and social and religious duties. In general, people in higher castes had more stringent religious duties and were expected to be more strict in their daily lives and observances, including diet, washing and worship. Many Hindus believe that the caste into which a person is born is determined by their karma (see above). Other Hindus – for example, followers of Swaminarayan (see above) – see caste as a purely social phenomenon. It is now illegal in India to discriminate on grounds of caste.

For thousands of years different castes and sub-castes lived almost completely separately, mixing little except in certain defined roles, and intermarrying rarely. Despite the pressures and demands of modern life, the system is slow to change; sub-caste identity and feeling often remain even when people move away from their roots. The sub-caste system also has clear benefits as well as disadvantages. People within a sub-caste often form a supportive community with strong mutual responsibilities and a sense of kinship. The family and the sub-caste are traditionally the two most important groups to which people belong. People may also turn to other members of their sub-caste for financial help or money for a good cause.

In Britain, caste awareness is particularly likely to remain among older people. Sub-caste bonds were often helpful during the early years of migration and settlement and many sub-caste organisations were set up to help members in need. Although other traditional differences to do with occupation and wealth are increasingly blurred, sub-caste is still likely to be important in marrying and socialising. It may also influence how strictly people observe food restrictions and other religious practices.

Dietary requirements

Many Hindus restrict what they eat and drink, on religious grounds. Although there is a good deal of variation, in general, older people, women, members of the Swaminarayan faith and people of higher castes are more likely to be careful about what they eat. Although food restrictions vary a good deal within Hinduism, for each individual they are not flexible. It is important to find out from each patient what they can and cannot eat (see also Chapter 11 *Planning and choosing from menus*).

A vegetarian diet Hinduism teaches that all forms of life are interdependent, and that all living creatures are sacred and subject to the laws of rebirth. Vegetarianism is generally highly regarded as an indication of spirituality. Many devout Hindus avoid all food that involves violence to any living thing. They do not eat meat, fish, eggs or anything made from or containing them. A strict Hindu vegetarian who eats any of these, even inadvertently, is likely to feel revolted and spiritually polluted.

Some Hindus who do not eat a vegetarian diet follow other food restrictions, based on community tradition and personal choice. Hindus whose families originated in the south-west coast of India may, for example, eat fish but not meat. Many Sri Lankan Hindus eat meat but not eat pork or beef. However, meat is also considered difficult to digest and some older people are vegetarian on health grounds.

The cow The cow is traditionally sacred. It symbolises the gentleness and unselfish love of a mother, and is generally revered and protected. Many Hindus who eat other meat do not eat beef. Some also refuse pork because the pig is a scavenging animal in India and its meat is generally considered dirty and easily spoilt.

Some Hindus eat only vegetarian cheese – cheese that is not made with animal rennet. (Some South Asians also dislike the taste of European cheese.)

Other restrictions Some conservative Hindus, including members of the Swaminarayan faith, regard onions and garlic as harmful stimulants and do not eat them. Some avoid tea and coffee. Members of the Swaminarayan faith and some other Hindus neither drink alcohol nor smoke.

Very strict restrictions – a minority

A few Hindu patients will eat only food brought in from home. This is because in the strictest Hindu tradition cooked food is regarded as easily polluted; it cannot be eaten if it has been in contact with a prohibited food or with utensils or plates that have been used for prohibited foods, or if it has been touched by another person since it was cooked. A few people may therefore feel able to eat only food that has been prepared on the same day by a member of their own family or community.

A very few people also refuse to drink water outside their own home and may carry drinking water with them. Some always drink filtered water to avoid pollution and to avoid accidentally taking the lives of small organisms in the water. In such cases it may be possible for families to bring in a jug-type filter. Glass, Pyrex and metal are believed to retain pollution less than china or plastic; some people may prefer to drink tea and other drinks out of a glass or a metal cup.

Medication

Most Hindus have no religious objection to opiates and other symptom-controlling medication; it is generally considered wrong to let a person suffer unnecessarily. Some people may refuse or prefer to avoid medication containing alcohol or any animal products. (See also Chapter 41 *Traditional South Asian medicine*.)

Fasting

Some Hindus fast during certain festivals. Some also fast regularly on certain days; for example, on the days of the new moon and the full moon, or on the 11th and 26th day of each lunar month. Some fast once a week on the day dedicated to a particular deity. Men, for example, may fast on Saturdays. Members of the Swaminarayan faith observe five major fasts each year.

Fasting is believed to bring both physical and spiritual benefits, and may also help to ensure good fortune in the future. Close relatives, especially women, often undertake strict fasts and say special prayers for the recovery of someone who is ill. Some may fast in thanksgiving for a successful operation or some other blessing.

The details of Hindu fasts vary. Some people take no food or liquid from dawn to dusk. Some drink only water. Most people eat one meal in the day consisting of foods that are considered pure, such as fruit, yoghurt, nuts or potatoes. Some people eat a vegetarian diet once a week, avoiding meat, fish and eggs. Some women eat a salt-free diet for one month each year.

Some patients may wish to maintain their regular pattern of fasts. People who are ill and older people do not have to fast but some may choose to do so. Some may refuse medication when they are fasting. If this is likely to affect a patient's well-being, discuss it with them.

Practical care

(see also Chapters 12 and 41)

Modesty and clothing

For many Hindus, modesty is a religious requirement.

Washing and cleanliness

Keeping clean is very important to most people and has spiritual as well as physical significance. Showers may be preferred to baths. Some people always wash with running water after using the lavatory.

Purity and pollution

The concepts of purity and pollution are important to many Hindus and are part of their way of life. Purity and impurity are both spiritual and physical, and physical impurity has spiritual consequences. Certain things, mainly to do with bodily emissions, death and decay, are intrinsically impure and spiritually polluting. Before they pray or touch holy things, most Hindus purify themselves by washing under running water, traditionally a particularly effective purifying agent.

Some Hindus consider all bodily fluids polluting (see Chapter 12 *Bathing and showering*). Their presence may cause distress to some patients and they should be removed as quickly as possible. Find out what is important to each individual.

Hair care

The head is traditionally regarded as sacred and is not touched by others without permission. Patting someone, even a child, on the head or ruffling their hair may be intrusive. Hindu women traditionally wear their hair long. It is kept loose until after marriage, when it is fixed up in a bun. A few people may not want to wash their hair on certain inauspicious days when they are considered vulnerable.

Make-up

Many Hindu women place a small coloured dot (called, for example, bindi, chandlo or tilaka) on their forehead every morning after they have prayed. Married women in some communities wear a streak of red powder (sindur) in the parting of their hair, especially in the early years of their marriage or on special occasions. Some Hindu women will wish to apply their bindi and sindur fresh every morning. They may ask relatives to help them if necessary.

Men in the Swaminarayan community (see above) may apply a tilak, a red dot surrounded by a yellow U shape.

Religious jewellery and other items

Relatives sometimes place blessed items of jewellery round a Hindu patient's arm, neck or body, often on a black string. This is intended to protect and help the patient and should not be removed. Some Hindu women wear a wedding necklace of gold and black beads, a mangal sutra. Other wedding jewellery may include glass or gold bangles, rings (sometimes with precious stones) or nose jewels. Wedding jewellery is generally removed only if a woman is widowed.

In some Hindu families a boy receives a sacred thread when he is about seven or eight, the age at which he is regarded as beginning to reason and to distinguish right from wrong. The thread is put around his upper body and over his left shoulder. Some men wear a thread round their right wrists. Sacred threads are never removed, even when bathing. If a thread must be removed, it is wrapped round a sacred tulsi plant.

Initiated Swaminarayan men and women (see above) wear a necklace (kanthi) made of sandalwood, sometimes threaded with gold. This is not normally removed. Some people leave the kanthi on after death; others replace it with a thread.

Visiting a Hindu home

The traditional Hindu greeting is to join the palms of the hands at about chin level. Older people, in particular, may prefer this to shaking hands, especially with members of the opposite sex.

In many Hindu homes, shoes are removed at the front door or at the bottom of the stairs to avoid bringing dirt and pollution into the house. Shoes are always removed when entering a room containing a shrine (see earlier).

It is important not to bring any food into the home that the family regards as unacceptable. Check before going into the kitchen, as this is often regarded as a particularly pure room.

When someone is ill or dying

Families and illness

Large numbers of relatives may wish to visit (see also Chapters 17 and 41). It may be particularly important to the patient that all the closest members of their family are there. Some families may bring clothes or money for the patient to touch. These will be given to the poor later to symbolise the dead person's generosity.

Physical comfort

A dying person's last few days should be as comfortable as possible, both physically and mentally. All pain and symptom-relieving measures are usually acceptable (see also *Medication*, above). Some people may very much want to die at home so that they can be sure that everything is done correctly. Others may want to go to India to die. Relatives may be very concerned to follow the person's last wishes as far as possible and staff should, wherever they can, try to help the family achieve them.

Prayer and religious rituals

A Hindu patient may receive comfort from hymns and holy books, especially the Bhagavad Gita. Relatives may wish to pray round the bed. If possible, a person should die thinking of God and with a prayer on their lips and in their heart.

'And he who at the end of his time leaves his body thinking of God, he in truth goes unto Him only.'

Bhagavad Gita 8: 5

For many families it is essential to be present to support the patient, to ensure that they do not die alone and that the religious rituals are carried out correctly. The last words of a dying person may be regarded as very significant, and someone should always be there to hear them.

Families who have not carried out the essential rituals may be very distressed and anxious, both about the long-term well-being of the soul of the dead person and about the spiritual consequences for themselves. It is most important, whenever possible, to make sure that family members know that death is imminent and to allow them to be present.

'There are many important procedures to be carried out when a person dies. And these things must be done correctly in order to permit the onward passage of the soul in peace and to prepare it in peace for the next habitation. This is both our duty and an act of love for the dying person.'
Hindu grandmother

Prayers may be said, hymns (bhajans) sung, or passages from a holy book read to try to ensure that the last words the dying person hears are holy. A sacred thread may be tied around their neck or wrist. Water from the River Ganges (Ganga), the most sacred river in Hinduism, may be sprinkled over them or used to wet their lips or mouth in order to wash away sins. A coloured mark may be made on the forehead. Most families do this themselves; some may wish to call on a pandit. Wherever possible, privacy should be ensured.

Traditionally, a dying person is placed on the floor on a sheet or a clean mat. This symbolises their closeness to Mother Earth, frees them from all physical constraints and may be believed to ease the departure of the soul. A few families may very much want to do this and should be accommodated if possible. When necessary, they should be provided with a mattress (Laungani 1997, Firth 1996).

A death for which people have been unable to prepare, such as accidental, sudden or violent death, may be regarded as very unlucky and may cause particular distress (see also Chapter 19 *Sudden death*). Some Hindus believe that a person who had no time to prepare for their death will be reborn almost immediately. Additional prayers may be said and special rituals carried out for the soul of the person who has died and for their family (Firth 1996).

Organ donation

There is no religious prohibition against organ donation. Nevertheless, many relatives will feel able to allow organs to be donated only if they know that the donor was willing. Some Hindus may refuse to donate organs because they believe that it is very important that the body is complete at cremation.

After the death

Last offices

Some Hindu families are extremely concerned about who touches the body after death. Real distress may occasionally be caused if a non-Hindu touches the body without disposable gloves. Washing the body is traditionally part of the rituals carried out by close family members immediately before the funeral, and families may wish to do this themselves. (See also Chapter 20 *Immediately after the death and last offices*.)

Unless the family wishes otherwise, close the eyes and straighten the legs. Do not cut the nails or trim the hair or beard without checking first. Place the hands on the chest with the palms together and the fingers just under the chin, in the traditional Hindu sign of greeting. Do not remove any jewellery or other religious objects. Wrap the body in a plain sheet without religious emblems.

Some families may wish to light a lamp or a piece of cotton wool soaked in ghee (clarified butter) in a bowl. The light symbolically leads the soul towards God. If the body is in a mortuary, most families are prepared to keep the light burning at home. Some may wish to burn an incense stick near the body.

Post mortems

There is no specific religious prohibition against post mortems but many Hindus find them abhorrent and disrespectful. They may be especially upset if the post mortem delays the funeral. The body should traditionally be complete when it is cremated or buried, and some families may be very concerned that all the organs are returned to the body after a post mortem. In addition, if the family intends to wash the body themselves before the funeral, it must be well repaired and carefully stitched to prevent additional distress (see Chapter 20 *Post mortems*).

Timing

Cremation traditionally takes place within 24 hours. For some families it is therefore important to register the death as soon as possible. They may appreciate help in dealing with the necessary documentation urgently. Sometimes there are unavoidable delays because the crematorium is fully booked and this can increase a family's grief. Some people believe that the spirit cannot be released as long as the physical body remains whole (Green and Green 1992).

In Britain some Hindu families delay the cremation so that people from abroad can attend. Traditionally, as a mark of respect, family members do not cook, eat or drink between the death and the funeral. If the funeral is delayed, other relatives may bring them food.

Preparation for the funeral

Large numbers of family members may wish to come to pay their last respects before the funeral. This is a binding duty and should be accommodated as far as possible. Immediately before the funeral, close relatives of the same sex traditionally wash the body. Sacred water from the Ganges may be used. The body is usually dressed in normal clothes and wrapped in a white cotton shroud.

The funeral

Adults and older children are traditionally cremated. Stillborn babies, babies, young children and monks are usually buried. All members of the Swaminarayan faith are cremated.

The eldest son or another male relative traditionally takes charge of the funeral arrangements. Before the cremation or burial there is usually a service, often held at home. All family members and friends and other people who knew the dead person attend to pay their respects and to commiserate with the family. In some communities failure to do so may be considered unforgivable. Depending on the size of the family and the community in the UK, several hundred people may attend. In India the body is normally placed on an open bier. In Britain the coffin may be kept open until the journey to the crematorium.

In India a pandit normally chants passages from the holy scriptures; in Britain families cannot always arrange this. The chief mourner (usually the eldest son) performs certain religious rituals. Herbs, sandalwood and ghee (clarified butter, which purifies the body and traditionally helps it burn) are placed on the body. (In Britain, some crematoria prefer ghee not to be used because it is unnecessary with modern cremators and could be dangerous.) Ganges water, grains of rice and a real or symbolic sacred tulsi leaf may be placed in the mouth, together with a small coin that symbolises the paying of the ferryman crossing the river of death. The mourners walk anti-clockwise around the open coffin to symbolise the unwinding of the thread of life. The coffin is then closed and taken to the crematorium for further prayers (Firth 1993). It is an honour to help carry the coffin.

Traditionally the eldest son has the special duty of lighting the funeral pyres of his parents, sometimes helped by close male relatives. Because this is not usually possible in Britain, he may instead place camphor in the coffin to aid combustion. In some British crematoria, family members are allowed to press the button or to help push the coffin into the cremator. Prayers are said during the cremation. The ashes may be taken to India to be scattered on a sacred river, often the River Ganges, depending on the wishes of the dead person. Alternatively, they may be scattered on a local river or on the sea around Britain, because all rivers and seas eventually flow together.

In many Hindu communities women traditionally do not attend the cremation in order to spare them unnecessary distress. In Britain, however, the actual cremation is hidden and more women attend. In some communities, people whose parents are still alive do not attend cremations. White is the traditional colour of mourning for men and women.

Mourning

In the days following the death, relatives and friends sit with the immediate family and share their grief. Everyone has a binding duty to visit, men visiting men and women visiting women in some communities. They traditionally talk about the person who has died, his or her good qualities and achievements and the sadness of the death. Crying and the overt expression of grief may be encouraged as healthy. In some communities people are encouraged to pray and chant rather than grieve loudly.

Family members traditionally wear white for the first ten days after the death. They say special prayers and eat simple food. A full reading of one of the holy books may be held. The widow and the eldest son of the dead person sometimes shave their heads.

Around the twelfth day after the death the family may hold an important religious ceremony, Kriya Pani. This releases the departed soul – which until this time is believed to have remained nearby – from all its attachments to the family and other people it loved. It marks the time when family members are expected to begin to re-engage in the world and to get on with their lives. Hymns and songs about the good qualities of the dead person are sung. In some communities, special rice balls are symbolically cut to symbolise the separation and release of the soul. For some people this ceremony may be particularly distressing because it severs their last links with the dead person.

Another ceremony may be held on the 40th day after the death. (The precise timing varies between families and communities.) This marks the end of the period of strict mourning, during which family members often remain at home and may be avoided by other people because of the impurity of death.

Some bereaved families and, in particular, widows may lead restricted lives for several months, possibly staying away from festivals and community events. Special ceremonies may be held on the anniversaries of the death to pray for the soul of the dead person.

44 Islam

The information below will apply only to certain Muslim patients and their families. Never assume. Always check everything with the person concerned.

Islam has over 1 billion adherents throughout the world (Weller 1997). Although the basic beliefs and practices of Islam are universal, there are different branches and denominations, each of which also has its own traditions and practices. The two main branches are Sunni (about 90 per cent of all Muslims), and Shia. Each branch has become, over time, divided into different denominations. Some denominations emphasise the literal meaning of the Qur'an (the Muslim holy book). Their members are generally more conservative and adhere more strictly to traditional practices and external observances. Members of other denominations may focus more on the internal aspects of religion and be less concerned about external practices.

Although, in general, all Muslims regard themselves as part of the great Muslim community, and accept and respect the differences between different traditions, there is sometimes disagreement. For example, a group originating in Pakistan, the Ahmadiyas, is often rejected by other Muslims and this may give rise to mutual hostility.

Muslim communities in Britain

In the early nineteenth century, seamen and traders from the Middle East began to settle around major UK ports such as South Shields, Liverpool, London and Cardiff. A number of Muslims from the Indian subcontinent who had fought with the British Army in Europe during the First World War settled in Britain afterwards.

The main period of Muslim immigration occurred in the decades after the Second World War. Most people came from rural areas of Pakistan and Bangladesh, and a few from India (see Figure 41.1). During the 1970s a small number of Muslims of South Asian heritage came from East Africa, most as refugees.

Smaller British Muslim communities originated in other parts of the world, including the Middle East, Malaysia, different parts of Africa, Cyprus,

Turkey, Indonesia, the Philippines, Singapore and Sri Lanka. More recently a number of Muslim refugees from Somalia (see Chapter 40) and the former Yugoslavia have come to Britain. In addition, some people of white and African-Caribbean British heritage have converted to Islam. There are now approximately 1.5 million Muslims in Britain, about two-thirds of them of South Asian origin (Weller 1997).

Diversity Because the families of British Muslims originated in many different countries, they are influenced by different cultural and local religious traditions. As in all religions, there is also a tremendous range of devotion and practice within Islam. In general, the practices described here are those of more conservative Muslims. **It is important never to assume that someone who says they are Muslim will adhere to everything set out in this chapter. Always check.**

Languages

Muslims in Britain speak a range of other languages, depending on their heritage. These include Punjabi, Bengali, Urdu, Pashto, Somali, Gujarati, Arabic, Turkish, Malay and Farsi. (See also Chapter 41 *Languages*.)

Names

The traditional naming systems used by Muslims in Britain vary, depending on where their families originated. In general, it is most acceptable to use title plus full name if you are not sure of the correct form of address (see also Chapter 30 *Recording people's names correctly*).

Islam – a brief description

Islam was established by the Prophet Muhammad (570–632 CE*) through revelations from Allah. In the first hundred years after the Prophet Muhammad's death, the message of Islam spread from the area that is now Saudi Arabia all over the Middle East, North Africa and into Spain, much of Central Asia and China, and into and beyond the Indian subcontinent.

'Islam' means submission and peace. A Muslim is someone who obeys Allah's will and so is at peace with Him and with other people. To become

---

* Common Era, used as an alternative to AD.

a Muslim, a person must say sincerely and with true belief in front of two witnesses: 'I bear witness that there is no god but Allah and that Muhammad is the messenger of Allah.' Most Muslims use Allah, the Arabic word for God. As a sign of respect, many Muslims always follow Muhammad's name with the phrase 'Peace be upon him'.

The recorded words and actions of the Prophet Muhammad show him as a man of great gentleness, kindness, humility, good humour and common sense, who loved all people, especially his family (Maqsood 1994). Muslims regard Muhammad as a model of goodness, piety and courage. They believe that he was the last of a line of human prophets and that he completed and perfected everything that had gone before. Abraham, Moses, David, Job, John the Baptist and Jesus, among others, are regarded by Muslims as forerunners of Muhammad. Islam teaches that their messages were changed and distorted in the process of transmission by those who came after them. Jesus is particularly revered in the Qur'an, though the idea of his divinity is rejected. Much of the teaching of the Old Testament is shared by Muslims, Jews and Christians. Muslims believe that Islam is the ultimate and most complete of all religions, the timeless, perfected, revealed Truth.

Beliefs and practices

Allah is revealed in the Qur'an and in His created world as loving, merciful, just, all-knowing, all-powerful, all-creating and all-judging. Being a Muslim involves following a complete way of life in accordance with Allah's wishes as revealed to the Prophet Muhammad. There is no separation between the religious and the secular; everything has a religious aspect.

Most practising Muslims follow five main duties or pillars of Islam:

- faith in one God;
- prayer at five set times every day;
- giving a required amount to charity each year;
- fasting during the holy month of Ramadan; and
- making a pilgrimage (hajj) once in their lives to the sacred city of Makka (Mecca) if they can.

They aim to be just, compassionate, honest, generous, humble, modest, patient and brave (Maqsood 1994). They are to use the worldly goods that Allah has entrusted to them responsibly in His service.

'It is not righteousness that ye turn your faces towards East or West; but it is righteousness to believe in God and the Last Day, and the Angels, and the Book, and the Messengers; to spend of your substance, out of love for Him, for your kin, for orphans, for the needy, for the wayfarer, for those who ask, and for the ransom of slaves; to be steadfast in prayer, and practice regular charity; to fulfil the contracts which ye have made; and to be firm and patient, in pain (or suffering) and adversity, and throughout all periods of panic. Such are the people of truth, the God-fearing.'

The Qur'an 2: 177 (Trans Ali)

Muslims believe that the entire universe is under Allah's direction; nothing can happen unless He wills it. There is no such thing as a random or chance event. At the same time, each individual has free will and is accountable for the way in which they respond to the challenges of life (Maqsood 1994). Each individual should live as perfectly as they can, doing Allah's will in whatever circumstances they find themselves. Muslims believe in the immortal soul and life after death. After death, each soul awaits the Day of Judgement, when everyone will be resurrected and judged (see below).

Personal difficulties and tragedies are a natural and inescapable part of life and enable each person to develop their inner strength and their capacity to cope. Most Muslims believe that Allah never puts a greater burden on a person than she or he has the capacity to bear (Qur'an 2: 23). Illness and death are not punishments from Allah, any more than health is a reward. They are part of Allah's plan for mankind. People who are ill are expected to seek treatment and to maintain their faith and obedience to Allah. They are expected to accept difficulties and sorrows patiently and without resentment, knowing that they are part of Allah's plan and that He will support them and will reward them both in this life and after their death. What matters is steadfastness in the face of adversity. For many Muslims, their faith is a vital source of support, comfort and strength.

Angels In Muslim belief there are a large number of angels, beings made of pure light, who carry out the tasks assigned to them by Allah. Among the four most important angels are Jibril (Gabriel) and Mika'il (Michael), also mentioned in the Old Testament. Each person has two angels who record all their deeds and thoughts: one records everything good, the other everything bad. When a person dies, Allah will judge them and reward or punish them with heaven or hell. The other angels have a variety of tasks: some are present whenever prayers are said and the Qur'an is read, others pray and glorify Allah.

The Muslim code of behaviour

Many of the practical rules that Muslims follow in relation to their personal, family and community life are laid down in the Qur'an. Muslims also follow the recorded precepts and sayings of Muhammad, the Hadith. Muslim law (Sharia) has evolved over time based on the Qur'an and the Hadith, and continues to evolve. Although there is variation in the way that Muslims express their faith, there are some areas where many Muslims feel that no variation or compromise is possible.

Many Muslims reject certain aspects of modern Western culture and lifestyles, which they see as conflicting with Allah's law. For example, the free mixing of the sexes, aspects of dress, current attitudes towards sex and marriage, non-religious music, gambling and alcohol may all be seen as un-Islamic, especially by conservative Muslims, though this also depends on which denomination they belong to. Many observant Muslims feel that to adopt a Western lifestyle would require them to go directly against their faith and would damage them.

'We are ordinary people trying to live by our faith sincerely, as best as possible, and our faith has lots of responsibilities for us ... but we are trying our best.'
Muslim head teacher (Parker-Jenkins 1995)

Western hostility towards Islam

The expression of anti-Muslim opinions and feelings has become common and is increasingly seen as respectable and acceptable. The views expressed have become more explicit, more extreme and more dangerous. Anti-Muslim sentiments are now part of the fabric of everyday life in modern Britain, in much the same way that anti-Semitic views were socially acceptable earlier in the century (Runnymede Trust 1997).

Anti-Muslim feeling in Europe has historical roots, including the Christian crusades in the eleventh century and the Turkish (Muslim) siege of Vienna in the seventeenth century. Recently it has become stronger, encouraged by the media focus on conflict involving Muslims, terrorism, extremism and oppression rather than on the everyday attempts of most Muslims to live responsible, moral lives. Islam is increasingly portrayed as fanatical, monolithic, violent and aggressive, and all Muslims as 'fundamentalists'.

The term 'fundamentalism' arose from US Protestantism in the nineteenth century and referred to people going back to the fundamentals of their religion, in that case to the Bible. It was first applied to Islam in the 1970s, to denote fanaticism and violence. Islamic fundamentalism is, strictly speaking, a Western idea, because all practising Muslims agree with the fundamental principles and tenets of Islam. There are also moves in many Muslim communities to return to the basic principles of Islam. This is often a reaction to Muslims' realisation of how far 'Western values' such as materialism and secularism have penetrated their societies.

Islam does not legitimise the use of violence any more than Christianity, Judaism or Hinduism. The term 'Jihad' (often translated as holy war) means striving, and usually refers to the daily struggle of each individual to live according to Allah's law and to be pure in spirit. Muslims are, however, permitted to use force to a limited extent in defence of Islam and against tyranny (as in the generally accepted Christian concept of a just war) (Maqsood 1994).

Some of the movements described as Islamic fundamentalist are attempts to combat injustice and corruption by calling on basic religious principles. Others use the label of Islam in a local battle for power. Sometimes the name of Islam, like other religions, is used by terrorists and fanatics to justify violence and cruelty that mainstream Muslims regard as utterly unacceptable. Many of the oppressive practices associated in Western minds with Muslim societies are South Asian or Middle Eastern cultural traditions, or minority interpretations of Muslim scripture.

Most British Muslims are horrified when Islam is used to justify violence and terrorism, and deplore the abuse of their faith in this way. At the same time, they are deeply offended by the assumption that all Muslims are fanatical and uncivilised, and by the denigration of their faith. Many have become reluctant to discuss Islam with non-Muslims, because of the ill-informed and hostile responses they often encounter. Recent research (Modood, Berthoud et al 1997, Runnymede Trust 1997) concluded that Muslims in Britain suffer even more from racist violence and harassment than other minority communities.

'I can hardly watch or listen to the news any more. It makes me so angry. The term 'Muslim', which is so precious to me, and which encapsulates the values of integrity, compassion, humility, patience and generosity that I am teaching my children, is used by the media as a synonym for cruelty and insane acts of terrorism. Nobody calls the Hiroshima bomb the Christian bomb, nobody calls massacres in central Africa Christian massacres. But everything to do with Islam, and every Muslim, is regarded as bad, or at least suspect.'
British Muslim woman

Religious observance

Islam requires formal practices such as the five daily prayers, fasting and pilgrimage. At the same time, the Qur'an and the Hadith stress that it is people's awareness of Allah and their obedience to His will that really matter. Different denominations have different requirements.

Worship

Prayer keeps Muslims in regular contact with Allah, reminds them of their duties and produces feelings of peace and contentment (IQRA Trust 1997). Most adult practising Muslims say formal prayers (salat) in Arabic five times a day: at dawn, just after mid-day, in the mid-afternoon, immediately after sunset, and at night before going to bed. Extra formal prayers may be said after sunset during the holy month of Ramadan (see *Fasting*, later) and at other times. Shia Muslims may combine some of the prayers and pray three times a day. This is also permitted to Sunni Muslims if it is very difficult or impossible to fit in five separate prayer times. Shia Ismaili Muslims – who regard the Agha Khan as their living imam or leader – pray formally twice a day.

The most important Muslim prayer is taken from the opening of the Qur'an:

'In the name of Allah, Most Gracious, Most Merciful
Praise be to Allah
The Cherisher and Sustainer of the Worlds
Most Gracious, Most Merciful,
Master of the Day of Judgement
Thee do we worship
And Thine aid we seek.
Show us the straight way
The way of those on whom
Thou hast bestowed Thy Grace
Those whose (portion)
Is not wrath
And who go not astray.'

The Qur'an 1 (Trans Ali)

It is considered beneficial, and to promote a sense of fellowship, for people to say formal prayers together, though men and women usually pray in separate groups. People praying alone usually whisper. In a group, one person may recite parts of the prayer out loud. Women who are menstruating or in the 40 days after childbirth do not say formal prayers. Children and people who are mentally ill are not obliged to, but may wish to. Muslims may also say individual personal prayers at any time, and some carry a string of prayer beads.

Place and times of prayer Formal prayers are said in Arabic, standing on a clean surface – often a prayer mat or a towel – and facing the Ka'ba, the sacred shrine in Makka (Mecca), Saudi Arabia. This direction, called the

Qibla, is south-east in Britain. While praying, people who can, perform a series of movements, including standing, kneeling, bowing and touching the ground with their forehead.

In Britain and other northern countries the times of prayer vary depending on the season and are published in Muslim newspapers and in local mosques. In winter the mid-day, mid-afternoon and early evening prayers run very close together. In midsummer the first prayer is at 3.15 am and the last at 10.15pm (IQRA Trust, personal communication 1998). Many Muslim men try to attend mid-day prayer at the mosque every Friday. This is not obligatory for women.

Dress and cleanliness Physical and spiritual cleanliness are closely linked. Before praying or reading the Qur'an as part of worship, Muslims wash according to a set pattern. The hands, face, ears, forearms and feet are washed three times under running water, and the nose and mouth rinsed out. The perineal area must also have been washed with running water after using the lavatory.

Both men and women must be suitably dressed and in clean clothes. Shoes are removed. Women normally cover their heads with a scarf or cape; men may wear a prayer cap, often of white lace.

When someone is ill Many Muslims will want to maintain their normal prayer routines when they are ill. Patients in hospital or other residential accommodation who are mobile should, if possible, be offered a clean, quiet room where they will not be disturbed. This can also be used by Muslim visitors and staff. It is helpful to mark the Qibla with an arrow. Chairs can be supplied for the old and infirm. If possible, two rooms should be provided so that men and women can pray separately. If only one room is available, men and women usually feel able to pray together if it is large enough and they are modestly dressed. A curtain or screen could also be provided to ensure privacy between the sexes. Men usually stand at the front of the room and women at the back. Larger rooms may be needed for Friday congregational prayer.

To help people who cannot get out of bed, the Qibla could also be marked by discreet arrows on the ceilings of wards, side wards and so on (McIntosh and Andrews 1992). Some religious shops sell compasses that indicate the Qibla. People who cannot get out of bed can pray sitting or lying down. They may prefer their curtains drawn. It is important not to interrupt or walk just in front of a person who is praying except in an emergency. Consultations, tests and treatments should normally be delayed for a few minutes until prayers are over (Gatrad 1994a).

Some Muslims may need help with washing before prayer. Patients who are confined to bed may wish to make a symbolic wash using a small quantity of running water. They may need a bowl of water and a cup for pouring before each formal prayer. The perineal area should also have been washed with running water after using the lavatory or bedpan, or after breaking wind (see Chapter 12 *Practical care*). In addition, discharging wounds, colostomy bags and so on must be as clean as possible so that patients feel able to pray. Find out each person's needs and how these can best be met.

The Qur'an

The Muslim holy book, the Qur'an, is regarded as the sacred revealed word of Allah dictated to the Prophet Muhammad. It is the ultimate source of guidance, and its principles can be applied to all situations and at all times. The Qur'an is always treated with great care and kept in a clean place. It is touched only by people who have washed in the prescribed manner. If a non-Muslim needs to move the Qur'an, they should wrap it in a clean cloth to avoid touching it.

Nothing may be placed on top of the Qur'an, and it is never placed on the floor or near, for example, shoes or dirty clothes. Muslims normally cover their heads during a reading of the Qur'an. Full attention is paid and no one eats, drinks, speaks or smokes.

The mosque and the imam

In Britain there is usually an imam in charge of each mosque, who performs religious functions and teaches the children. Although every Muslim makes their own decisions about religious observance, people may also ask an imam for information and guidance. Usually, each Muslim community, based on national origin, language and denomination, worships separately, though any mosque is open to all Muslims. All formal prayer is in Arabic, but people use their own first language for talks and social occasions at the mosque.

Visiting the sick, praying with the dying and supporting those in trouble are traditionally done by ordinary Muslims, women for women and men for men. The imam does not traditionally have a pastoral role, though this is changing in many British communities.

The hajj

People who have performed the hajj to Makka (see *Beliefs and practices*, earlier) are given the title Haaj or Hajji (men) and Haajjah, Hajjah or

Hajjiani (women). (Different titles are used in different countries.) Muslims in some communities use this title all the time as a mark of honour. A few may use it instead of their own personal name (see Chapter 30 *Recording people's names correctly*).

Sometimes relatives bring holy water from the well of Zamzam in Makka for the patient to drink (Gatrad 1994b). Sharing Zamzam water is like sharing the blessing of the person's pilgrimage; it may bring healing or may simply bring comfort and strength to the dying person (see also Chapter 10 *Holy water*).

Festivals

Friday The Muslim holy day is Friday. Men in most communities, and women in a few communities, are expected to attend the mosque at noon to say a special additional Friday prayer. In some Muslim countries Friday is also the official day of rest. Some male patients may very much want to attend the mosque for Friday prayers; this should be arranged if at all possible.

Other festivals The religious calendar plays a large part in the lives of devout Muslims. The two most important festivals are Eid-al-Fitr (marking the end of the holy month of Ramadan), and Eid-al-Adha (commemorating the willingness of the Prophet Abraham to sacrifice his son at Allah's command). 'Eid' means festival. (The Turkish word is 'Bayram'.) Both festivals are joyful and begin with special prayers. Many people visit friends and relatives, and exchange sweets and gifts. The precise date of the eids depends on the sighting of the new moon (the eid is the following day) and so can be predicted only roughly in advance (see the SHAP Calendar, listed in the References).

Patients may want to bathe and put on clean clothes on the morning of an eid. If there are several Muslim patients in hospital, they may be grateful if a room is provided where they can pray together in the morning (see *Worship*, above). Visiting restrictions should be lifted wherever possible.

Families and relationships

The family is central to Muslim life. In the Qur'an, Allah gives specific guidance on the responsibilities and rights of every Muslim in his or her family, and stresses the family as a source of support, love and security. The Prophet Muhammad also emphasised the special duty of looking after one's parents as they grow older and when they are ill.

Younger Muslims are generally expected to show courtesy towards older people, addressing them respectfully, helping them without being asked, waiting for them to sit down first, not interrupting or hurrying them when they are speaking, and not arguing with them even if they disagree. They should also not draw attention to the care and support they are giving, in case the older people feel that they are a burden (Maqsood 1994). Families who cannot care for frail or dying relatives as they feel they ought may feel distressed and guilty (see also Chapter 4 *Traditional expectations*).

Women

The treatment of women in Arabia at the time of the Prophet Muhammad was appalling. Under Islam major reforms were introduced: women and girls were no longer commodities, to be bought, sold and inherited; female infanticide, common at the time, was forbidden. Instead, Islam gave women legal status and economic rights. Under Islamic law women can control and dispose of their own money and property without reference to husbands or fathers. They can run their own businesses and are not required to contribute to family expenses. (Women in England and Wales received these rights only in the nineteenth century. Until then they had a status similar to children in law.) A Muslim marriage contract is valid only if the husband has covenanted a sum of money to be given to the wife if he dies or divorces her. Under Islamic law, daughters inherit only half of what sons receive. But daughters can keep what they inherit for themselves; sons have to spend a portion discharging other responsibilities (Vallelly 1997). Muslim women in many male-dominated communities have successfully used the Sharia (Islamic law), the Qur'an and the Hadith to argue for equal education, fair treatment and respect (Maqsood 1994, Dearden 1983).

At the same time, many Muslims believe that the identical role demanded by many Western women is against the fundamentally different natures of men and women as ordained by Allah. Many consider that, although women and men are spiritually and morally equal, they have complementary rather than identical roles and responsibilities. In some Muslim communities, men are expected to be responsible for all matters outside the home, including shopping, contact with non-family members and financial support. Women's lives are centred around the family. They are responsible for the atmosphere and conduct of the home, the comfort of family members, the upbringing and moral education of children, the care of the sick, housework, cooking and other practical domestic tasks. Their work is accorded high status in the Qur'an.

Physical separation Segregation of men and women – often described by the South Asian word purdah – is the norm in certain Muslim communities. The degree of segregation varies but purdah is traditionally seen in these communities as promoting orderly relationships and preserving family stability. It gives women privacy and protects them from molestation and abuse. To many conservative Muslims, free and easy relationships between unrelated men and women are signs of moral corruption and disrespect. It may be seen as the duty of a good family to protect women by keeping them at home and not, for example, sending them out to work. Although not every family can afford this, some men and women prefer to live in respectable poverty than to put the women at risk.

In some communities men and women customarily lead segregated lives in the home. Women and children spend their days in one area and men in another. Unrelated men and women in conservative communities rarely meet, and do not normally touch or sit together. They may keep their eyes down in each other's presence.

In some Muslim families and communities in Britain, though not all, strict purdah is regarded by both men and women as the right way to live, and is a matter of pride and family honour. A good husband is expected to try to enable his wife to live in purdah. Many women in these families rarely leave their homes, going out only to visit other family members, either on foot or by car (rarely by public transport). Family visits are often a very important part of their role, and at certain times – illness, a death, a birth, a wedding – visiting is an absolute obligation.

Some women in these communities, particularly older women, may see it as improper to attend a surgery or a clinic because they would have to sit in a waiting room with unrelated men and be seen by them. In a few very conservative families, therefore, the husband or another male relation may go to the doctor, describe the symptoms and ask for medication (Currer 1986). Some GPs provide a separate waiting room for women who prefer privacy.

Because the outside world is not sex-segregated and is very different, the observation of purdah causes major problems for British Muslim women who observe it. Those who have no relatives nearby whom they can visit on foot can be particularly isolated. However, the difficulties and inconveniences that such women experience are generally regarded as to do with life in Britain, and not as indicating the general undesirability of purdah (Currer 1986, Saifullah-Khan 1976).

Authority

In many conservative Muslim families, most non-domestic decisions are made by older people and by men. When serious decisions have to be made, older family members often expect to be fully informed and to be obeyed. A woman may be considered to be under the guardianship and protection of a man: her father, her husband, or her sons if she is a widow. This may be important, for example, when seeking consent or making decisions about surgery or other treatments (see also Chapter 15 *Informed consent*). In some communities it is considered good manners for the women to withdraw or remain silent when men or older people are talking to visitors or non-family members.

Some Muslim men from conservative communities are unused to any contact with women outside their own family. They may feel embarrassed and uncomfortable with other women, and may feel inhibited in dealing with women in positions of authority.

Marriage

Marriage in Islam is a civil contract, involving mutual consent and responsibilities. Conducting a responsible marriage and raising children well are religious duties. Marriage between first and second cousins is common in certain communities and is regarded as promoting family well-being and stability.

Sexual morality is very important, to protect the family and society. Sex is allowed only within marriage, in which men have specific and clear responsibilities to protect and provide for women and children. Casual social interaction between the sexes is not permitted. Deep shame for the whole family usually follows the discovery of illicit relationships.

Divorce is permitted in Islam but severely disapproved of. Before a divorce is granted, at least three attempts must be made by three different parties over several months to reconcile the couple. Divorced men and women are generally encouraged to remarry.

Polygamy At the time of the Prophet Muhammad, local men often had large numbers of wives as well as extramarital relationships. Limited polygamy was intended to protect women and to restrain male excesses (Dearden 1983). Under certain clearly defined conditions, a Muslim man can have up to four wives: he must be able to treat them all exactly the same and to support them all equally at a suitable level. Each wife also has the right to a separate home.

Some Muslims regard polygamy as preferable to the situation they observe in the West where men may father children outside marriage and take little or no responsibility for them, or where families split up and mothers are left to carry the burden of providing for themselves and the children.

In many Muslim countries, polygamy is forbidden unless permission is obtained from a special court. This is normally granted only if the wife is permanently infirm or infertile. Most Muslim men nowadays have only one wife. In Britain, a polygamous marriage is recognised in law provided it was contracted in a country where such marriages are legal.

Dietary requirements

Restrictions on what Muslims can eat are laid down in the Qur'an and are regarded as the direct command of Allah. They are based on the belief that the health of body and soul are connected. Many Muslims follow dietary restrictions even if they do not, for example, say formal prayers every day. Ismaili Muslims (see *Worship*, earlier) follow only some restrictions.

Pork Most practising Muslims do not eat pork, or anything made from pork (eg sausage, ham, bacon) or made with pork products (eg food fried in bacon fat, food containing lard, some biscuits and bread).

Halal meat and fish Muslims can eat all other meat and meat products, provided they are halal (which means permitted) – that is, killed as laid down in Islamic law. They can eat seafood of any kind. Fish is considered to have died naturally when taken out of the water, so the question of a special method of killing does not arise.

Eating away from home Many Muslims eat a strict vegetarian diet when they are away from home, unless they can be absolutely sure that other foods are completely halal. They may avoid all processed and other foods that could contain non-halal products (eg rennet in cheese, gelatine in jelly, animal fat in cakes, ice creams and soups). Many food additives with E numbers contain substances that are haram (forbidden). E471, for example, is a fatty acid derived from animal (usually pig) fat, widely used as an emulsifier in bread, cakes and other confectionery (IQRA Trust 1997). Because it is very difficult to be absolutely sure that prepared or processed food contains nothing forbidden, many Muslims avoid anything whose ingredients they are not absolutely sure of (see also Chapter 11 *Providing food in hospital and other residential care*). If a patient requires a liquid diet supplement, it is important to check the contents carefully to ensure that there are no prohibited substances or derivatives.

Like orthodox Jews and some very strict Hindus, a few Muslims will refuse all food that has not been prepared in separate pots and with separate utensils, on the grounds that equipment that has been used for prohibited food contaminates all other food it comes into contact with. Some Muslims may refuse any food prepared outside their own home, for this reason.

Alcohol

Alcohol is forbidden in the Qur'an because it causes people to quarrel and to forget about Allah. Most Muslims do not drink alcohol, but it is permitted as a constituent of essential medication if there is no alternative.

Tobacco

Smoking is not specifically forbidden in the Qur'an, as it is a more recent habit. Many Muslims regard smoking as forbidden in view of the Qur'anic injunction to do nothing that is self-destructive.

Medication

Practising Muslims may try to avoid prohibited substances in medication – for example, capsules with gelatine coatings, additives derived from animal fat, and oral medicines containing alcohol. Nevertheless, in an emergency or when there is really no alternative, most people will accept medication containing prohibited substances (see also *Medication during the fast*, below, and Chapter 14 *Religious dietary restrictions and fasting*).

There is no prohibition against opiates or other symptom-relieving drugs. However, a few people might refuse pain relief, believing that whatever they suffer in this world will reduce their punishment for their sins in the next. This may help them to bear even extreme pain patiently (IQRA Trust, personal communication 1998).

Fasting

Most practising healthy Muslims over the age of ten fast during the holy month of Ramadan, the ninth month of the Muslim year (pronounced Ramzaan by most South Asian Muslims). People who are ill, pregnant or on an arduous journey need not fast but may wish to (see below). Women who are menstruating or who have given birth within 40 days are not allowed to fast. The dates of Ramadan and of other Muslim festivals vary each year, because they are based on the lunar year (see the SHAP Calendar, listed in the References). Muslims of certain denominations do not fast.

Fasting is generally regarded as a valuable form of worship, enabling people to come closer to Allah, to practise self-denial, and to share and understand the suffering of hungry people all over the world. The shared hardship of fasting and the celebrations at the end of the fast bring families and communities together. Many Muslims are keen to observe the fast properly. Extra prayers are said throughout the month, the Qur'an is read from beginning to end, and many people abstain from frivolous pleasures and try to behave particularly well. The end of Ramadan is marked by a very important and joyful festival, Eid-al-Fitr (see *Festivals*, above).

Fasting means taking no liquid or food at all between dawn (about one and a half hours before the sun rises) and when darkness falls. The fast begins every day when it is light enough to distinguish a black from a white thread, and ends when the sun sinks below the horizon. Timetables are printed and distributed by local mosques to help people keep the fast correctly (Gatrad 1994a). When Ramadan occurs during the summer in Britain, people spend many hours without any liquid or food. Toothpaste and tobacco are forbidden during fasting hours.

Muslim household routines during Ramadan

During Ramadan, people usually get up an hour or two before dawn to eat and drink before the fast begins. The early morning meal ends at least ten minutes before dawn. When darkness falls, they end the fast with traditional food, for example a sweet drink, dates, a little salt, milk or yoghurt. They then say the sunset prayer. This is followed by a meal with plenty of fluid, often including milk, fruit juices and carbonated drinks (Aslam and Healy 1986). Relatives and friends are often invited to share the breaking of the fast.

The routines of many Muslim households change drastically during Ramadan (depending in Britain on the time of year). Women, who usually get up early to prepare the first meal and stay up late to clear up the last one, may spend much of the day in bed. They can become very tired as Ramadan progresses. It may be necessary to adjust the times of morning home visits so as not to disturb sleeping families. Outpatient and GP appointments should also allow for late rising.

Many people feel faint, dizzy or nauseated, especially in the first week of Ramadan while their body adjusts. They may also feel irritable and develop headaches, and may feel the cold more. By the fourth week people who are fasting may have little energy or strength and be very tired because of the broken nights. They may find it difficult to cope with additional stress and worry.

During Ramadan, Muslims who are not fasting do not eat or cook in front of other people, because this might lead someone to break their fast. It is considered a grave sin for anyone to break the fast of Ramadan without a compelling reason.

People who could not make the full fast during Ramadan, possibly because they were travelling, ill, menstruating, pregnant or breast-feeding, are required to make up the days they have missed as soon as possible. Some Muslim patients and visitors may therefore be fasting at times other than Ramadan.

Muslim patients during Ramadan

The sick and infirm are not obliged to fast, nor are people who have chronic illnesses or who must take medication regularly throughout the day. People who are too ill or frail ever to fast can give a set amount of money to the poor instead.

Some Muslim patients, even if they are seriously ill, will wish to fast whatever the circumstances, deciding that the shared experience and the spiritual benefits outweigh any physical risks or problems, especially if the fast has always been very important to them. Cline (1995) quotes a terminally ill Muslim woman who said that she knew that food could not help her recover and she would feel nearer to Allah if the hospital authorities allowed her to fast. For every patient the decision is an individual one and should be respected. It is helpful to find out the dates of Ramadan in advance each year so that Muslim patients can be given appropriate care and advice, and that possible problems can be discussed.

Providing for fasting patients

Every effort should be made to provide patients with adequate and acceptable meals during the hours of darkness, including at least one cooked meal. Relatives staying with patients will also be fasting and will need to eat after dark and before sunrise. Ramadan mealtimes will rarely coincide with hospital mealtimes, except, perhaps, when Ramadan falls in mid-winter. Discuss with Muslim patients and relatives who plan to fast how best their needs can be met.

In the morning, well before sunrise, people will need a meal with plenty of fluid before the fast begins. They will then not normally eat or drink until sunset. It is important that they get something to eat and drink as soon as it gets dark; people become extremely hungry and often feel weak towards the end of the day. If possible, therefore, schedule doctor's visits, tests and other interventions so as not to delay the breaking of the fast. At mealtimes, people who are fasting may prefer to go and sit in a day room, away from people who are eating. Those who are bed-bound might like to have their curtains drawn.

Some people, both patients and visitors, avoid swallowing any saliva during the hours of fasting and may spit it out. If necessary, sputum pots should be provided.

Medication during the fast

A fasting patient will normally not take any medication by mouth, nose or suppository between dawn and sunset. Some Muslims may refuse pain relief while fasting. Some may accept injections and intravenous infusions. A study of 44 Muslim patients attending their GP or an outpatient clinic found that only seven continued to take their medication as prescribed during Ramadan. Some missed one or more doses every day and a few took all their medicines for that day in a single dose (Aslam and Healy 1985).

Wherever possible, medication should be adjusted to fit in with the fast. For example, it may be possible to prescribe tablets to be taken twice a day, or at sunset, midnight and before dawn. In some cases slow-release preparations or preparations with a longer half-life can be prescribed in order to maintain therapeutic effects while fasting and to prevent toxic side-effects (Aslam and Healy 1986). It may also be necessary to consider the effects of medication on an empty stomach (Gatrad 1994a). In some cases enteric-coated preparations help to prevent gastric irritation. If the fast is long, people may become dehydrated and this should also be taken into account when prescribing. Discuss with each patient whether and how they plan to keep the fast, what they are likely to eat and drink and when. It is important to recognise that a patient's decision to fast and/or to refuse medication during Ramadan is not an issue of non-adherence or ignorance but one of different priorities. (See also Chapter 14 *Religious dietary restrictions and fasting*.)

> 'They think we don't understand that they are worried about us fasting. We do, but our ways are different.'
> Pregnant woman fasting during Ramadan

Some people do not like to have blood taken during Ramadan, possibly because they fear it may further exhaust them. A few women may refuse vaginal examinations (Gatrad 1994a).

Practical care

Modesty and clothing

Modesty in dress and behaviour are religious obligations for Muslim men and women. To avoid temptation and immorality, Islam forbids unmarried adults of the opposite sex to be alone together or to touch each other. Many Muslim women always wear high-necked clothes that cover their arms to their wrists and their legs to their ankles. Some always cover their heads. Men are covered at least from the navel to the knees. Nudity, even in the presence of other people of the same sex, is humiliating. Many Muslim women and men undress only when they are alone.

For many Muslims, it is very important that the doctors and nurses who care for them are of their own sex. Many conservative Muslim women, and some men, feel that they should never be touched by a doctor or nurse of the opposite sex, except in an emergency.

'I would rather die than be examined by a male doctor or cared for by a male nurse.'
Female Muslim health professional

For these patients, all possible efforts should be made to provide same-sex doctors and nurses. When this is not possible, the reasons should be clearly explained and consent obtained. A few people may refuse any examination or treatment by a member of the opposite sex whatever the medical consequences (see also Chapters 12 *Modesty* and 13 *Modesty and physical examination*).

Women In some communities, women's clothes (eg a burqa or chador) traditionally cover them from head to ankle, and also conceal the shapes of their bodies. Some women wear these clothes all the time, others only when they leave their homes or in public. Conservative South Asian Muslim women, for example, may put on a burqa or chador over their everyday clothes when they leave their homes. Some very conservative Turkish women wear a similar garment called a charshaf. Although, strictly speaking, these are cultural rather than Islamic requirements, many women welcome this form of dress because it enables them to leave their homes in complete privacy, free from intrusive glances. Nowadays it is also often a positive statement of their Muslim identity.

Some Muslim women simply wear a headscarf (hijab) in all public places, including hospital wards. Muslim women who wear Western dress often wear trousers or long skirts to cover their legs.

If it is not possible to provide gowns and other garments that cover the body completely, advise women to bring suitable clothes or invite them to keep their own clothes on. Because of the requirement to preserve modesty in front of men, some Muslim women in hospital may wish to keep their curtains drawn at visiting times, or throughout the day.

Men Most Muslim men in the UK wear a Western-style shirt and trousers. Some wear traditional dress, especially to relax in at home or to go to the mosque. A few Muslim men keep their heads covered at all times. In some communities, men who have performed the hajj (have made the pilgrimage to Makka) dye their beards red.

Washing and cleanliness

Cleanliness is a religious duty for Muslims as well as a matter of hygiene. Traditionally, only running water is considered truly cleansing. It is also necessary to wash before praying (see earlier). For some Muslims, fears about not having private and adequate washing facilities in hospitals are greater than their fears about their illness (see Chapter 12 *Personal hygiene*).

Some Muslim men and women remove their pubic hair for hygienic reasons. Some people use a razor; others use wax or sugar syrup, or a depilatory cream.

Religious jewellery and other items

Many people, especially women, wear jewellery signifying marriage or religious adherence or devotion. Some men and women wear jewellery to protect them when they are ill. This may be a medallion or a small amulet made of cloth, leather or metal containing words from the Qur'an. It is often worn on a black string around the waist, arm or neck. Jewellery should never be removed without discussion and consent.

> 'One family [of a patient] had paid £50 for a locket from a Muslim leader. Nursing staff had removed the locket and thrown it away, without realising its religious significance. The family was distressed, not because of the cost but because they would be unable to replace the holy verses from the leader who had been visiting and had returned home.' (Slater 1993)

Visiting a Muslim home

Muslims are required always to seek (and get) permission before entering a home, and to greet everyone in the home when they visit (Qur'an 24:

27–28). Visitors should also try to observe this. Family customs vary in different communities, and visiting professionals should try to take their cue from family members. Visitors should be modestly dressed. Older people should always be greeted as a sign of respect. If there are shoes by the front door, it is polite to remove one's own. Because it is very important to visit anyone who is seriously ill, there may be a large number of people with the patient. In some homes it may be polite for professionals to avoid eye contact and physical contact with members of the opposite sex.

When someone is ill or dying

Beliefs about death and dying

Islam teaches that there is life after death and that death is part of Allah's plan for humanity (see also *Beliefs and practices*, earlier). In Muslim tradition, a person who is dying does not fear death, because it is only temporary; nevertheless, people who are dying may need support in coming to terms with the reality of death and with whatever harm they have done in their lives. It is regarded as the duty of a devout Muslim to strive to accept whatever Allah sends. Lamenting one's fate may be interpreted as questioning His will.

A Muslim who knows that they are dying is required to prepare for death. Debts should be paid, arrangements made for dependants after one's death, forgiveness sought and efforts made to heal damaged relationships. Many Muslims believe, therefore, that it is right to tell someone if they are likely to die so that they can make the necessary preparations. At the same time, it is wrong to take away all hope: whatever the doctors' opinions, the time of death is always decided by Allah, who is all merciful. It is in Allah's power either to cure a person who seems to be dying or to take their life. Nothing can change the time appointed for a person's death; whatever Allah decides is for the best (see also Chapter 15 *Telling patients the truth*).

'Say: "O my servants who have transgressed against their souls! Despair not of the Mercy of God: for God forgives all sins: for He is Oft-Forgiving, Most Merciful".'

The Qur'an 39: 53 (Trans Ali)

Families and illness

A dying person should never be left alone. Because, in an extended family, many people may feel very close to the patient, and because it is a very important religious duty to visit the sick and dying, there may be large numbers of visitors at all hours. Wherever possible, their obligation to visit and their grief should be respected, and arrangements made to accommodate them (see Chapter 17).

Physical comfort

Everything possible should be done to alleviate the suffering of a seriously ill person, though nothing should be done with the intention of shortening life. Many Muslims believe that the time of death is ordained by Allah and that it is wrong to try to prolong life once Allah's will is clear (Firth 1993). 'Heroic' and 'unnatural' measures to preserve someone's life at all costs may be unacceptable.

The dying Muslim may wish to lie on their right side with their face towards the Qibla in Makka (south-east in Britain – see above) or with their head slightly raised so that their face is looking in that direction. This may require moving the bed.

Many Muslims prefer to die in their own homes in familiar surroundings where their religious and personal needs will be understood and met. However, it is also possible to create such an atmosphere in hospital. Comfort can be provided by familiar people reading to the patient from the Qur'an. The patient will also trust them to deal respectfully with their body after death.

Some patients may find the playing of secular music, intended to soothe and possibly distract, unacceptable. It is always important to check with the patient or their relatives.

Prayer and religious rituals

It is very important that the dying person dies in a state of faith. Family members may quietly recite verses from the Qur'an. An imam is not required. Someone may gently prompt the dying person to say the Muslim declaration of faith (kalima): 'There is no god but Allah and Muhammad is the messenger of Allah'. These are among the first words that any Muslim hears and the last words that they utter. If the person is too weak to speak he or she may raise a finger to indicate agreement, or may simply listen. In some communities, women who are menstruating or in the 40 days after childbirth do not visit if a person is known to be dying, because they cannot read the Qur'an (see above).

Muslims believe that at the time of the death the angel of death (Izra'il) descends from Allah to take the person's soul. Traditionally, the soul is believed to hover around the body for some time after death, and only gradually to distance itself.

Organ donation

The question of organ donation has been much discussed by Muslims around the world. In general it is officially regarded as permitted, though the need to define a person as dead while their body is still functioning, and to remove organs and therefore in some senses mutilate the body, cause problems for many Muslims. In 1982 organ donation after death was declared halal (permitted) and desirable by the Senior Ulama Commission, the highest religious authority in such matters, in Saudi Arabia (Lamb 1993). In 1995 the Muslim Law (Sharia) Council in Britain, which consists of scholars from all the major Muslim Schools of Law, issued a statement accepting brain stem death as constituting the end of life for the purpose of organ transplantation, and supporting organ donation as a means of alleviating pain or saving life. If the donor themselves has not expressed a wish to donate their organs, the next of kin may give permission. Organs must be given freely and without reward. Donation should be carried out only when it is likely to be successful. Trading in organs is prohibited (Muslim Law (Sharia) Council 1995).

The issue of organ donation, however, remains problematic for many. At the time of the Prophet Muhammad, dead bodies were often mutilated by their enemies. Anything that resembles mutilation arouses horror and disgust in many Muslims. Some believe that organ donation is not permissible on religious grounds. Others feel unable to agree for personal and cultural reasons. (See also Chapter 19 *Organ donation and transplantation*.)

After the death

Last offices

The human body is regarded as sacred in Islam. The dead person should be treated as if still alive – with love, modesty and respect. For many families it is important that the body is not touched by non-Muslims after death. Non-Muslim nursing staff and others should check with the family before carrying out any procedures. Some families might ask non-Muslim staff to wear disposable gloves.

Traditional Muslim procedure is to straighten the body, close the eyes, tie the feet together with a thread around the toes, and place a bandage round the chin and head so as to keep the mouth closed. Some families will wish to do this themselves.

If the family wishes, health professionals should simply do the following: close the eyes and mouth, straighten the limbs, remove medical equipment, lines and drains and seal wounds. If possible, turn the head towards the right shoulder so that the body can be buried with the face towards the Qibla (the direction of Makka). Do not cut the hair and nails. Wrap the body in a plain unstitched sheet without emblems. The body should not normally be washed, because this is done by the family or other members of the community when preparing for the funeral. (See also Chapter 20 *Immediately after the death and last offices*.)

Timing

Muslims are buried, not cremated. According to Islamic law and practice, burial takes place as soon as possible, on the same day or within 24 hours. Delay can cause great distress, and all efforts should be made to release the body as soon as possible so that the family can make funeral arrangements.

In some communities, close family members do not eat until after the burial, as a sign of respect. It is also an extremely important religious duty for all friends and relatives to visit a bereaved family and to attend the funeral. In Britain, where most Muslim communities are close knit, large numbers of relatives and community members may come to stay or to spend their days at the family's home from the moment they hear of the death until after the burial. Delay can therefore put a great practical and financial burden on the family (Gatrad 1994b). Families may also worry that the body of the person they loved will decay. (Embalming to preserve the body is prohibited in Islam unless required by law, for example, when a body is sent overseas for burial – see Chapter 20 *Repatriating the body*.)

Post mortems

There is a strong prohibition against any form of mutilation for any purpose (see also *Organ donation*, above). Post-mortem examinations are therefore forbidden in Islam and most families will refuse. When Muslim families are asked for permission, this should be done with an awareness that it is likely to be a sensitive issue.

If a post mortem is legally required, the reasons must be clearly explained to the family. Every effort should be made to treat the body with respect, preserving the person's modesty throughout. The body should be returned for burial as soon as possible. All the organs should be replaced and the body should be repaired very carefully so that the family is not distressed unnecessarily when they wash the body in preparation for burial. (See also Chapter 20 *Post mortems*.)

Preparation for the funeral

Many families are members of a local Muslim funeral committee. Members of the committee may collect death certificates and arrange funerals in order to take pressure off the family (Gatrad 1994b). Some families prefer not to use a funeral director. They may, for example, arrange all transport themselves and keep the body at home or at the mosque until the funeral.

Formal funeral preparations are usually carried out at home or at the mosque. The body is washed carefully and gently several times according to a set procedure, so that it is as pure as possible for the funeral prayers. Modesty is carefully preserved, because the person can no longer protect themselves. Women usually wash a female body and men a male body, though a husband may wash his wife's body and a wife her husband's. Voices are kept low and the Qur'an may be read. Jewellery is removed. The arms are placed across the chest and the body is usually wrapped in a plain white shroud. Muslims in some communities prefer to dress the body in formal daytime clothes. This is especially likely among Muslims who have lived in Communist countries where religious rituals and traditions were not permitted (Jonker 1996). A cloth is placed over the face in such a way that it can be folded back for people to say their last farewells. Camphor or other scented materials may be put under the armpits and around the orifices (Firth 1993). In some communities, women who are menstruating or in the 40 days after childbirth do not go near the body

Burial and the funeral

If the family has enough room, the short funeral procedures usually begin at the dead person's home. Passages from the Qur'an are recited. The coffin may be kept open so that people can say their farewells. It is then taken to the mosque or to the graveside for prayers. In most communities only men attend the burial. Women may go to the mosque or attend the final formal prayers but under Islamic law are discouraged from going to the graveside in case they become too distressed.

According to Islamic law the area above the grave should be slightly raised and the grave aligned so that the face of the dead person is towards the Qibla. Some denominations believe it is wrong to mark the grave in case this leads to idolatry. Some local authorities provide special areas for Muslim burials where Islamic law can be followed.

Funerals are often very large, with several hundred people attending. The most qualified man present usually officiates. Flowers are not traditional in most communities, though practice is changing in Britain.

Some families may wish to take the body back to their home country to be buried, especially as it is not always possible in Britain to follow Qur'anic prescriptions concerning burial. Some communities have saving schemes for this purpose (Currer 1986).

Mourning

Traditions and beliefs about 'correct' behaviour at a time of sadness vary. The Prophet Muhammad said that Allah accepts tears and private grief but that wailing and excessive public grieving were wrong. Muslims are required therefore to try to contain their grief and to exercise self-discipline. However, the pre-Islamic custom of loud wailing is still common in some communities. Sometimes improvised poems are said, describing and praising the dead person (Jonker 1996).

The initial period of formal mourning lasts three days, during which prayers are recited continuously (Gatrad 1994b). Traditionally the close family stay indoors and do not cook. Food is brought by relatives and friends. The widow may remain secluded. The full period of mourning lasts several weeks or months. It is very important to visit and sit with bereaved family members.

The grave may be visited every Friday for 40 days after the funeral and alms given to the poor. Special prayers may be said on certain days. A widow is traditionally expected to modify her behaviour for 130 days, wearing plain clothes and no jewellery, and staying at home during this period unless absolutely necessary.

Suicide

The Qur'an forbids Muslims to destroy themselves. Muhammad spoke of a man who had killed himself as being in hell. Suicide by a person who is in his or her right mind may therefore be regarded as lack of faith in Allah and a grievous sin.

45 Jainism

The information below will apply to only some Jain patients and their families. **Never assume. Always check everything with the person concerned.**

Jain communities in Britain

There are about 30,000 Jains in the UK (Weller 1997). Almost all are Indian in origin and most of their families originated from:

- East Africa (see Figure 39.1). A number of Jains moved there from Gujarat (see below) one or more generations ago. Most Jain families from East Africa came to Britain in the late 1960s and the 1970s, many as refugees.
- The state of Gujarat in north-western India (see Figure 41.1). A few Jain families from Gujarat came to Britain in the 1950s and '60s.

Because the families of most British Jains originated in the Indian state of Gujarat, they share many aspects of traditional north-west Indian culture with other families of Gujarati origin (see Chapter 41). The religious practices and customs of Jains from other parts of the Indian subcontinent may differ to some extent.

Jainism and Hinduism, the majority religion in India, have existed side by side for thousands of years. Although they have different origins and histories, they share some common traditions and practices. Some Jains may give their religion as Hindu, as they may not expect people to have heard of the Jain religion.

Languages

The first language of most older Jains in Britain is Gujarati (see Chapter 41 *Languages*).

Names

In general it is most acceptable to use title plus last name when addressing people, especially if they are elderly. Names must also be recorded correctly to prevent dangerous confusion in records (see Chapter 30 *Recording people's names correctly*).

Jainism – a brief description

Jainism teaches that every single living thing has an individual eternal soul – jiva – and a temporary physical form or body. In Jain belief, all souls have an equal potential and an equal capacity for infinite knowledge, energy and bliss; however, these capacities are hampered by karma. Jains understand karma as a negative influence that is attached to and obstructs the soul. Karma arises from previous wrong-doing and actions that go against important Jain principles.

Because of its karmic attachment, each soul must go through many cycles of birth and rebirth in different forms order to achieve liberation from karma and from the cycle of transmigration. Liberation is attained through right living and good actions, and can be achieved only from the human form. The soul will then exist in an eternal state of bliss and perfect knowledge at the 'top of the universe'. Jains do not believe in a supreme or creator god; the universe has always existed.

Jains honour 24 teachers, the Tirthankaras or pathfinders, for their faith. They worship them (see below) as examples of right living. They especially honour Mahavira (599–527 BCE*), the twenty-fourth and most recent Tirthankara, who revived Jainism. Mahavira taught in the language of the people rather than in Sanskrit. Jains also worship the guardian deities who possess 'right perception' and who help Jains to meditate on the teaching of the Tirthankaras. Some people pray to the guardian deities for special causes and in times of distress.

Jains are encouraged to follow certain important principles. These include:

- Non-violence, not hurting any living creature, even the smallest life forms, physically or mentally. As part of non-violence, most Jains eat a strict vegetarian diet (see later). Jains are also encouraged to show friendship and love towards everyone, to hold malice towards nobody, and to practice forgiveness and self-discipline.

---

* Before the Common Era, used as an alternative to BC.

- Truthfulness, including not harming another by one's speech, and honesty, not taking things that belong to another.
- Non-materialism, not attaching importance to material things.
- Chastity and sexual continence, not being sexually promiscuous.
- Non-one-sidedness, the belief that no one perspective on any issue carries the whole truth. Jainism encourages tolerance and acceptance of other people's beliefs.

The following Jain prayers, both of which form part of daily worship, express the essence of Jain belief and practice. The first, the Vanditu sutra, is a prayer of forgiveness and friendship, and forms part of the daily ritual of penitential retreat (see below):

I forgive all living beings
Let all living beings forgive me
All are my friends
I have no animosity towards anyone.

The second, part of Shanti stotra, is a prayer for the happiness of all the beings in the universe:

Let the cosmos be happy
Let all beings act for the welfare of others
Let all miseries be destroyed
Let human beings be happy and peaceful everywhere.

Religious observance

Worship

Most Jains worship three times a day: in the morning, around noon and just before sunset. The most important is the morning prayer or Navkara mantra, the recitation of surrender and obeisance to the five supreme beings. This is believed to remove all sins and to be the most auspicious prayer for the happiness of all living beings.

I pay homage to the persons who have conquered themselves
I pay homage to the spiritual victors
I pay homage to the spiritual leaders
I pay homage to the spiritual teachers
I pay homage to all saints throughout the universe.

Some Jains also perform the morning and evening ritual of 'penitential retreat'. This lasts for about 48 minutes, during which the person will not respond to others.

People usually stand, sit or kneel to worship. It is not necessary to bathe beforehand. Some women cover their heads with one end of their sari while worshipping. People may chant, usually silently but sometimes out loud, sometimes using a string of beads, a mala. They may read from a holy book. Some people may listen to tape recordings of prayers and holy readings.

When someone is ill Although Jains are unlikely to ask, most would prefer privacy and not to be disturbed when they are praying. The offer of a quiet room or to draw bed curtains would be much appreciated. In times of stress, anxiety or pain, it may be helpful to ask Jain patients if they would like their mala, to recite the Navkara mantra or to listen to their tapes. These can bring comfort and reassurance and are believed to lessen the need for pharmacological treatment of pain and distress.

Relatives and friends visiting a seriously ill or dying person will also appreciate privacy and freedom from disturbance during worship.

Holy articles and books

Jain patients away from home may bring religious books, a mala and cassette tapes of prayers and chanting. They may also bring photographs of Jain temples and holy places, and pictures or statues of one or more of the 24 Jain teachers which they may use as a focus for worship and meditation. All holy items and books are kept clean and safe. They are often wrapped in cloth for protection. The mala may be kept in a small wooden or tin box with a miniature book of prayers.

It is important that holy items are never put on the floor or near the feet or near shoes, leather articles or dirty clothes, and that nothing is put on top of them. If it is necessary for staff to touch or move holy items, they should ask permission and wash their hands before doing so.

Worship at home

Most Jain worship is performed at home, privately, within families or in small groups. Most Jain families have a family shrine containing images of the Tirthankaras. This may be in a special room or a specially designed cupboard. People may wash and anoint the images and make offerings to them of flowers, incense or fruit before beginning their worship. Jains worship the images of the Tirthankaras only in order to focus their minds on their virtuous qualities and to concentrate on the values of Jainism. The Tirthankaras are not thought to be present.

If a home has a separate room for worship, this is kept pure and is not entered without an invitation. Everyone who enters takes off their shoes at the door. Women cover their heads and should be modestly dressed. They should not be menstruating. No one touches anything on a shrine unless specifically invited to.

The temple and religious leaders

There are very few Jain temples (mandirs) in Britain. Some people worship at Jain centres that contain consecrated images on which they focus to meditate.

There are at present no official Jain religious leaders in the UK, though some members of the community teach, advise and have a pastoral role. In India, Jains are advised and guided by monks and nuns who are highly respected and lead a life of detachment and spiritual endeavour. As far as is humanly possible, they try to do no harm to any living being. Jain monks and nuns do not keep money, travel only on foot and do not use any form of transport because by doing so they might destroy living beings. This means they cannot come to Britain.

Astrology and good and bad events

Some people believe in astrology and may select auspicious times for ceremonies and other events. It is also believed that chanting the Navkara mantra removes potential harm from inauspicious times. Some people may pray and chant before surgery and at other worrying times.

Festivals

Jain festivals follow the lunar calendar, so the dates vary slightly each year. (See the SHAP Calendar, listed in the References.) The traditional Jain greeting (see *Visiting a Jain home*, below) is suitable for all festivals. The main festivals are as follows.

Mahavira Jayanti *March/April* Celebrates the birthday of the teacher Mahavira.

Diwali *October/November (same day as the Hindu festival)* Commemorates the day when Mahavira left this existence. Lamps are lit as a symbol of 'right knowledge', and family celebrations held. The second day of Diwali is the Jain New Year's Day and celebrates the attainment of omniscience by Gautam, Mahavira's chief disciple.

On the fifteenth day of Diwali, Jain holy places open for pilgrimage. Jains who cannot visit them often display a very large picture of a holy place and perform prayers and rituals as if they were actually there.

Paryushana parva *August/September* The most important Jain festival; it lasts for eight days. A time of penance, reflection, fasting (see below), confession and seeking forgiveness. Alms are given to the poor and for animal welfare. Many patients will want to observe as much of this festival as possible in order to become spiritually more pure and to shed negative karma (see earlier).

Families and relationships

Jain families are expected to be close knit, co-operative and mutually supportive. (For more on traditional family structure and values, see Chapter 41.) The caste system does not apply to Jains.

Dietary requirements

A vegetarian diet Because of the emphasis on non-violence towards any living thing, most Jains are vegetarians and do not eat meat, fish or eggs or anything made from or containing them. Although most Jains drink milk, some do not eat butter or cheese because of the micro-organisms they contain. For the same reason, most Jains avoid alcohol. Honey is not eaten because it deprives the bees and may also contain small organisms. Many devout Jains also avoid root vegetables, including onions, garlic, potatoes and carrots, and some eat a vegan diet. Jains who break dietary restrictions, even unwittingly, are likely to feel revolted and also spiritually polluted and damaged.

Times of eating Some Jains eat only during daylight hours. In the days before electric lighting it was impossible to see what one was eating after dark and there was a risk that some living organism might be damaged (Weller 1997). Eating during daylight hours is also a form of self-discipline. Check with Jain patients whether they follow this practice and discuss how it can best be accommodated.

Food and health Some Jains also follow traditional South Asian beliefs about food and health (see Chapter 41 *South Asian foods*). They may eat or avoid certain foods at certain times of the year to strengthen and restore harmony to the body. Tobacco is forbidden.

Fasting

Fasting is important in Jain life, because all eating and drinking is bound to harm some life forms, however tiny. Women are especially likely to fast.

Some people fast regularly on the eighth and fourteenth days of each lunar month. Many also fast during the festival of Paryushana parva (see above).

Jains sometimes perform a partial fast in which they take restricted amounts of food. Some do not eat but will drink boiled water. Others avoid all food and liquid for a given period. Some people may make a partial fast as a penance and to shed negative karma, sometimes for up to 30 days. This may be particularly important for people who are ill or near death. Most people who fast will be willing to take essential medication (see below).

A *holy death*

In rare cases a Jain who is old, very ill or for whom no further treatment is appropriate may decide gradually to withdraw from the world. They may fast for long periods of time, reducing their food intake until only fluids are taken, and then reducing and finally eliminating fluid intake. They may refuse all medication. During this time the person meditates and works towards complete detachment from this world. The decision to undergo a holy death is not taken lightly and should be respected.

Food away from home

If an Asian vegetarian diet is provided, ask Jain patients if this is acceptable to them or if they need special foods. Indian vegetarian food that does not contain root vegetables is generally acceptable. Some people will prefer freshly cooked food from home so that they can be sure that it does not contain prohibited ingredients. If they can, most families are willing to bring in freshly prepared food (see Chapter 11 *Relatives bringing in food*). Most Jains do not eat any cooked food that has been kept overnight.

When preparing or serving meals, it is extremely important to keep meat, fish, eggs and other prohibited food away from food intended for Jain patients (see also Chapter 11 *Religious considerations*). Some older, more conservative, Jains may also be distressed if meat, eggs or fish are served to others in their presence. They may prefer to eat alone with drawn curtains or in another area.

Medication

Because of the prohibition against killing or harming any form of life, some Jains prefer not to take antibiotics. If antibiotics are essential, most Jains will accept them but often with regret. Most people prefer to avoid drugs that contain animal or other prohibited substances, but will usually accept them if life is at stake. Some Jains may also be reluctant to take opiates because of the emphasis in Jainism on endurance and non-attachment to worldly and physical things and the importance of shedding negative karma through self-discipline and suffering. They may prefer to rely on human support and comfort and on spiritual endeavour, prayer and chanting rather than medical means of alleviating pain. (See also A *holy death*, above.)

Practical care

For information about practical care, see Chapters 12 and 41.

Visiting a Jain home

Jains will appreciate receiving the traditional greeting. Join the palms of the hands at about chin level and bow slightly, saying Jai Jinendra (pronounced Jigh, as in high, Jenendra). This means 'Honour to the person who conquers themselves'. Visitors should dress modestly and normally remove their shoes at the door.

Jains value cleanliness and tidiness highly. It is important to leave things neat after a visit or the patient may feel impelled to get up and tidy them later. No prohibited foodstuffs should be brought into a Jain home.

When someone is ill or dying

Prayer and religious rituals

A Jain who is very ill or dying may receive comfort from meditation, worship, prayer beads, prayer books and recordings of chanting and prayers (see above). Some may want to make a final visit home or, if there is one nearby, to a temple. If possible, this should be arranged.

Repentance, confession, penance and asking forgiveness are very important. The patient may ask for certain people to visit in order to confess and to ask forgiveness for any conscious or unconscious harm they may have caused. Privacy and time for this will be appreciated. The patient may also want to make donations to charity.

At the time of death

For many families it is extremely important that everyone be present when a loved one is approaching death. A large number of people may need to be accommodated (see also Chapter 18 *The needs of relatives*).

> 'We would like you to understand how important it is for us to keep our diet, to recite the Navkara mantra and listen to our religious tapes. It is also very important to us to be with a person when they are dying and we would like to be welcome to be there.'
> Jain doctor

It is considered ideal for a Jain to die in a state of auspicious meditation, reciting mantras and prayers or listening to relatives chanting and praying. Even if the person is unconscious, families may wish to play religious tapes quietly. A relative may also wish to chant into the dying person's ear, as they may be able to hear at some level. Some people may wish to burn incense sticks.

Organ donation

There is no religious objection to organ donation or transplantation. Jains may regard the chance to preserve the life of another as the greatest gift they can give. Provided clear explanations are given, many Jains are likely to consent.

After the death

Last offices

Jain families are unlikely to be concerned about who touches the body after death and issues such as removal of jewellery but it is always wise to check. Sometimes family members may wish to help wash the body. The arms are placed alongside the body, which should then be wrapped in a plain sheet without religious emblems.

In some cases, large numbers of family members will wish to gather immediately after the death to see the person who has died. They may appreciate it if the body is washed and tidied beforehand. Ask the relatives what they would prefer. (See also Chapter 20 *Immediately after the death and last offices*.)

Post mortems

There is no religious prohibition against post mortems. Jainism regards the body as being like a piece of clothing which is discarded at death. Most people will agree to a post mortem if the reasons are explained clearly.

Timing

It is traditional to hold the funeral soon after the death, within 24 or 48 hours of the death. Families may appreciate help in dealing with documentation as fast as possible. Until the day of the funeral, the whole community usually gathers every evening at the home of the person who has died to worship, chant, pray for peace and offer condolences to the bereaved family.

Funeral and cremation

It is customary for the body to be taken home for prayers immediately before the funeral. The mourners, both men and women, then proceed to the crematorium. If numbers are very large, the women may remain at home. All Jains are cremated, partly because unburned bodies are a medium for bacterial growth and may present a source of infection and harm to other people.

Traditionally, the eldest son has the special duty of lighting the funeral pyres of his parents, sometimes helped by close male relatives. In some British crematoria family members are allowed to press the button or help push the coffin into the cremator.

Following the cremation most people simply dispose of the ashes, though a few families may fly them home to India. It is believed that scattering the ashes in a designated place would go against the principle of non-attachment by making the place special to family members and others.

46 Jehovah's Witnesses

The information below will apply only to certain Jehovah's Witness patients and their families. Never assume. Always check everything with the person concerned.

Jehovah's Witnesses in Britain

There are Jehovah's Witnesses in about 230 countries throughout the world. In the UK there are around 132,000 baptised and committed adult Jehovah's Witnesses with an additional number of children and associates (Watch Tower 1997).

The families of Jehovah's Witnesses in Britain originated in many parts of the world, including the UK, the West Indies, the Indian subcontinent, Greece, Italy and Spain. Individuals are likely to be influenced by their family's cultural heritage as well as by their religious faith.

Jehovah's Witness beliefs and values

Jehovah's Witnesses accept the whole of the Bible, both the Old and the New Testament, as inspired by God. They are expected to try to live their lives according to God's commands and requests as written in the Bible. Jehovah's Witnesses regard Jesus Christ as the Son of God. Their highest priority is faithfulness to God and this transcends earthly considerations. They have a strong commitment to spreading their faith. Jehovah's Witnesses regard the cross as a pagan symbol and shun its use.

Jehovah's Witnesses are baptised when they have reached 'the age of understanding'. Each Witness must make their own baptismal commitment, which they describe as a personal dedication. This commitment cannot be made on their behalf. The conscience of the individual is very important. Everyone makes individual decisions taking official Jehovah's Witness rulings and biblical teachings into account.

Jehovah's Witnesses believe that when a person dies there is a period of rest until resurrection when the Kingdom of God will rule the earth. An individual's life after death depends entirely on God remembering and resurrecting them.

> 'I don't fear death because I know in my heart that I would just cease to exist. There would be a time of rest and then God would re-create me and I would continue to exist as myself. Actually death could be my friend, a release from pain, suffering and indignity.'

Jehovah's Witness Elder

Religious observance

Prayer and the Bible

Both silent and congregational prayer are important for Jehovah's Witnesses. Patients may wish to pray silently before eating and at other times. They may also pray quietly with visiting Elders, and with relatives and friends who share their faith. They may prefer to draw their curtains for privacy while praying.

Bible study is very important, and patients may have a Bible and other religious literature with them.

The congregation and the Elders

Most Witnesses belong to a local congregation of around 100 people. This is often regarded as an extension of the family. There are no salaried ministers, because all Jehovah's Witnesses are ministers in a similar way to the apostles at the time of Jesus (Green and Green 1992). However, each congregation has lay Elders who have pastoral and spiritual responsibilities and authority within the community. They may play a special role in the emotional and spiritual support of a seriously ill person and should be given the same respect, privileges and access as are accorded to ministers of other faiths (Green and Green 1992).

The Jehovah's Witnesses' meeting place is called the Kingdom Hall. Patients may wish to listen to tape recordings of meetings of their local congregation.

Religious festivals

Jehovah's Witnesses do not observe Sunday as a holy day and do not celebrate Christmas or Easter. People in hospital during these festivals may not want to participate actively in celebrations. Jehovah's Witnesses do not celebrate birthdays.

Once a year, Jehovah's Witnesses hold an important ceremony, the Memorial, at which a very small number of Witnesses with a special heavenly calling take bread and wine, representing Christ's body and blood. A Witness with a heavenly calling who is too ill to attend the Memorial may be brought bread and wine.

Blood transfusions

Jehovah's Witnesses seek alternatives to blood transfusions because of their strong religious belief that a human must not sustain his or her life with another creature's blood (Acts 15: 20, 28–29). This is a deeply held core value. Jehovah's Witnesses believe that if they knowingly allow transfusion of blood they damage their personal relationship with God, and risk losing eternal life under the Kingdom of God. They are likely therefore to refuse a blood transfusion, whatever the possible consequences (Butler Sloss 1992).

'For me, accepting blood would be comparable to the sin of committing adultery.'
Jehovah's Witness Elder

Most Jehovah's Witnesses carry a small personal advance directive card that directs medical staff not to use blood or blood products as a means of treatment, and releases them from responsibility in this regard. Hospitals should have a standard form for refusal of blood which a Witness will sign when necessary (Green and Green 1992). Some Witnesses also sign more detailed health-care advance directives specifying what is and is not acceptable to them in terms of blood products and end-of-life decisions, in case they later become unable to make or communicate their health-care decisions themselves. Jehovah's Witnesses are advised to discuss their wishes and the full implications of the decisions they make with their GP before completing the directive (Watch Tower 1995).

'Other people besides Jehovah's Witnesses refuse blood transfusions, but it seems that we are pre-judged and treated with greater intolerance, more prejudice and less understanding.'
Adult Jehovah's Witness

Most Jehovah's Witnesses are well informed both about their religious teaching and about their right to determine their own treatment.

'Many negative myths and semi-truths have been propagated about their beliefs. Their desire to co-operate in treatment as fully as their conscience allows is often underplayed.' (Malyon 1998)

It is not a doctor's job to question Jehovah's Witness principles, but they should discuss with patients the medical consequences of non-transfusion in the management of their specific condition (Royal College of Surgeons 1996). It is important to find out sympathetically and respectfully from each patient what they regard as prohibited and to plan optimal care, taking the patient's requirements into account.

> 'Before I went in for major surgery I said to the surgeon, "I would rather die than have a blood transfusion, but I want to live. So please do your best for me." He said he would. And he did.'
> Middle-aged woman

If the doctor or surgeon is unable to accept the restrictions placed on them, they should refer the patient for a further opinion (Royal College of Surgeons 1996). It may also be helpful to contact the local Hospital Liaison Committee for Jehovah's Witnesses (see below).

Clinical implications The prohibition on blood transfusions includes whole blood, red cells, white cells, platelets and plasma. Blood fractions such as factor VIII, anti-D and globulins are considered to be substantially different from whole blood and from the basic constituents that nourish and sustain the body. These are not mentioned in the Bible and are therefore not universally regarded as prohibited. It is up to individual Witnesses to decide whether to accept them. Jehovah's Witnesses with haemophilia, for example, may accept factor VIII. People with hereditary conditions affecting the blood, such as sickle cell disease and thalassaemia (see Chapter 33), need special consideration. Jehovah's Witnesses are able to receive all medical treatment and care that does not include receiving blood (see also *Medication and treatment*, below).

Auto-transfusion

Auto-transfusion during surgery is acceptable to some Jehovah's Witnesses provided that the blood is returned to the patient immediately through a continuous and constant link. This method is acceptable because it is seen as an extension of the patient's own circulation, whereas blood that has been stored before infusion is not. Haemodialysis and heart bypass surgery are acceptable to many Jehovah's Witnesses provided that no blood prime is used.

Blood sampling

Blood is generally seen to represent life itself and should always be handled with respect. It should not be stored or re-used. Blood samples may be taken for testing, provided any unused blood is disposed of and not re-used (Green and Green 1992).

Children

Most Jehovah's Witness parents will refuse blood transfusions for their children. In extreme cases, parents' wishes may be over-ruled by a court order. In such a case it is important that the parents – whose sincerely held beliefs and concerns must be respected – should be represented in court, so that justice can be seen to be done (*re O* 1993, *re R* 1993).

Further help and advice

The Royal College of Surgeons' publication (1996) lists considerations for clinicians in the management of surgery on Jehovah's Witness patients. Medical alternatives to transfusion and bloodless surgery techniques are increasingly available and should be sought whenever possible. Local Elders are often very knowledgeable about medical issues and especially about possible alternatives. There is also a country-wide network of 36 Jehovah's Witness Hospital Liaison Committees, whose members are well informed about medical and surgical procedures. They have detailed information about alternatives to blood transfusion, and some are in regular contact with physicians and surgeons who are experienced in giving medical and surgical treatment without the use of blood. For more information and, on a case by case basis, for names of clinicians who are prepared in principle to accept Jehovah's Witnesses, contact the Hospital Information Services at Watch Tower (see *Useful address*, below).

Dietary restrictions

Jehovah's Witnesses believe that the Bible forbids the eating of blood or blood products. Foods such as black pudding are therefore unacceptable. Because animals are bled after slaughter, meat is usually acceptable. Some Witnesses are vegetarian.

When someone is ill or dying

Visitors

Congregational support is often important, and a seriously ill or dying patient may be visited by Elders and by other members of the community. If there are too many visitors for the patient to cope with, it may be best to talk to one of the Elders and ask him to have a word with community members.

Medication and treatment

Except for blood transfusions, all normal curative and palliative medical treatment is permitted. There is no restriction on pharmacological methods of pain relief. Each person makes their own informed choices, depending on their own situation.

Euthanasia is forbidden but most Jehovah's Witnesses will agree to the withdrawal or withholding of treatment if there is no hope of a meaningful life. This is a question of individual conscience.

At the time of death

There is no formal religious ritual when a person is dying. A Jehovah's Witness who is close to death might appreciate the opportunity to pray quietly with an Elder or with relatives. Privacy and quiet for this should be ensured as far as possible.

Organ donation

There is no religious prohibition against organ donation. However, some Jehovah's Witnesses may refuse to receive an organ because the transplanted organ might contain residual blood.

After the death

Last offices

Last offices are performed as normal, provided the family has no special wishes. The body should be wrapped in a shroud without religious symbols. In the chapel of rest, crosses and other religious symbols should be removed.

Post mortems

There is no religious prohibition against post mortems but, unless there is a compelling reason or a legal requirement, Witnesses generally prefer that the body of a loved one is not subjected to dissection. Relatives may sometimes grant permission for a limited autopsy to determine the cause of death.

Funerals and mourning

Jehovah's Witnesses may be buried or cremated. The aim of the funeral is to bring comfort to the bereaved. Funerals are usually led by an Elder who addresses the congregation and leads the singing of hymns. It is regarded as perfectly normal and acceptable and as sanctioned in the Bible for people to weep and mourn and to express their sorrow (Watch Tower 1994).

Useful address

Hospital Information Services
Watch Tower
The Ridgeway
London NW7 1RN

Tel: 0208-906 2211 (8am–10pm)

Information and, on individual cases, names of clinicians who are prepared in principle to accept Jehovah's Witnesses.

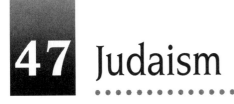

47 Judaism

The information below will apply to only some Jewish people. Never assume. Always check everything with the person concerned.

The Jewish communities in Britain

History and heritage The origins of the Jewish religion and people lie in the Middle East. Even before the Roman occupation of Judea in the middle of the first century BCE, the Jewish people suffered frequent periods of occupation and exile. A number left Judea and settled in Asia and southern Europe, including Spain and Portugal. In CE 70 the Romans destroyed Jerusalem and took Jewish prisoners of war to Rome. A large number migrated from there to western Europe, including England and Scandinavia. However, in the thirteenth and fourteenth centuries, Jews were expelled from Britain and most other western European countries after repeated persecution and massacres, often in the name of Christianity. Many fled to eastern Europe, where they were accepted and allowed to live in freedom.

During the following centuries, the situation of Jews in western Europe gradually improved, though with periods of renewed intolerance and persecution. They were sometimes urged to settle by local rulers, though often restricted to certain occupations and areas. Jews were invited to live in Britain in the seventeenth century. Meanwhile, in eastern Europe, the previous policy of tolerance was reversed and governments began officially persecuting Jews and imposing fierce restrictions. Massacres (pogroms) were encouraged and in some cases financed to divert local people's attention from their own discontent (Encarta 1996). Despite repeated repression, exclusion and insecurity, Jewish communities have made major contributions to European culture, intellectual life and prosperity.

The main periods of recent Jewish immigration into Britain occurred between 1880 and 1914, during pogroms in Russia and Poland, and in the 1930s and '40s when Hitler's Third Reich in Germany systematically attempted to murder all European Jews. A number of Israelis have made their homes here, as well as some Jews of other Middle Eastern origins.

Diversity and difference The term 'Jewish' is a cultural as well as a religious label. In the British Jewish communities there is a very wide spectrum of belief and different degrees of observance. Some Jews are secular and have no religious beliefs. Among religious Jews there are several denominations, including Orthodox, Masorti, Reform and Liberal Jews (the last two sometimes referred to as Progressive). Each group attends their own synagogues and follows their own religious practices. Both secular and religious Jewish families may also be influenced by customs and cultural traditions that are part of the strong Jewish heritage. These vary to some extent, depending on the family's background.

> 'Because we speak English, health professionals assume we are part of the indigenous population and that we have the same needs and attitudes as everyone else. But this is not true. We may sound the same and maybe look the same but we have specific needs and wishes that are different.'
> Orthodox Jewish woman

Only a few strictly Orthodox Jews will observe all the religious practices and obligations described in this chapter. In varying degrees, other Orthodox and Masorti Jews will observe many of them and most Reform and Liberal Jews will observe some of them. The term 'observant' is used when referring to aspects of Jewish law that **may** be important to Jews of all denominations.

It is important never to assume that someone who says they are Jewish will adhere to everything – or anything – set out in this chapter. There are also variations of observance and practice within the different denominations as well as between them. **It is essential to find out what is and is not appropriate and relevant to each individual patient and their family.**

Languages

Most British Jews under 60 were born in the UK and therefore speak English as a first language. Older people born on the continent of Europe may speak German, Polish, Rumanian or another eastern European language better than English. In some communities people speak Yiddish at home and to each other. Yiddish is a central European language derived mainly from Old German, Polish and Hebrew. Israeli families speak modern Hebrew (Ivrit) as their first language.

Where Hebrew words are transliterated in this chapter, the colloquial pronunciation common in many Jewish communities in Britain is used, rather than the modern Hebrew pronunciation.

Names

The naming system is the same as the British system. Some people have a religious name as their first or second personal name. Health professionals should find out how each patient would like to be addressed. In some communities it is traditional for a person who is seriously ill to be called by a different first name in order to deceive evil spirits. This tradition persists occasionally.

Judaism – a brief description

Jewish beliefs and values

Religious Jews believe in one God who created and governs the universe and is merciful and just. Humankind's purpose on earth is to worship and serve God, and to sanctify their lives by living justly according to God's laws and submitting to God's will. Jews are also required to do good, to give a proportion of their income to charity and to study. For some Jews the whole of life and every act and thought form a continuous act of worship. Judaism teaches that the human soul is immortal but that it is also important for people to concentrate their religious efforts on creating a better world for the living on earth.

Written and oral Jewish law

The main Jewish holy book is the Bible, which Christians call the Old Testament. The most sacred part is the Torah or Humash – the first five books. The Torah is known as the Written Law and reveals God's will for humankind. The Oral Law consists of detailed commentary on the Written Law by distinguished rabbis over many centuries, on how it should be applied in daily life and on other legal and ethical issues. The Oral Law was written down between 1,500 and 2,000 years ago and is called the Talmud.

'Jewish Law has developed over a period of several thousand years, and there has been continuous tension between the need to maintain strict traditions and the need to modify the tradition to suit changing circumstances – whether of climate, geographical location or advances in technology. This tension continues today, which is why rabbis from different groups within Judaism may have very different attitudes to some of the traditions.'
Rabbi

Religious observance

Worship

Most Orthodox men and a few Orthodox women pray three times a day – in the morning, afternoon and evening. Some people say their first prayers before rising, eating or drinking in the morning. Morning prayers usually take about 30 minutes and other prayers about 10 minutes. Most observant Jews pray once a day. People will appreciate privacy while praying. In hospital and other residential care they may want bed curtains drawn, and will need help with this if they cannot get out of bed.

During certain prayers it is important to stand, though someone who cannot stand unaided can sit or lie. Ritual bows are made during certain prayers and some men make rapid, rhythmical bowing movements, sway or rock back and forth to help concentration. People should not be disturbed while praying except in an emergency. If they are disturbed they may seem to ignore the interruption; this should not be taken as offensive. (See also *Visiting*, later.)

> 'Hear O Israel: the Lord is our God, the Lord is One.
> We praise His name Whose glorious kingdom is for ever and ever.
> And you shall love the Lord your God with all your heart,
> With all your soul, and with all your might.'
> And these words, which I command you this day, shall be upon your heart; and you shall teach them diligently to your children and you shall talk of them when you sit in your house, and when you walk by the way, and when you lie down, and when you rise up. And you shall bind them as a sign upon your hand, and they shall be like frontlets between your eyes. And you shall write them on the doorposts of your house, and upon your gates.
>
> Jewish prayer: the Shema

Observant Jews may keep a prayer book (a siddur) and a copy of the Torah or the Book of Psalms by their bed (see also Chapter 10 *Religious items*).

Men Observant men wear a tallith or tallis (prayer shawl) during morning prayer. This is wrapped round the shoulders and sometimes covers the head. It is usually white with blue or black stripes at the edges, and fringes (tsitsith or tsitsis) at the four corners. The fringes are a perpetual reminder to obey God's commandments. When a man dies he is buried in the tallith he has worn all his life. The tallith is usually kept in a special bag when not in use.

Orthodox men may 'lay tefillin' (pronounced t'_fill_in) before they pray. ('Laying' here means putting on.) This is usually done for morning prayers though some men also do it for later prayers. Tefillin (phylacteries) consist of two small boxes, each of about one cubic inch, attached to leather thongs. The boxes contain passages from the Torah (see above). One box is placed on the forehead above and between the eyes with a thong round the head to hold it in place. The other is placed on the left upper arm near the heart (the right arm in left-handed people). The thong is wound in a precise pattern down along the arm and onto the hand where it forms the first letter of the Hebrew word for Almighty (see the Shema, above). When not in use, tefillin are kept in a special box or bag. It is customary to stand when laying tefillin.

Traditionally, there should be a minimum of ten men (minyan) for formal prayers, and at certain times and festivals. Very occasionally, an Orthodox Jewish patient may want nine men at the bedside to pray with him.

Some Orthodox men also wear a miniature tallith (tallith katan, sometimes called tsitsith or arba kanfot) under their shirt during the day. The fringes can sometimes be seen hanging down, and again act as a reminder. Some men might want to wear a miniature tallith in hospital during the day. It is often removed at night.

Washing before prayer Many Orthodox men and some Orthodox women perform ritual cleansing by pouring water over their hands with a cup before all prayers, especially the first morning prayer. People who pray before rising and those who are bedbound will appreciate having a cup of water and a bowl by their bed overnight as well as being offered a cup and a bowl before other prayer times.

The synagogue and the rabbi

Most observant Jews belong to a synagogue (sometimes called a shul). Most synagogues have a full- or part-time rabbi. Many have visiting committees that organise hospital visits and support people who are ill and their families.

A Jewish religious leader is called a rabbi (teacher). Rabbis are highly educated in Jewish law. They teach and advise the community on religious issues and may visit people who are ill. Observant families may want to consult their rabbi when decisions must be made about initiating or maintaining treatment that could be dangerous, about discontinuing treatment or about resuscitation (see also *Attitudes to life and illness*, below). There is no single central authority in Judaism. Each community generally looks to its own rabbi for guidance on religious issues.

Shabbat

> 'Religious Jews take a delight in trying to live in accordance with the commandments. The delight comes from the sense of obeying God's will.' (Cross 1974)

Shabbat (pronounced shabb<u>at</u> or <u>shabb</u>us) or the Sabbath, is on Saturday, the seventh day of the Jewish week. It is the day ordained by God for rest and spiritual joy, removed from the cares of the outside world. It starts just before sunset on Friday and ends at nightfall on Saturday. Shabbat is traditionally a major and joyful festival, a day of relaxation and refreshment, family prayers and religious study, when Jews celebrate the goodness of life.

For many families, Shabbat begins with the ritual lighting of candles and a special family supper at which a blessing is recited over wine and bread. The candles are left to burn down. Shabbat ends with a ceremony called Havdalah at which a wine glass is filled to overflowing, the perfume of a special spice box is inhaled, and a braided candle is lit and then extinguished in wine.

The traditional Shabbat ceremonies and prayers are very important to many observant Jews. Patients who wish should be helped to celebrate them if at all possible. Any visiting restrictions should be lifted (though some Orthodox families may be unable to visit – see below).

Some Orthodox Jewish patients or their visitors may wish to light candles just before Shabbat begins. This can be especially important for married women, single people and widowers who have nobody to light them for them at home. If candles are forbidden for safety reasons, some patients may want to keep their bedside light on throughout Shabbat (Feldman and Rosner 1984). (It is important to check. They might have left the light on simply because they cannot switch it off – see below) In the USA, candle-shaped plugs (similar to night-light plugs) that glow when plugged into ordinary electrical sockets are sometimes used as substitutes for Sabbath candles. These may become available in the UK.

Shabbat and festival restrictions The degree to which people observe the following restrictions varies a good deal. Observant Jews do no work on Shabbat or on certain festivals (see below). They may avoid many activities, for example carrying anything outside the home, driving or using any form of transport, handling money, cooking, writing, or any activity that involves initiating the use of electricity or gas (eg running a hot water tap, cooking, opening a fridge door that activates an internal light, using a lift, a telephone or an electric lamp). Some Orthodox Jews may also be unwilling to sign papers or consent forms on Shabbat unless it is a matter of life and death. Patients may also not want to use the bell to call a nurse except in a real emergency (see below). Some people prefer to avoid surgery on Shabbat unless it is essential to preserve life (see *Attitudes to life and illness*, later.)

Strictly observant Jews may avoid tearing paper on Shabbat and may prefer interleaved lavatory paper. They may be unwilling to open paper packages, for example for dressing wounds. Some people also avoid altering the shape of anything (other than food) and may prefer to use liquid soap rather than a bar, tooth powder rather than toothpaste. They may avoid using creams or ointments.

The prohibition against using transport may mean that Orthodox families who do not live within walking distance cannot normally visit on Shabbat or on certain festivals. If Orthodox patients are going home for the weekend or for a festival, it is important to have everything organised and prepared early for them so that they can travel and reach home well before sunset.

In emergencies Any necessary activity is permitted on Shabbat or on festivals if life or health are threatened. For example, a patient's relative can telephone for an ambulance in an emergency and can go with them, but might walk home from the hospital afterwards. Prohibitions on, for example, travelling and receiving phone calls can also be overridden if the presence of a relative might sustain a dying person (Feldman and Rosner 1984). Families of critically ill patients in hospital may wish to make special arrangements so that they will know if a phone call is important. For example, staff could agree with the family that, if they telephone, they will first let the phone ring three times and then ring off. This would let the family know that the call is from the hospital and that they should pick up the phone when it rings again.

Note that the prohibitions on using transport and receiving phone calls are not lifted when an Orthodox Jewish person dies on Shabbat or on a festival. If the family follows Shabbat restrictions, the phone call informing them of the death should be delayed until after nightfall on Saturday. If death is anticipated, staff should discuss with the family beforehand what they should do. Funerals are not held on Shabbat.

If the family's views on receiving calls on Shabbat have not been ascertained beforehand, it is important to phone as normal when a patient deteriorates or dies; the family may wish to know immediately. If they observe Shabbat prohibitions they will anyway not answer the phone. In this case it is important to phone again immediately after nightfall on Saturday.

Other festivals

Festivals are very important in Judaism. Most commemorate biblical events and involve cultural traditions as well as religious rituals. They have great emotional significance for many Jews of all levels of observance. People who are in hospital during a festival may want to partake as far as possible. Some may very much want to go home for all or part of a festival if they can.

The most important Jewish festivals are Rosh Hashanah and Yom Kippur. Some people observe all the festivals strictly; others observe only some and may be less strict in their observance. Jewish patients should be asked if they have any special wishes or requirements. The dates of Jewish festivals are based on the lunar calendar. (See the SHAP Calendar, listed in the References.)

Jewish festivals start just before sunset on the eve of a festival, and last until after nightfall the next day. The main festivals are as follows.

Rosh Hashana (rosh ha<u>sha</u>na) the Jewish New Year. *September/October* Lasts for two days though some people observe only one day. It is a solemn festival, a time for reflection rather than celebration. Like Shabbat, it is a day (or days) of rest; many people observe the same restrictions.

The New Year is announced by blowing the shofar (<u>sho</u>far; a ram's horn) which proclaims the need for spiritual revival. Because it is important for Orthodox Jews to hear the shofar every New Year, a visitor may bring one in and blow it for Jewish patients in hospital. If possible, a small room could be set aside for this.

Yom Kippur (yom ki<u>poor</u>) the Day of Atonement. *September/October* Yom Kippur falls ten days after Rosh Hashana. It is a day of repentance and the most solemn festival in the Jewish year. No work is allowed and many activities are avoided. Observant Jews fast strictly from just before sunset the previous day until nightfall on the day of Yom Kippur (see *Fasting*, later).

Sukkot (su<u>kkot</u>) *October* The festival of tabernacles, a joyful festival of harvest and thanksgiving, lasting eight or nine days. On the first two and the last days (sometimes only one day), observant Jews may follow the same restrictions as on Shabbat. Men traditionally eat their meals in a temporary booth or hut, a sukkah (<u>sukkah</u>), symbolising the Jews' 40 years of wandering in the wilderness. Although hospital patients will not expect a sukkah to be built, for some men it may be very important to be allowed to go home to eat in their sukkah.

During Sukkot, observant Jews wave a palm branch bound with willow and myrtle leaves in a specific ritual with a lemon-like fruit, an etrog. They remind people of their dependence on the earth and their debt of gratitude to God who created it. These may be brought into hospital for Orthodox patients. People may wish for privacy while the ritual is performed.

Chanukah (<u>han</u>nooka) *December* The feast of lights. Lasts eight days. Each night people light an increasing number of candles on an eight-branched candlestick (a cha<u>nu</u>kiah). Normal daily life and work continue.

Purim (<u>pu</u>rim) *February/March* A joyful festival. Children dress up and the story of Purim, as told in the Book of Esther, is read. It is important for Orthodox Jews to hear the story every year, so an Orthodox Jewish patient may be visited by someone who will read it to them from a special scroll. Normal daily work and life continue.

Pesach (<u>pay</u>ssah) or **Passover** *March/April* Eight-day (sometimes seven-day) festival commemorating the flight (Exodus) of the Jews from Egypt under the leadership of Moses. Pesach starts with a ritual meal, the seder (<u>say</u>der). A second seder is often held on the second day. On the first two and the last two days (or, in some families, the first and last days) of Pesach observant Jews follow Shabbat restrictions (see above).

During Pesach observant Jews do not eat foods containing flour or yeast, to commemorate the fact that there was no time to make proper bread before the flight from Egypt. Instead, people eat unleavened bread (matzo or matzah) and special cakes and biscuits.

Observant Jews may wish to avoid all foods other than those that are specifically permitted and have been prepared under supervision during the week of Pesach. As well as flour, yeast and their products, prohibited foods include fermented and brewed substances and anything containing them, such as vinegar and ketchup. Some people avoid rice and pulses. The Hospital Kosher Meals Service provides specially labelled Pesach (Passover) meals. During Pesach people may also refuse medication that contains prohibited ingredients. This restriction is lifted if life or health are threatened.

Before Pesach, many observant Jews spring clean their homes thoroughly to ensure that no breadcrumbs or other leaven remain. Observant Jews also use a completely different set of cutlery and china during the festival so that there is no possible contamination from prohibited foods. Preparations for Pesach involve a great deal of cooking, baking and cleaning, and can be a very tiring and busy time for women. This may affect women who are caring for patients at home or who normally visit frequently. Observant patients in hospital may want to clean their lockers before Pesach begins and may be grateful for help with this.

Shavuot *May/June (seven weeks after Pesach)* Two- (or one-) day festival commemorating the giving of the Torah (see above) by God to Moses on Mount Sinai. Orthodox Jews may observe Shabbat restrictions (see above). It is traditional to eat dairy foods such as cheesecake.

Tish'ah B'av (tisha ba-av) *July/August* The ninth day of the month of Av; concludes the Jewish year. It is a solemn day of mourning and fasting (see *Fasting*, below) to commemorate the destruction of the first and second temples in Jerusalem and other tragedies that have occurred throughout the ages.

Families and relationships

Family structures and relationships vary in different Jewish communities and from family to family. Broadly speaking, marriage and the family are the centre of traditional Jewish life and it is the duty of a married couple to create a peaceful home. In most Orthodox families, male and female roles are clearly delineated, the mother taking primary responsibility for the home and the children though she may also work outside the home. Fathers take particular responsibility for the religious education of the children. Mutual respect between husband and wife are very important. Sexual morality is central to traditional Jewish values. In some communities men and women socialise separately.

Marriage

In some Orthodox Jewish communities marriages are guided; families consult a marriage broker who suggests potentially suitable partners. The final decision is made by the couple themselves. In some Orthodox communities people marry in their late teens.

Divorce, though considered very undesirable, is permitted if a marriage is very unhappy and cannot be rescued.

Older Jewish people

Responsibilities to parents are strong, particularly as they grow older. For many people the commandment to 'Honour thy father and thy mother' extends to all older people. Many Jews now reaching old age have lived through the dislocation and trauma of the Holocaust. Many lost some or all of their family.

Dietary requirements

Jewish culture and food

It is traditionally important to offer food and drink to anyone who is ill or distressed. Some families may be anxious that a person should eat properly and may regard reluctance or inability to eat as a very bad sign. They may bring special delicacies to tempt or comfort patients.

Religious requirements

'For an observant Jew to be deprived of the opportunity to practise his or her faith, or to be compelled to do something which Judaism actually prohibits, is a very real hardship, which could create a conflict of conscience.' (Berkovits 1992)

The aims of Jewish dietary laws are to sanctify the act of eating, to follow the teachings of the Torah and to preserve health. Observant Jews eat only food that is kosher, meaning ritually correct and fit as laid down in the Torah:

- Only certain meats are permitted: beef, lamb, mutton, chicken and turkey. All meat must be slaughtered according to ritual Jewish law, cleaned, soaked to remove the blood, and salted. Any meat not prepared in this way is not kosher.
- Pork, game, shellfish, any fish without fins and scales, and anything made from or containing extracts of them, are forbidden.
- Milk or milk derivatives are not eaten at the same meal with meat or meat derivatives.

For many observant Jews, religious dietary laws are fundamental to their lives. However, the precise level of dietary observance varies from family to family and individual to individual. Some people follow only certain dietary laws (eg no shellfish or pork) and so may be able to select carefully from hospital menus (see also Chapter 11 *Providing food in hospital and other residential care*). Others need specially prepared and packaged kosher food ordered for them at every meal (see below). It is important to ask each person about their personal dietary needs and never to make assumptions.

Meat and meat products Many observant Jews are very careful to eat only kosher meat, to avoid pork and to avoid anything that might contain or have come into contact with non-kosher meat products or pork products. Some eat only kosher cheese to avoid non-kosher animal rennet. Some eat only bread that has been prepared under religious supervision to ensure that no non-kosher animal fat has been used in the preparation or to grease the baking tins.

Milk and meat In order to keep milk and meat and anything made with them completely separate, many people leave a gap of several hours – from one to six – after eating meat foods and before eating dairy foods. An observant Jew cannot have, for example, a cup of tea with milk or a milk pudding after a meat meal. Cheese and meat are not eaten together. At home, some people keep a kosher kitchen with two complete sets of cutlery, china and cooking utensils – one used for meat foods and one for dairy foods. These are always washed and stored separately. Kosher kitchens have two sets of washing-up equipment and drying-up cloths, and some have two sinks. If using the kitchen in an Orthodox Jewish home, it is important to find out if the family keeps a kosher kitchen and which equipment and surfaces are kept for dairy foods and which for meat foods.

Milk Some Orthodox Jews drink only milk that has been produced and processed under religious supervision. Traditionally this was to ensure that the milk came only from cows and had not been contaminated by other substances. Some patients may bring in their own milk, packaged under the supervision of the Rabbinate. Space will be needed to store this in the fridge. Because it is forbidden to turn electrical appliances on or off on Shabbat and on certain festivals, some ambulant patients may ask for the milk to be taken out of the fridge for them if the fridge has an internal light. Alternatively, the internal light bulb can be removed, or a piece of tape put over the switch to prevent the light coming on when the door is opened (see *Shabbat and festival restrictions*, earlier).

Other considerations

- With an increasing amount of processed food whose ingredients and methods of production are unknown, it is becoming very difficult for people to be sure of what they are eating. Even if the ingredients are kosher, the product may still be non-kosher because of other unlisted agents used in its manufacture, such as grease. Any processed food containing, for example, edible fats, glycerides, polysorbates, stearates, casein, emulsifiers, stabilisers or shortenings, as well as a variety of E-numbers is non-kosher, because it may contain prohibited animal or other products (London Beth Din 1998).
- Strictly observant Jews do not eat food that, during preparation or serving, has come into contact with saucepans, dishes or utensils that are also used for non-kosher food. They may prefer disposable plates, cups and cutlery for breakfast and tea if kosher meals are not supplied. Some (both patients and relatives) may refuse a cup of tea made in a non-kosher kitchen. This is not intended to cause offence but is because of strict observance of dietary laws.

- To be acceptable, wine and grape juice must also come from a rabbini-cally approved source. Foods made of or containing wine, grape juice or their products such as wine vinegar, many jams, brandy and sherry are avoided unless they are rabbinically approved. Many Orthodox Jews are extremely careful that all the fruit and vegetables they eat, whether fresh, cooked or processed, are scrupulously clean and do not contain any insects (London Beth Din 1998). Some people may refuse vegetables that are difficult to clean thoroughly, such as brussels sprouts (Berkovits 1992).
- Some people eat only white-shelled eggs to avoid the risk of eating a spot of blood in the egg. Blood spots are more easily detected in white eggs during candling (before the eggs are packed for sale) and so white eggs with blood spots are rarely sold (London Beth Din 1998).
- During the festival of Pesach people may avoid foods containing wheat or yeast (see above).
- Orthodox men may want to wash and pray before meals.

Because of the complexity of Jewish dietary requirements and the processes of modern food production and mass catering, many Orthodox Jews do not eat any food prepared outside their home unless it has been produced under the supervision of the Rabbinate using special cooking utensils.

When someone is ill

Once a patient's level of observance has been established, every effort must be made to try to meet their nutritional needs while observing religious dietary laws. If required, prepacked frozen kosher meals made under rab-binical supervision are available from the Hospital Kosher Meals Service. These should be ordered through the catering department. They come in disposable wrappers wrapped in double aluminium foil. They can be heated in any oven (not microwave) provided the packs remain sealed, and should be given to the patient still sealed in the container together with the dis-posable cutlery. Help the patient open the packs if necessary. Kosher meals should not be placed in normal crockery as this renders them non-kosher. If for some reason a kosher meal cannot be provided, ask the patient if a vegetarian meal, though usually without cheese, or a cold fish meal such as tinned sardines or salmon, is acceptable (Van den Bergh 1997).

For breakfast most cereals are acceptable to Orthodox Jewish people, with milk, fruit, vegetables, tea or coffee. Some may not eat bread unless it is kosher.

If an Orthodox patient cannot eat solid food, kosher meals can be liq-uidised provided that the liquidiser is kept solely for kosher food. Separate liquidisers should be used for meat and non-meat dishes. Proprietary high-calorie liquid food supplements may be unacceptable for patients who drink only kosher milk (see above), as most contain dried skimmed milk. However, many people would accept such supplements if they are medically indicated and there is no suitable alternative.

Medication

Some people who observe strict dietary laws may prefer to avoid any oral medication containing prohibited products such as animal-derived glycerine or gelatine. However, all dietary restrictions are lifted if health or life are endangered. If a particular drug is considered medically necessary and there is no suitable substitute, most people will accept it. If there is a problem, discuss this with the patient and the relatives. When medication is given by injection, issues of religious acceptability do not generally arise. (See also *Symptom control*, later.)

Fasting

There are two major religious fasts each year, on Yom Kippur and Tish'ah B'av (see *Other festivals*, above). All food and drink, including water, are forbidden from just before sunset on the eve of the fast until after nightfall the next day. The dates of these fasts vary from year to year, depending on the moon. (See the SHAP Calendar, listed in the References.)

People who fast usually eat a good meal before the fast begins, and provision should be made for this. The pre-fast meal should end about 15 minutes before sunset. Another meal should be served to end the fast after nightfall.

Judaism discourages fasting if it is likely to endanger health. However, the major annual fasts are very important and some observant Jewish patients may be extremely reluctant to miss them. Some people may ask for their usual medication to be prescribed by suppository during a major fast. Some may want to ask their rabbi for advice; the rabbi will normally discuss the issue with the patient's doctor. If a patient is on essential medication, it is important to explain the need to keep taking it during a fast. A person who misses a fast does not have to make up the fast at a later date.

There are several minor fasts during the year. These start just before dawn and end after nightfall the same day. They are not considered as important as the two major fasts and most people will not fast if they are seriously ill. However, visiting relatives and friends may be observing a strict fast.

Practical care

Modesty and clothing

Observant Jews are required to dress modestly at all times. The way in which this is interpreted varies between communities. For strictly observant women and men physical exposure, especially in front of someone of the opposite sex, may be offensive and humiliating. It is important to help all patients preserve their dignity and self-respect as far as possible during investigations and treatments, and to avoid any unnecessary exposure (see also Chapter 13 *Examination, investigation and treatment*). Invite people who find hospital gowns inadequate to wear clothing of their choice. Mixed sex wards are likely to cause considerable distress to Orthodox Jews of both sexes and especially to women. Some patients on mixed-sex wards will want to keep their bed curtains drawn at all times (see also Chapter 12 *Modesty*).

Men Jews traditionally cover their heads when praying, as a gesture of respect to God. Consequently, many Orthodox Jewish men keep their heads covered all the time in recognition of God's constant presence. Most wear a kippah (skull cap), called a yarmulke in Yiddish. Some men wear a kippah only to eat and pray. If a man who keeps his head covered can no longer care for himself, staff should help ensure that his kippah is kept in place unless removal is required for clinical reasons.

Some Orthodox Jewish men wear a tsitsith under their shirt during the day (see *Worship*, earlier). Many Orthodox men wear sedate colours such as black and navy blue.

Women Many Orthodox Jewish married women cover their heads with a headscarf or a sheitel (wig), especially outside the home. If a woman normally wears a wig or a scarf, staff should help her keep her head covered at all times (unless removal is required for clinical reasons), even when she is unconscious or very ill.

Some women wear a shawl, a headscarf or a hat when praying. Strictly observant women usually wear high necklines, long sleeves and skirts that cover the knees.

Health professionals It is important to dress modestly when caring for Orthodox Jewish clients or visiting them at home. Women should keep their arms covered to the elbows and their legs to the knees, and should normally wear a skirt rather than trousers. The rules of modest behaviour and physical contact outlined below should be observed wherever possible.

Modesty and physical contact

In Orthodox Judaism, touch between a woman and a man is forbidden unless they are married. The prohibition against touch is waived when physical contact is strictly necessary as part of a medical examination or treatment. Nevertheless, some strictly observant women and men strongly prefer to be cared for by nurses and doctors of their own sex. They may also prefer to discuss intimate matters with health professionals of the same sex. Some women may not wish to be examined in their husband's presence.

Orthodox Jews of both sexes may be unhappy to be alone in a closed room or a lift with a member of the opposite sex. This should not be taken personally. Some people feel more at ease if the door of the room is left slightly ajar. In some communities, Orthodox Jewish men and women may be more comfortable if they sit separately.

Some Orthodox men avoid all physical contact with unrelated women, and may prefer not to shake hands. A few avoid eye contact or looking at an unrelated woman. An Orthodox Jewish man may feel extremely uncomfortable if a female nurse or doctor puts her arm round him or takes his hand to comfort him. An Orthodox Jewish woman is likely to feel the same with a male nurse or doctor.

Husbands and wives Jewish law forbids any physical contact between man and wife while she has any uterine blood loss. During menstruation and after birth, Orthodox couples avoid touching each other until the woman has had seven days with no loss and has been to the ritual bath (mikvah). Some couples also avoid any physical contact during labour and the puerperium or if the woman has uterine bleeding due to illness.

Washing and cleanliness

Orthodox Jews may want to wash their hands and say a blessing before meals in which bread is eaten. If they cannot get out of bed, they will appreciate being offered a cup of water and a bowl. They may also want to wash their hands before praying (see earlier).

Shabbat and festivals Some Orthodox Jews do not bath or shower during Shabbat or the other major festivals (see earlier) because running hot water activates the heating system. These prohibitions are overridden if there is a medical need for washing. Some people may prefer the hot water to be turned on and off for them. Some may prefer to use a mouth wash rather than toothpaste, in order not to break the prohibition on not changing the shape of anything. Some Orthodox Jews do not clean their teeth on fast days (see *Fasting*, above). However, all laws are overridden in Judaism when there are medical reasons. Whatever is necessary can always be done for a person who, for example, is incontinent or in need of frequent mouth care.

Men Orthodox men may want to wash their hands by pouring water over them with a cup first thing in the morning before getting up and before all prayers. They may ask for a bowl with a tumbler of water to be left by their bedside each night to enable them to do so.

Some Orthodox men do not shave at all; others shave every day except Shabbat, on certain festivals and when in mourning. Some men who shave usually use an electric razor because it is forbidden to use a blade on the head. If an Orthodox man cannot shave himself, an electric razor should therefore be used. Most men will accept a safety razor if they are being shaved for medical reasons, for example before a clinical procedure.

Some Orthodox men wear side locks, either loose or wound round their ears. These are not cut unless there is a clear medical need. If a person cannot care for himself, his beard and side locks should be kept clean and tidy as part of normal nursing care.

When a person is critically ill or dying

Beliefs about life after death

'The Lord is my shepherd; I shall not want. He maketh me to lie down in green pastures; He leadeth me beside the still waters. He restoreth my soul; He leadeth me in the paths of righteousness for His Name's sake. Yea, though I walk through the valley of the shadow of death, I will fear no evil; for Thou art with me; Thy rod and Thy staff they comfort me.'

Psalm 23: 1–4

Most observant Jews believe that the spiritual part of a person, the soul, is immortal. Although the body dies, the soul will be reunited with God in the world to come. Some Jews also believe in bodily resurrection; this is one reason why some people feel strongly that a body must be complete and whole at burial. Many Jews believe that immortality exists through those who have known us and been influenced by us. A person lives on especially through their children, and so the family has an additional special significance.

Attitudes to life and illness

'I acknowledge before Thee, O Lord my God and God of my fathers, that my life and my death are in Thy hands. May it be Thy will to heal me. But if death is my lot, then I accept it from Thy hand with love.'

Jewish prayer recited when critically ill

Judaism values life above all else. Human beings are created in the image of God and therefore each moment of life, regardless of quality or usefulness, is of infinite value. There is an obligation to seek medical help, to accept treatments that are known to be effective and to preserve life if at all possible. In Jewish law a doctor should use all available means to treat a patient (Bleich 1996, Daniels 1996). The dietary laws and restrictions normally observed by strictly observant Jews on Shabbat (see earlier) and other festivals are disregarded when necessary to save or maintain life (Feldman and Rosner 1984). Euthanasia is strictly forbidden.

Medicine and technology are generally regarded with great respect. Many people will want to know that every available treatment has been tried and that everything possible is being done to maintain life, whatever the age or condition of the patient. Some may be anxious to continue active treatment even when there is no apparent chance of recovery (see also Chapter 18 *Making decisions at the end of life*). This can create dilemmas for health professionals, especially when there are resource implications or when pressure to continue treatment comes from the family rather than from the patient. When medical decisions, especially about discontinuing treatment or life support, must be made, some families may seek the advice and views of their rabbi.

Jewish intellectual and cultural traditions

Great value is placed on study and intellectual understanding in Judaism. Traditionally, people reach an understanding of religious texts through questioning, discussion, argument and debate. Asking questions and arguing in order to reach a deeper understanding of issues is therefore an important part of Jewish heritage. This may encourage Jews to question in a way that can seem challenging to people unaccustomed to this style of communicating.

Throughout their history Jews have fought for survival against repeated persecution (see earlier). This has perhaps heightened 'a strong grip on life' (Neuberger 1987). It has almost always proved unwise for Jewish people to trust those in power; what they were told was for their own good frequently turned out to be disastrous, and they have too often been attacked, betrayed and used.

'It was hard for our parents and grandparents to trust anyone in authority. Asking searching and difficult questions was a matter of survival.'
Retired secular Jewish man

The Jewish emphasis on the value of life, the tradition of religious questioning and Jewish history explain why some people may be seen, by

English standards, as over-anxious, demanding and vocal in their contacts with health professionals.

Discussing a poor prognosis

Many people of Jewish heritage consider it essential to help people who are ill to maintain hope, because no one can know for certain what is going to happen. It is traditional to soften the implications of the confessional prayer for people who are critically ill by reminding the patient that many people who have confessed have lived, while many who have not confessed have died (Katz 1995). People of Jewish heritage may therefore strongly prefer the phrase 'critically ill' when others might say 'terminally ill' or 'dying'.

In Jewish law it is permissible not to tell a person that they are dying if there is good reason to believe that knowing the truth would hasten their death or raise intolerable anxiety or fear. Hope should never be taken away. Relatives who worry about the effect on the patient may therefore urge health professionals not to divulge the prognosis even if the patient asks directly. This can create ethical dilemmas. Each situation should be considered individually, trying to take the patient's own wishes and best interests as the guiding factors. The needs, concerns and fears of the relatives should also be fully explored. If relatives continue to insist that the truth would hasten the patient's death, it may be acceptable to agree as long as the patient shows no signs of wanting or needing to talk about the reality of their situation (see also Chapter 15 *Telling patients the truth*).

Visiting

Jewish tradition stresses the importance of visiting the sick to offer practical help, concern and encouragement and to pray for their recovery. In some families this results in large numbers of visitors by the bedside for many hours. The obligation to visit should be understood and the family's needs accommodated wherever possible. However, some religious authorities state that the duty to visit should be set aside if the patient finds it embarrassing or distressing (Zwebner and Shofnos 1989, Jakobovits 1975) (see also Chapter 17).

Traditionally, no one who is near death should be alone. In most cases one or more family members will want to stay with a patient. Some people may want a rabbi to be present though this is not generally regarded as essential. If the patient is too ill to read prayers and psalms, a family member may read them on their behalf. Some families help a dying person to recite a confessional prayer or, if the patient is too ill, may recite it quietly on their behalf (Katz 1995). Traditionally, visitors sit so that they are lower than the sick person.

Symptom control

In Jewish law it is considered legitimate and laudable to alleviate distressing symptoms and pain, provided that the methods used do not in themselves hasten death (Bleich 1996). Opiates are acceptable though some people may be concerned about respiratory depression. The dying must be treated with exactly the same dignity and respect as the living.

The last few days

In Jewish law, both life and death are God's prerogatives. The preservation of human life is a divine commandment. Nothing should be done that might cause a person's death or hasten it by even a few minutes.

However, Jewish law also deals specifically with the situation when death is clearly inevitable and is likely to take place within three days. When a person is clearly in the process of dying (at which time they may be described by the Hebrew word goses), nothing should be done that might influence the process or disturb the patient in any way. Some Jewish authorities state that a goses should not be touched or moved at all, because this might hasten their death. At the same time, everything possible should be done to alleviate the dying person's suffering and to maintain their comfort, peace and dignity (Bleich 1996, Daniels 1996).

In practice, especially in the context of modern medical care, it can be difficult to identify the point at which the patient becomes a goses. Individual families are likely to have very different views about what treatment or care they feel is appropriate. Some consult their rabbi for advice. A few relatives who accept that death is imminent will want the person to be left completely undisturbed. Most will want professionals to continue symptom control and essential and gentle nursing care. This is likely to include mouth and wound care and dealing with incontinence, as failure to do so may increase the dying person's suffering. People who believe strongly in the requirement to preserve life at all costs may press for continued treatment, even if this is futile from a medical point of view, and may be distressed if treatment is stopped. They may want hydration and nutrition to continue. Because the duty of care is to the patient, it is important to explore the family's wishes and concerns and to explain the advantages and disadvantages of possible courses of action from the patient's point of view.

Organ donation

Jewish communities have generally followed the accepted practices of the country in which they live with regard to organ donation. However, attitudes among Orthodox Jews are changing in response to changes in Jewish medico-ethical views and practices in Israel and elsewhere. People's views will vary but may be strongly influenced by the prohibitions in Jewish law against hastening death and against desecrating corpses, and the importance of burying the body complete and whole. Some find both giving and receiving tissue or organs unacceptable. It is therefore essential to deal with each situation individually and to find out exactly what recipients, potential donors and their families want and will accept (see also Chapter 19 *Organ donation and transplantation*).

Issues for potential recipients Most Orthodox Jews accept the idea of receiving blood, blood products, bone marrow, corneas and kidneys. Some may express concern about the transfer of infection or disease; in Jewish law a doctor has an obligation to screen donors before using donated blood, tissue or organs.

A transplant may be unacceptable to some patients on religious grounds if the procedure involved endangers the recipient's life, for example when the recipient's own heart or liver must be removed before the new organ is inserted. Some people reject the idea of removing organs from animals that are still alive on grounds of cruelty. Receiving animal organs removed after slaughter is likely to be acceptable.

Issues for potential donors For some observant Jews, the importance of burying the body complete and whole precludes the donation of any tissue or organs except blood and bone marrow which are replaced naturally. Some may be unwilling to donate bone marrow because this involves a general anaesthetic, which is potentially life-threatening.

Other observant Jews are willing to donate organs because they consider that the religious duty to sustain life outweighs the importance of the body being complete and whole when buried. Religious views on the removal of vital organs and the definition of death are the subject of continuing debate among Jewish medical ethicists in Israel and elsewhere (eg New York). Changes there are likely to influence the views of Orthodox Jews in Britain. One influential rabbinical authority in the USA accepts the concept of brain stem death and therefore considers the subsequent removal of organs ethical. Others define death as the cessation of all breathing and circulation. This definition makes organs unsuitable for transplant.

Disposal of diseased tissue and organs Because of the importance of burying the body whole and complete, some Orthodox Jews may ask for all tissue to be packaged and handed over to the Chevra Kadishah (see below) for burial.

After the death

Immediately after death

Customs when an observant Jew dies vary a good deal. In some families it is traditional to wait for about quarter of an hour to be sure that the soul has departed. Then the son or the nearest relative closes the eyes and mouth and covers the face. If no family member is available, this should normally be done by a nurse or doctor. It is considered disrespectful to the dead to look on their face. Jewish men who are descended from the priesthood are forbidden to be under the same roof as a dead person, other than a close relative. For this reason, some men may leave abruptly when death occurs or seems imminent.

Relatives who are present at the death may perform the ritual tearing of clothing as a sign of mourning (see *Mourning*, below). For cultural reasons, some people may want any water that was standing in the room at the time of death to be poured away. Some may want the windows opened and then closed and all mirrors covered (see Chapter 20 *Possible cultural and religious wishes*).

Last offices

Families will vary in the way they wish the body to be handled, depending on their degree of observance and personal preference. It is therefore important always to check with the family, if possible in advance, what staff should do and what is and is not acceptable to them.

Some may wish the body to be prepared and washed by the Jewish Burial Society, the Chevra Kadishah (<u>h</u>evra ka<u>d</u>eesha) (see *Preparation for the funeral*, below). If the family does not wish the Burial Society to be called, they should be asked about their wishes concerning last offices. (See also Chapter 20 *Immediately after the death and last offices*.)

A few Orthodox families may ask that the body is not touched at all by non-Jews; however, this may not always be practical or desirable. If the body must be moved, it should be done with the minimum disturbance. In most cases it is acceptable for staff to do the following before members of the Chevra Kadishah arrive (Visitation Committee 1997):

- Close the eyes and mouth (but see above).
- Cover the face.
- When necessary, clean orifices and remove all drains, infusions, catheters and other equipment.
- Seal all wounds and incisions.
- Do not cut the hair or the nails.
- Deal with jewellery in the usual way unless the family request that a particular item be left.
- Straighten and lay the body flat with arms by the sides and hands open.
- Wrap the body in a plain white sheet for removal to the mortuary or chapel of rest.

It is traditional to place the body with the feet facing the door. A few families may want this. It is also customary to keep a vigil by the body; one or more people may want to remain with the body until it is handed over to the Chevra Kadishah. They may recite psalms and keep a lighted candle beside the body both at the bedside and in the mortuary. If the funeral is delayed and the body is placed in a mortuary fridge, some sitters may wish to remain nearby. The family's wishes should be accommodated wherever possible, and when necessary a compromise should be reached (see Chapter 20 *Spending time with the body*).

Post mortems

In Orthodox Jewish tradition the body should be disturbed as little as possible after death and should remain whole and intact. Post mortems are therefore forbidden. Orthodox Jews are likely to be distressed if a post mortem is legally required, both because they fear that the body will be desecrated and because it is likely to delay the burial. In such a case, the post mortem should be carried out as soon as possible, and special care taken to ensure that all organs and tissue are replaced afterwards. If appropriate, a partial post mortem should be performed. It is also important that the body is repaired as well as possible to avoid causing distress and offence to the members of the Chevra Kadishah (see above).

Timing

It is customary and, for some people, a religious obligation to hold the funeral within 24 hours of the death. Delay may be seen as disrespectful to the person who has died. It is therefore important for a doctor to issue a Cause of Death Certificate as soon as possible. In some areas the Registrar of Births, Deaths and Marriages makes special arrangements to issue death certificates out of normal hours and at weekends. Funerals are not held at night, on Shabbat or on certain days of major festivals (see earlier) so, if a person dies on a Thursday night, early on a Friday or just before a festival, there may be special urgency to hold the funeral (see also Chapter 20 *Paperwork and certificates*). (A few families may decide to delay the funeral if a close relative has to come from abroad.)

Preparation for the funeral

Preparing the body for burial is generally considered a religious duty. In Orthodox Jewish communities, the ritual washing and purification of the body is carried out by the Burial Society, the Chevra Kadishah. This is a group of respected community members whose duty is to prepare the body for burial with care, love and dignity. Members perform their duties voluntarily and anonymously so that the bereaved family does not feel under any obligation to them. Women prepare the bodies of women and children; men prepare the bodies of men. If there is a post mortem, the preparation for burial takes place afterwards.

Members of the Chevra Kadishah should be advised to take routine universal infection control precautions in order to safeguard their own health. If the body is known to pose a high risk of infection or is severely mutilated, the Chevra Kadishah should be advised not to open the body bag (see Chapter 20 *Infection control issues*). The safety of the living overrides all other considerations in Jewish law.

For some Jews it is very important that every bit of the body should be buried; following an accident, for example, some people will wish to bury the person with the clothes they were wearing to ensure that no blood or tissue remains unburied. (See also *Post mortems*, above, and Chapter 19 *Sudden death*.)

Embalming

Embalming is unacceptable to some observant Jews because the body should remain intact and whole. It is therefore particularly important that people who want to see the body do so as soon as possible. However, families who wish to transport the body to another country for burial have to accept embalming, because it is required by international law (see Chapter 20 *Repatriating the body*).

The funeral

By tradition Jews are buried. It is considered respectful to allow the body to revert naturally to the elements of which it was composed. Some Reform and Liberal Jews accept cremation. Some Jews, especially those who survived the Holocaust and those who lost family members in the Holocaust, find the idea of cremation particularly abhorrent. Those whose families were killed in camps and who therefore have no grave, may feel strongly that it is important to have a grave that surviving family members can visit. Sometimes there are differences of opinion in the family, especially if some members are more observant than others.

Funerals are traditionally simple, signifying that everyone is equal at death. A few Orthodox families have the body at home before the funeral. Mourners may follow the coffin on foot for a short distance when the cortege leaves. In traditional Orthodox communities, the men then go by car to the graveyard while the women return home, though this is changing. It is not customary to send flowers to a Jewish funeral. Some families suggest that charitable donations are made instead.

Mourning

Traditional Jewish mourning rituals recognise the trauma and grief that people suffer when a loved one dies. They provide a structure to support the bereaved by encouraging them to express their grief, and gradually to readjust to everyday life. Relatives and friends usually play an important role in supporting the bereaved through this process.

It is traditional for close relatives – the parents, siblings, spouse and children of the person who has died – to symbolically perform kri'ah (kri'<u>ah</u>; 'rending the garment'). This is done by cutting and then making a small tear in, for example, a jacket lapel or a tie. People perform kri'ah before the funeral.

After the funeral, the immediate members of an observant family – the parents, siblings, spouse and children – sit shivah (<u>shi</u>vah; the Hebrew word for seven). They stay at home, secluded and protected from the outside world and from work, for seven days. Traditionally, people sit on low stools. Relatives and friends visit to express their condolences, to offer comfort and to talk about the person who has died. When visiting a bereaved person it is customary to say, 'I wish you long life'.

Friends and relatives usually bring food for the family and offer help in other ways. There may be communal prayers each morning and evening. Sitting shivah is suspended on Shabbat and on other festivals, as it is considered that communal rejoicing should take precedence over private grieving. Some people also suspend expressions of personal grief.

'Some might consider the shivah an out-of-date custom. For me it was the bridge between trauma and normalcy, when, surrounded by a wall of comfort and concern, I was able to draw from the strength offered to me by those who cared.'

Jewish woman (New North London Synagogue 1997)

After the first seven days, the bereaved return to daily life and work but lead a quiet life for the next 30 days during which close male relatives may choose not to shave. After 30 days, the official period of mourning ends except for children mourning a parent. They continue to lead a quiet life, avoiding joyful gatherings. In Orthodox families the nearest male relatives attend synagogue every day for the next 11 months to recite the kaddish, a special prayer praising God.

Within a year of the death a stone-setting ceremony may be held at the graveside. The end of the first year of mourning is traditionally marked by the nearest male relative leading prayers in the synagogue or being 'called' to the reading of the Torah. Every year the anniversary or Yahrzeit of the person's death is commemorated similarly by lighting a candle that burns for 24 hours. The nearest male relatives attend synagogue to recite the kaddish (Goldberg 1991).

Useful addresses

Visitation Committee of the London Jewish Community
735 High Road
London N12 0US

Provides visitors for Jewish people in hospitals and offers bereavement counselling. Can also refer to people who visit in other parts of the UK.

Jewish Medical Ethics Group
c/o 80 East End Road
London N3 2SY

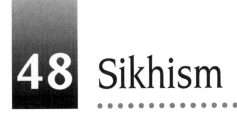

48 Sikhism

The information below will apply to only some Sikh patients and their families. Never assume. Always check everything with the person concerned.

Sikh communities in Britain

The Sikh communities have a long-standing military tradition and more recently a tradition of emigration for work, mainly to countries with links with Britain such as Singapore, Hong Kong, East Africa and Canada. There have been small Sikh communities in Britain since the First World War, when a number of Sikh servicemen who had fought in the trenches in Europe settled here after being demobbed. Between the two world wars. Sikh traders settled in the ports. During the Second World War, 36,000 Sikhs died fighting for Britain (Hiro 1991). Afterwards a few Sikh ex-servicemen stayed in Britain. Many others were recruited to work here by private industrial companies whose staff had fought beside Sikhs in the War.

It is estimated that there are almost half a million Sikhs in the UK (Weller 1997). Sikhism is now the third-largest faith in Britain, after Christianity and Islam.

- The families of most British Sikhs originated in Punjab in northern India (see Figure 41.1). Most of these families arrived in Britain in the 1950s and '60s.
- A few Sikh families came to Britain from East Africa (see Figure 39.1), to which their forebears had emigrated from Punjab. They came mainly in the 1970s, often as refugees and as whole families.

Diversity The very different backgrounds and experiences of these two groups mean that, at least among older people, there is a tendency to live, worship and socialise separately, and to see themselves to some extent as separate communities.

Languages

Most Sikhs in Britain speak Punjabi. Sikh holy books are written in Punjabi (in the Gurmukhi script) and Punjabi is the language of worship (see also Chapter 41 *Languages*).

The Sikh naming system

Many Sikhs do not use a family name, for religious reasons (see *Guru Gobind Singh*, below). Instead, they use a religious second name, Kaur or Singh (see Chapter 30 *Recording people's names correctly*). In general, it is most acceptable to use title plus the first two names or the full name, especially with older people. Names must be recorded fully and correctly to prevent dangerous confusion.

Sikhism – a brief description

The Sikh religion was founded in the sixteenth century in Punjab in northern India. Almost all Sikhs are Punjabi in origin (see also Chapter 41).

Sikh beliefs and values

Sikhs believe in one personal God who is the eternal creator and the source of all being. Sikhs stress the need for each person to develop their own individual relationship with God, seeking truth and leading a virtuous life. Prayer and meditation, congregational worship, family duties and community involvement are all important. Many Sikhs give ten per cent of their income to charity and other good causes.

Sikhs believe that each soul must go through many cycles of birth, death and rebirth in the world. The ultimate aim of each soul is to break this cycle by reaching a state of perfection and so becoming united with God. Being born as a human being is a great privilege and opportunity, because only human beings can break the cycle. Devout Sikhs may see death as the door to unity with God and eternal bliss.

Belief in rebirth is linked to belief in karma, the natural moral law of reward and punishment for all thoughts and deeds. Belief in karma leads to a strong sense of personal responsibility: a person's current situation is the result of their past actions and thoughts. Their actions and thoughts now will determine their future in this life and in the next. Sikhs also believe that a person's karma can be improved through prayer and by the grace of God.

Guru Nanak (1469–1539 CE*), the founder of Sikhism, wanted to end the divisiveness of the caste system, and the excessive ritual and priestly domination of the Hindu and Muslim societies of his time. He is regarded by Sikhs as a great spiritual leader and a messenger from God, reminding people of God's name and of the possibility of spiritual liberation (Cole 1994). The word 'Sikh' means disciple.

Sikhism stresses community and equality between all people, whatever their caste, class, occupation or financial situation. It also stresses religious tolerance. Men and women are considered equal, though they may have different traditional roles. Sikhism has no ordained priesthood or official priestly hierarchy, and all the members, male and female, of each community play a part in worship and in running their own temple (gurdwara).

Guru Gobind Singh There were nine living Sikh gurus after Guru Nanak. All are greatly honoured and revered. The tenth and last, Guru Gobind Singh (1666–1708 CE*), wanted to make the Sikhs into a visible community and to strengthen them as a fighting force against the Muslim Mughal emperors who were persecuting them at the time. He instituted five symbols, including uncut and unshaven hair and a steel bangle, which all initiated Sikh men and women wear (see *The five symbols of the Sikh faith*, below). All the Sikh gurus had uncut hair and wore turbans. The turban has become the best-known mark of a Sikh man.

In order to eradicate caste-consciousness, Guru Gobind Singh also required Sikhs to stop using their family names, which indicated their traditional position in the Hindu caste system. Instead, all Sikh men were to use the last name Singh (Lion), and all women the last name Kaur (Princess) (see also Chapter 30). Nevertheless, caste awareness and divisions, which were as deeply rooted in society as class awareness and divisions in Britain, proved difficult to destroy. Awareness of caste status still influences many Sikhs, particularly older people, with regard to social life and obligations and to marriage.

The ten Gurus are seen as divine teachers who conveyed God's word. They are not worshipped. Guru Gobind Singh stated that there would be no human guru after him. Before he died, he handed spiritual authority over to the Guru Granth Sahib (the Sikh holy book), and secular authority to the community of initiated or Amritdhari Sikhs (see below).

Amritdhari Sikhs Some adult Sikhs devote themselves more closely to their religion and go through an initiation or confirmation ceremony known as

---

* Common Era, used as an alternative to AD.

taking amrit or amrit pahul. This was first performed by Guru Gobind Singh in 1699. A Sikh man or woman who has taken amrit is likely to be particularly careful about spiritual and practical discipline, including wearing the five symbols, not using a family name and eating a vegetarian diet. An Amritdhari Sikh who breaks any of the prohibitions except when absolutely necessary, may have to go through the amrit ceremony again and to perform a penance.

Religious observance

Prayer

The time before sunrise is considered a good time to pray without distraction, and many devout Sikhs, especially older people, like to wake up early to pray. People also pray in the evenings and before they go to sleep. Privacy during prayer (eg with bed-curtains drawn) is appreciated. Some people may prefer the quiet of a separate room if one is available.

The japji, or the meditation
(Morning prayer)

As He was in the beginning: the Truth,
So throughout the ages, He has ever been: the Truth,
So even now He is Truth immanent, so for ever and ever He shall be
Truth eternal.

There is one God,
Eternal Truth is His Name:
Maker of all things,
Fearing nothing and at enmity with nothing,
Timeless is His Image;
Not begotten, being of His own Being:
By the Grace of the Guru, made known to men. *

It is important to be physically clean and in a clean place when praying; people normally wash or shower beforehand. If patients cannot have a full wash, they may wish at least to wash their hands and face. If they are bed-bound they need a towel and a bowl of water, and they may also like a cup for pouring the water. Find out if and when a Sikh patient wishes to pray and what they will need.

---

* Trans Singh T, Singh BJ, Singh K et al, 1960. The Guru here refers to God, the True and Perfect Guru.

The Guru Granth Sahib

The Sikh holy book, the Guru Granth Sahib, contains devotional hymns, meditations and the teachings and sermons of the Sikh gurus and other holy men. It is treated with great reverence and when not being read it is covered with a special cloth or 'robe'. Sikhs may turn to the Guru Granth Sahib for comfort, support and guidance at difficult times. A few families have a complete copy of the Guru Granth Sahib at home, but a special room must be set aside for it. Everyone covers their head and removes their shoes before entering. Visitors enter only if invited.

Sikh patients may use a book of prayers and hymns called the Nit-Nem Gutka for their daily prayers. This is wrapped in a cloth and opened only with clean hands. Nothing must be put on top of it and it should not be put near dirty clothes or shoes, nor at the foot of the bed near the patient's feet. It should never be allowed to fall on the floor.

Religious articles

Patients may have pictures of the ten Sikh gurus (see earlier) and prayer beads with them. These are treated with the same respect as a prayer book (see above).

The gurdwara

Sikhism is a community-based religion. Communal worship and social activities at the gurdwara (the Sikh temple) are very important. The main room is the diwan hall, the prayer room, in which the Guru Granth Sahib, the Sikh holy book, is kept on a covered throne. Any devout Sikh who can read the Guru Granth Sahib in the original can lead worship in the gurdwara. There is also a kitchen, facilities for washing, and a communal dining area where meals are served for the whole congregation after services. Sikhs in Britain generally hold their main services on Sundays. Sikh communities of different backgrounds may each have their own gurdwara. Some communities are more conservative than others.

Before entering the gurdwara, both men and women remove their shoes and cover their heads. Some people also wash their hands and feet. As is common in South Asian tradition, men and women usually sit separately. Everyone sits with the soles of their feet pointing away from the Guru Granth Sahib as a matter of courtesy. Non-Sikhs are welcome, provided they observe these customs.

At the end of a service everyone is given a small portion of karah parshad. This is a special sweet dish made of equal parts of sugar, butter and flour mixed with water, cooked and blessed. The sharing of karah parshad emphasises the equality and fellowship of all Sikhs.

When someone is ill Sikh families or community members may bring a small portion of karah parshad to patients who cannot attend the gurdwara. If a person is on a restricted diet for medical reasons, it may be important for them to eat only a tiny portion.

Some families may also bring holy water from a special ceremonial reading of the Guru Granth Sahib for a patient to drink (see Chapter 10 *Holy water*).

The granthi

Most Sikh communities in Britain employ a granthi, an elected caretaker, to lead services and look after the gurdwara. The granthi does not traditionally have a pastoral role. The job of visiting the sick and comforting the old and dying belongs primarily to the family and the community. In Britain, however, some patients may ask the granthi to visit.

Anniversaries and festivals

The dates of most Sikh anniversaries vary each year, depending on the date of the full moon (see the SHAP Calendar, listed in the References). In some cases the celebrations may be moved to the nearest Sunday. All are celebrated in a spirit of gratitude and thanksgiving. There are usually special prayers at the gurdwara, most commonly a 48-hour full reading of the Guru Granth Sahib, known as an Akhand Path, timed to end on the morning of the festival. Patients may have more visitors at this time. Patients who have no relatives to pray with them may ask for a granthi (see above) to visit. The main Sikh festivals are the following.

The birthday of Guru Gobind Singh, the last living Sikh guru (see earlier). *December/January*

Vaisakhi *Usually April 13th* The Sikh New Year festival. Celebrates the day on which Guru Gobind Singh founded the Khalsa, the community of initiated (Amritdhari) Sikh men and women (see above).

The martyrdom of Guru Arjan Dev, the fifth Sikh guru. *May/June*

Bandhi Chhord *October/November* Commemorates the release from prison of Guru Hargobind, the sixth Sikh guru, by the Mughal emperor Jehangir. Falls at the same time as Diwali, the Hindu festival of light, and many Sikhs celebrate both (see Chapter 43 *Festivals*).

The anniversary of the installation of the Guru Granth Sahib, the Sikh holy book, as the successor to the ten living Sikh gurus (see earlier). *August/September*

The birthday of Guru Nanak, the first Sikh guru. *October/November*

The martyrdom of Guru Teg Bahadur, the ninth living Sikh guru. *November/December*

The five symbols of the Sikh faith

Central to the Sikh religion are the five symbols or articles of faith. These were instituted by Guru Gobind Singh, the last living Sikh guru, to bind the Sikh community together and to give them a permanent reminder of the practical and spiritual discipline required of them. They are: kara – a steel bangle; kesh – uncut hair and unshaven beard; kangha – a special comb to fix the hair; kirpan – a short sword; and kacchera – special underpants. They are always worn and should not be removed.

In the early days of migration some Sikhs were persuaded to give up the five symbols in order to make it easier to get a job. Many have now re-adopted some or all of them as a sign of confidence and pride in their identity and religion. Most devout Sikhs wear all five symbols all the time and never remove them completely, even when they are ill, in bed or washing. Every care must be taken to treat them with respect and care.

Kara (bangle)

The kara symbolises the divine unity and infinity of God and reminds people to do good. Most Sikh men and women wear a thin steel bangle on their right wrist all the time. Left-handed people wear it on their left wrist. The kara is never removed.

A kara should normally be taped before an operation. If removal is essential, discuss this with the patient or the family if possible. The kara may perhaps be placed on the other wrist but in any case should normally be kept with the patient. It is not removed after death.

Kesh (uncut hair and beard)

In South Asian tradition the head is regarded as the most sacred part of the body. Long hair symbolises spirituality. Many devout Sikh men and women never cut their hair, and men never shave or trim their beards. The hair and beard should always be kept clean and tidy. It may be plaited (women only) or fixed up on the head in a bun (see *Hair care*, below). Some devout Sikhs may refuse to have hair on any part of their body cut or shaved (see also Chapter 12 *Practical care*).

The prohibition on cutting or shaving hair specifically bans the use of razors and scissors. If it is essential for clinical reasons to remove body hair, it may sometimes be more acceptable to use a depilatory cream.

Kangha (comb)

The kangha, a small semicircular comb used to fix the hair on the head, symbolises disciplined spirituality, neatness and cleanliness. When their hair is loose, people may keep their kangha in a pocket. A Sikh with short hair may carry a kangha in a pocket or wear a miniature one on a chain around their neck. If a kangha must be removed, it is usually acceptable to put in under the pillow or in a locker. Discuss this with the patient.

Kirpan (short sword)

The kirpan symbolises the Sikh's traditional readiness to fight in self-defence and to protect the oppressed and needy. Some devout Sikh men and women wear a 10–15 centimetre-long kirpan in a cloth sash with a sheath (gatra kirpan). The sash is worn under the clothes over the right shoulder and round the left side of the body. Many devout Sikhs never remove their kirpan. It is always kept clean and dry, wrapped around the head when bathing or showering, and around the waist when washing the hair.

In most cases, kirpans cause no practical problems for medical or nursing care. A person who needs a bed bath will usually be willing to take off their kirpan and hold it until it can be put on again. If a kirpan must be removed completely for any reason (eg before surgery), consent should be obtained and agreement reached as to where it should be kept for the time being. It is generally acceptable to place the kirpan beside the prayer book in the locker, or to give it to relatives for safe-keeping. A devout Sikh may want to say a special prayer before removing their kirpan. Relatives or the granthi may recite the prayer on behalf of someone who is too ill to do it themselves. Some patients may wish to wear a miniature kirpan under their turban or head covering until they return to their bed.

Kacchera (underpants)

Kacchera (pronounced ka<u>che</u>ra) are to remind Sikhs of the duties of modesty, restraint and sexual purity. Traditionally they are loose and tied with a draw-string. Most non-Amritdhari Sikhs in the UK wear conventional underwear as kacchera.

Most devout Sikh men and women never remove their kacchera completely. When changing, they usually put one foot in the new pair before completely removing the old pair. They wear them while showering and then put on a dry pair. Sikh women giving birth in Punjab are accustomed to keeping one leg in the kacchera all the time. Kacchera are worn during the day and at night.

Devout Sikh patients are likely to continue to wish to wear their kacchera and never to remove them completely. Health professionals should help with this as much as possible, taking patients' wishes into account when bathing them or changing their clothes, and during medical treatments or examinations. Incontinence may cause particular difficulties and possible solutions should be discussed with the patient or their family.

Families and relationships

Guru Nanak stressed that men and women could come closer to God by being active members of their families. Providing for the family (often the extended family) and caring for its members' spiritual and emotional well-being are religious duties for Sikhs (see also Chapter 41 *Traditional family structures and relationships*). Sons and their wives, especially the eldest son and his wife, are traditionally responsible for the care and support of parents when they are ill or old.

The Sikh gurus stressed the equality of status of women and men. Men and women participate equally in religious ceremonies. Sikh women are traditionally educated equally with men. Socially and within the family, women usually have a good deal of freedom and authority, though in practice, as in most communities, major decisions are often made by men. In the early days of South Asian settlement in Britain, Sikh women were often the first women who went out to work.

Marriage

It is generally believed that all Sikhs should marry and raise a family. Marriage is a sacrament as well as a social ceremony and is highly valued. Both men and women are expected to take an active part in bringing up children. Sexual morality is traditionally strict.

Divorce is generally regarded as shameful and occurs only when the marital situation is desperate. There is often a social stigma attached to divorced people, especially women.

Dietary requirements

'A devout Sikh will appreciate recognition of their religious needs concerning diet and the five symbols of our faith. Everyone feels better in their own mind if their wishes and needs are recognised.'
Sikh man

Although there is a lot of variation among the Sikh communities, the dietary practices of each individual are binding and must be respected. Amritdhari and older Sikhs are likely to be stricter and more concerned about what they eat.

A *vegetarian diet*

Most Amritdhari and some other devout Sikh men and women are vegetarian. They do not eat meat, fish, eggs or anything made with or containing them. Some may prefer to eat only food that is brought from home so that they can be sure of what they are eating. Some may feel that even if utensils, serving dishes and cooking pots are kept separate, vegetarian food served from the same trolley as meat is unacceptable (see also Chapter 11 *Religious considerations*).

Most non-vegetarian Sikhs do not eat beef. Some do not eat pork because the pig is a scavenging animal in India and pig meat is generally regarded as dirty. Sikhs do not eat halal meat (meat killed according to Muslim regulations).

Medication

There are no religious prohibitions affecting medication. Decisions about symptom control and other medication are a question of personal choice. Vegetarian Sikhs may wish to avoid products containing animal, fish or egg products if possible.

Fasting

Fasting is not required in Sikhism but is a matter of personal choice. A few devout Sikhs may fast for special causes such as the recovery of a sick family member. Fasting usually means eating only a few foods such as fruit, yoghurt or nuts.

Alcohol and tobacco

Most Amritdhari and other devout Sikhs do not drink or smoke. Some feel strongly about not being exposed to tobacco smoke. Alcohol is generally acceptable if it is a constituent of medication.

Practical care

(see also *The five symbols of the Sikh faith*, above)

Modesty and clothing
See Chapter 12.

Washing and cleanliness
See Chapter 12.

Hair care
Many devout Sikh men and women follow Guru Gobind Singh's require-ment never to cut or shave their hair (see above).

Men and boys A Sikh man with long hair wears it fixed in a bun (jura) on top of his head, usually covered by a turban during the day and in public. The hair is washed frequently, possibly daily. After washing, it is dried loose and combed out well before it is rolled up onto the head.

The head should always be kept covered. Most men wear an inner and an outer turban. The inner one (choti dastar) is smaller and keeps the large outer turban clean. It may be changed every day. The outer turban (dastar) is usually about five metres long and up to a metre wide. It is starched before tying to stiffen it into the correct shape. Some people change the outer turban every night. Others take it off at night, still starched, and wear it for two or three days.

In bed Sikh men remove their outer turbans and wear just the inner one or a scarf. The turban, like the hair it covers, is treated with reverence. If it must be removed, it should be handled carefully, with two hands, and placed somewhere clean and safe near the patient. A patient may wish to put his outer turban on again or cover his head with a scarf, towel or piece of clean cloth if he has visitors.

A Sikh boy with uncut hair usually wears it plaited and tied in a bun on the top of his head. Over the bun (jura) boys generally wear a small white cloth (a rumal) or a larger square of cloth, often muslin or poplin (a patka). Very young boys may wear their hair coiled in two plaits pinned at the back of the head.

Beards Long beards are combed daily and washed as necessary. Most Sikh men wear their beards rolled up. A proprietary hair fixer may be used to fix it. While this is setting a man may wear a piece of muslin to set the beard in shape. Some men always have their beards tied up neatly with a net, including when in bed. Others always wear their beards loose. A long beard must never be trimmed or shaved without permission.

Women and girls Most devout Sikh women never cut or trim their hair. They usually wear it fixed in a bun or in a single plait. Girls and young women before marriage traditionally wear their hair in plaits or loose.

Many Sikh women cover their hair with a scarf (called a dupattah or a chooni) as a sign of modesty. A few wear a tight black (or occasionally white) turban. A woman in bed may wish to cover her head with her scarf if visitors come to see her, especially men, or if she is in a public room or ward (see also Chapter 12 *Modesty*).

Make-up

A few Sikh women may wear a bindi, a small dot on the forehead. This has no religious connotations for Sikhs and is purely decorative.

Religious jewellery and other items

Most Sikhs wear a kirpan, a steel bangle (see earlier). Some wear a necklace with a medallion of Guru Nanak. Religious and other jewellery should always be treated with respect and never removed without consent.

Visiting a Sikh home

The traditional Sikh greeting is to join the palms of the hands at about chin level.

Older people, in particular, may prefer this to shaking hands, especially with members of the opposite sex.

In many Sikh homes, shoes are removed at the front door or at the bottom of the stairs. Visitors should not smoke or enter a Sikh home after drinking alcohol. It is traditional to offer all visitors something to eat and drink. Refusing politely does not usually cause offence.

When someone is ill or dying

Families and illness

When a family member is ill or dying, everyone has strong responsibilities towards them. It is a religious and a social duty to visit and to give comfort and support. Some patients may have a large number of visitors at all hours (see also Chapter 17).

Prayer and religious rituals

A devout Sikh who is very ill or dying may receive comfort from verses from the Guru Granth Sahib. Family members may read or pray with a dying person, and may also pray at home. There are no specific formal religious ceremonies or rites at the death of a Sikh, but some families may call on a granthi (see earlier) to pray with them.

'Continue to contemplate the True Name with thy every breath;
Life is an uncertainty; Do not delay your practice, my friend
Neither in childhood, nor in youth, nor in age is one safe.
No one knows when death is going to ensnare you with his noose.'

Guru Granth Sahib, p 1239

Organ donation

There is no religious prohibition against organ donation (see also Chapter 19).

After the death

Last offices

Most Sikhs are not concerned about non-Sikhs touching the body. Staff can usually perform the normal last offices after checking that the family has no special wishes. Do not remove any religious items or trim the hair or beard without permission (see *The five symbols of the Sikh faith*, above). If necessary, clean and tidy the face so that it looks peaceful and tranquil, especially if the coffin is to be open before the cremation (Green and Green 1992). Wounds should be sealed and the hair and beard combed and covered with a scarf or a head cloth. Some families may wish to help with the last offices. Some may wish to read passages from the Guru Granth Sahib while the last offices are carried out.

If the family wishes to wash the body later, do only the following: close the eyes and mouth and prop the jaw, straighten the limbs, seal any wounds and wrap the body in a plain sheet without religious emblems. (See also Chapter 20 *Immediately after the death and last offices*.)

Post mortems

There is no religious prohibition against post-mortem examinations but many people find them unacceptable. It may also be important to the family that a post mortem does not delay the funeral. During a post-mortem examination the symbols of the Sikh faith (see earlier) should not be removed and the hair, beard and other body hair should not be cut or shaved. If the family wishes to prepare the body for the funeral themselves it is very important that repairs are carried out carefully (see also Chapter 20 *Post mortems*).

Timing

Cremation takes place as soon as possible, normally within 24 hours of death. Families may sometimes need help to get the necessary formalities completed in time.

The funeral

The funeral begins at the family home or the gurdwara; hymns are chanted and prayers said. Often the coffin is kept open so that family and friends can pay their last respects. The mourners then accompany the coffin to the crematorium. Sikhs are cremated wearing the symbols of the Sikh faith and with uncut hair. Traditionally, the dead person's oldest son or another close male relative lights the funeral pyre. Some crematoria in Britain have adapted their practice so that family members can press the button to start the coffin moving, or help push the coffin into the cremator. The mourners may then go back to the gurdwara. Flowers are acceptable at a Sikh funeral.

After the cremation the ashes may be thrown into the sea or a river, or buried. Some families may wish to take them to India to deposit them in the River Ganges.

Mourning

In the days following the death, relatives and friends come to keep the family company and support them. Family members may wear white. In the days after the death there is often a complete reading of the Guru Granth Sahib.

References

Age Exchange (1991) *Remedies and Recipes: Caribbean reflections on health and diet*. Age Exchange, Blackheath, London

Age Exchange (1984) *A Place to Stay: Memories of pensioners from many lands*. Age Exchange, Blackheath, London

Ahmad WIU (1992) The maligned healer: the 'hakim' and western medicine. *New Community* 18 (4): 521–36

Ahmed S, Cheetham J, Small J (eds) (1986) *Social Work with Black Children and their Families*. B T Batsford, London

Aitchison C (1994) By prior arrangement. *The Independent* 12 Feb, p 47

Ali Y (trans) (1992) *The Qur'an*. Amana Corp, Brentwood MD

Amin K (1992) *Poverty in Black and White: Deprivation and ethnic minorities*. Child Poverty Action Group, London

Anwar M (1979) *The Myth of Return: Pakistanis in Great Britain*. Heinemann, London

Aslam M, Healy M (1986) Compliance and drug therapy in fasting Muslim patients. *Journal of Clinical Hospital Pharmacists* 11: 321–5

Aslam M, Healy M (1985) Drug regimens and fasting Muslim patients. *British Medical Journal* 290: 1746

Au WKL, Au KPKL (1992) *Working with Chinese Carers*. Health Education Council/King's Fund Centre, London

Barker J (1984) *Black and Asian Old People in Britain*. Age Concern England, London

Baxter C (1989) *Cancer Support and Ethnic Minority and Migrant Worker Communities*. CancerLink, London

Beishon S, Modood T, Virdee S (1998) *Ethnic Minority Families*. Policy Studies Institute, London

Berkovits Dayan B (1992) *A Guide to Jewish Practice for Nurses and Medical Staff*. Federation of Synagogues, 65 Watford Way, London NW4 3AQ

Blakemore K, Boneham M (1994) *Age, Race and Ethnicity: A comparative approach*. Open University Press, Buckingham

Bleich JD (1996) Survey of recent Halakhic periodical literature: treatment of the terminally ill. *Tradition: A Journal of Orthodox Jewish Thought* **30** (spring): 3

Bloomsbury Health Authority (1984) *The Health Care Needs of Chinese People in Bloomsbury Health District: The report of a survey*. Bloomsbury Health Authority, London

Boneham M (1989) Ageing and ethnicity in Britain: the case of elderly Sikh women in a Midlands town. *New Community* **15** (3): 447–59

Boston P (1993) Culture and cancer: the relevance of cultural orientation within cancer education programmes. *European Journal of Cancer Care* **2**: 72–6

Bowler I (1993) Stereotypes of women of Asian descent in midwifery: some evidence. *Midwifery* **9**: 7–16

Brown C (1984) *Black and White in Britain*. Heinemann, London

Butler Sloss, Lord Justice (1992) Re T. *All England Law Reports* **4**: 665

Chan JYK (1995) Dietary beliefs of Chinese patients. *Nursing Standard* **9** (27): 30–4

Cheung FM, Lau BWK, Wong S-W (1984) Paths to psychiatric care in Hong Kong. *Culture, Medicine and Psychiatry* **8**: 207–28

Chiu S (1989) Chinese elderly people: no longer a treasure at home. *Social Work Today* 10 Aug: 15–17

Church J (ed) (1997) *Social Trends 1997*. Office for National Statistics/Stationery Office, London

Cline S (1995) *Lifting the Taboo: Women, death and dying*. Little, Brown, London

Cole WO (1994) *Teach Yourself Sikhism*. Hodder, London

Cross C (1974) *What is Judaism?* Board of Deputies of British Jews, London

Currer C (1986) *The Mental Health of Pathan Mothers in Bradford: A study of migrant Asian women* (unpublished thesis). Department of Sociology, University of Bradford, Bradford

D'Alessio A (1993) Culture clash. *Nursing Times* **89** (38): 16–17

Daniels C (1996) Crisis and comfort: the Halakhah and the moribund patient. *Le'ela: A Journal of Judaism Today*

Dearden A (1983) *Arab Women*, revised edn. Minority Rights Group, London

Divided Families Campaign (1990) *Give us a Happy Ending: How families are kept apart by British immigration law.* Divided Families Campaign, London

Divided Families Campaign (undated) *The Right to Visit.* Divided Families Campaign, London

Douglas J (1989) Food type preferences and trends among Afro-Caribbeans in Britain. In JK Cruickshank and DG Beevers (eds) *Ethnic Factors in Health and Disease.* Butterworth Heinemann, Oxford

Edwards V (1986) *Language in a Black Community.* Multilingual Matters, Clevedon

Encarta (1998) *Encarta World Atlas.* Microsoft, Redmond WA

Encarta (1996) *Microsoft Encarta Encyclopaedia.* Microsoft, Redmond WA

Erriker C (1995) *Teach Yourself Buddhism.* Hodder and Stoughton, London

Feldman D and Rosner F (1984) *Compendium on Medical Ethics: Jewish moral, ethical and religious principles in medical practice.* Federation of Jewish Philanthropies, New York

Fenton S (1987) *Ageing Minorities: Black people as they grow old in Britain.* Commission for Racial Equality, London

Firth S (1993) Cross-cultural perspectives on bereavement. In D Dickenson and M Johnson (eds) *Death, Dying and Bereavement.* Sage, London, pp 254–61

Firth S (1996) The good death: attitudes of British Hindus. In G Howarth and PC Jupp (eds) *Contemporary Issues in the Sociology of Death, Dying and Disposal.* Macmillan, London, pp 96–107

Foner N (1979) *Jamaica Farewell.* Routledge and Kegan Paul, London

Fong LC, Watt I (1994) Chinese health behaviour: breaking barriers to better understanding. *Health Trends* 26 (1): 14–15

Fuller JHS, Toon PD (1988) *Medical Practice in a Multicultural Society.* Heinemann, London

Gatrad AR (1994a) Medical implications of Islam for women and children. *Maternal and Child Health* July: 225–7

Gatrad AR (1994b) Muslim customs surrounding death, bereavement, postmortem examinations, and organ transplants. *British Medical Journal* 309: 521–3

Godagama S (1997) *The Handbook of Ayurveda.* Kyle Cathie, London

Goldberg C (1991) *Mourning in Halacha: The laws and customs of the year of mourning.* Mesorah Publications, New York

Goonewardene AD (1996) Buddhism. In WO Cole (ed) *Six World Faiths*. Cassell, London

Gopaul-McNicol SA (1993) *Working with West Indian Families*. Guilford Press, New York

Gordon P, Klug F (1985) *British Immigration Control: A brief guide*. Runnymede Trust, London

Green J, Green M (1992) *Dealing with Death: practices and procedures*. Chapman and Hall, London.

Hebblethwaite M (1996) Britain's black churches. *Tablet* 23 Nov: 1538–40

Hiro Dilip (1991) *Black British, White British*, revised edition. Grafton, London

Hiro Dilip (1973) *Black British, White British*. Penguin, London

Hornsby-Smith MP (1991) *Roman Catholic Beliefs in England: Customary Catholicism and transformations of religious authority*. Cambridge University Press, Cambridge

Huang WWC (1989) Chinese perspectives on death and dying. In A Berger, P Badham et al (eds) *Perspectives on Death and Dying*. Charles Press, Philadelphia PA

IQRA Trust (1997; unpublished) *Meeting the Needs of Muslim Patients*. IQRA Trust, 24 Culross Street, London W1Y 3HE

Jakobovits I (1975) *Jewish Medical Ethics*. Bloch Publishing, New York

Jang Y (1995) Chinese culture and occupational therapy. *British Journal of Occupational Therapy* 58 (3): 103–6

Jonker G (1996) The many facets of Islam. In CM Parkes, P Laungani and B Young (eds) *Death and Bereavement across Cultures*. Routledge, London

Kahin M (1997) *Education Somali Children in Britain*. Trentham Books, Stoke-on-Trent

Katz J (1995) Jewish perspectives on death, dying and bereavement. In D Dickenson and M Johnson (eds) *Death, Dying and Bereavement*. Sage, London

Küng H, Ching J (1993) *Christianity and Chinese Religions*. SCM Press, London

Lamb D (1993) Organ transplants. In D Dickenson and M Johnson (eds) *Death, Dying and Bereavement*. Sage, London

Laungani P (1997) Death in a Hindu family. In CM Parkes, P Laungani and B Young (eds) *Death and Bereavement across Cultures*. Routledge, London

Lem IM (1994) Physical and social geography. *In Africa South of the Sahara*, 23rd edn. Europa Publications, London

Li P-L (1992) Health needs of the Chinese population. In WIU Ahmad (ed) *The Politics of 'Race' and Health*. Race Relations Research Unit, University of Bradford, Bradford

London Beth Din (1998) *The Really Jewish Food Guide*. United Synagogue Publications, 735 High Road, London N12 [Contains information about acceptability of processed foods and of some drugs]

Malyon D (1998) Transfusion-free treatment of Jehovah's Witnesses: respecting the autonomous patient's rights. *Journal of Medical Ethics* 24 (5): 302–7

Maqsood R (1994) *Teach Yourself Islam*. Hodder and Stoughton, London

Mares Penny (1982) *The Vietnamese in Britain: A handbook for health workers*. National Extension College, Cambridge

McIntosh V, Andrews I (1992) *Respect for Religious and Cultural Beliefs*. Mount Vernon Hospital NHS Trust, Rickmansworth Road, Northwood, Middlesex

Modood T, Beishon S, Virdee S (1994) *Changing Ethnic Identities*. Policy Studies Institute, London

Modood T, Berthoud R, Lakey J, Nazroo J, Smith P, Virdee S, Beishon S (1997) *Ethnic Minorities in Britain: Diversity and disadvantage*. Policy Studies Institute, London

Muslim Law (Sharia) Council (1995) *Organ Transplants*. Muslim Law (Sharia) Council, London

Nazroo J (1997) *The Health of Britain's Ethnic Minorities: Findings from a national survey*. Policy Studies Institute, London

Neuberger J (1987) *Caring for Dying People of Different Faiths*. Austen Cornish, London

New North London Synagogue (1997) *The Laws of Life: A guide to traditional Jewish practice at times of bereavement*. New North London Synagogue, The Manor House, 80 East End Road, London N3 2SY

Northwick Park and St Marks NHS Trust (1994) *Somali Foods and Dietary Habits*. Department of Nutrition and Dietetics, Northwick Park Hospital, Harrow, Middx

OPCS (1993) *1991 Census: Ethnic group and country of birth – Great Britain* (CEN 91 TM EGCB). Office of Population Censuses and Surveys, London

Pakenham T (1991) *The Scramble for Africa*. Weidenfeld and Nicolson, London

Parker-Jenkins M (1995) *Children of Islam: A teacher's guide to meeting the needs of Muslim pupils*. Trentham Books, Stoke-on-Trent

Peach C (1968) *West Indian Migration to Britain.* Oxford University Press, Oxford

re O (a minor) (medical treatment) [1993] **2** *Family Law Reports* 149

re R (a minor) (blood transfusion) [1993] **2** *Family Law Reports* 757

Refugee Action (1987) *Last Refuge: Elderly people from Vietnam in the UK.* Refugee Action, Derby

Refugee Council (1994) *Somali Refugees in the UK,* Somalia Factfile 5. Refugee Council, London

Rose EJB (1969) *Colour and Citizenship.* Oxford University Press, Oxford

Royal College of Surgeons (1996) *Code of Practice for the Surgical Management of Jehovah's Witnesses.* Royal College of Surgeons, London

Runnymede Trust (1997) *Islamophobia: A challenge for us all.* Runnymede Trust, London

Saifullah-Khan V (1976) Pakistani women in Britain. *Journal of the Community Relations Commission* **5** (1-2): 1–10

Shang Anthony (1986) Seeds of Chinatown: the Chinese in Britain. In V Coombe and A Little (eds) *Race and Social Work: A guide to training.* Tavistock, London

SHAP (published annually) *Calendar of Religious Festivals.* SHAP Working Party on World Religions in Education, c/o The National Centre's RE Centre, 36 Causton Street, London SW1P 4AU

Shukla K (1991) Nutrition and dietetics. In AJ Squires (ed) *Multicultural Health Care and Rehabilitation of Older People.* Edward Arnold, London

Sibley D (1997) Caring for dying Buddhists. *International Journal of Palliative Nursing* **3** (1): 26–30

Silveira E, Ebrahim S (1995) Mental health and health status of elderly Bengalis and Somalis in London. *Age and Ageing* **24**: 474–80

Singh T, Singh BJ et al (trans) (1960) *Selections from the Sacred Writings of the Sikhs.* Allen & Unwin, London

Slater M (1993) *Health for All our Children: Achieving appropriate health care for black and minority ethnic children and their families.* Action for Sick Children/National Association for the Welfare of Children in Hospital, London

South Glamorgan Race Equality Council (1994) *Towards a Good Old Age?* South Glamorgan Race Equality Council and South Glamorgan Social Services Department, Cardiff

Stopes-Roe M, Cochrane R (1990) *Citizens of this Country: The Asian-British*. Multilingual Matters, Clevedon

Sutcliffe D (1982) *British Black English*. Basil Blackwell, Oxford

Swaminarayan Hindu Mission (1995) *Understanding Hinduism*. Shri Swaminarayan Mandir, Neasden, London

Tandon Y, Raphael A (1978) *The New Position of East African Asians: Problems of a displaced minority*. Minority Rights Group, London

Tang M (1994) *Vietnamese Refugees: Towards a healthy future*. Deptford City Challenge, c/o UK Programme Department, Save the Children, Cambridge House, Cambridge Grove, London W6 0LE

Thorogood N (1989) Afro-Caribbean women and the NHS. *New Community* 15 (3): 319–34

Tong KL, Spicer BJ (1994) The Chinese palliative patient and family in North America: a cultural perspective. *Journal of Palliative Care* 10 (1): 26–8

Vadgama K (1982) *Indians in Britain*. Maddison Press, UK

Vallelly P (1997) Make room for Britain's Muslims. *Tablet* (London) 1 Nov

Van den Bergh M (1997) *A Guide for the Care of Jewish Patients in Hospitals and Nursing Homes*. Visitation Committee of the London Jewish Community, London

Visitation Committee (1997) *Care of a Dying Jewish Patient*. Visitation Committee of the London Jewish Community, London

Watch Tower (1997) *1997 Yearbook of Jehovah's Witnesses*. Watch Tower Bible and Tract Society of Pennsylvania

Watch Tower (1995) *Health-Care Advance Directive*. Hospital Information Services, Watch Tower Society, London

Watch Tower (1994) *When Someone you Love Dies*. Watch Tower Bible and Tract Society of Pennsylvania

Weller P (ed) (1997) *Religions in the UK: A multi-faith directory*. University of Derby/Interfaith Network for the UK, Derby

Wenzhong H, Grove CL (1991) *Encountering the Chinese: A guide for Americans*. Intercultural Press, Yarmouth ME

Williams RB (1984) *A New Face of Hinduism: The Swaminarayan religion*. Cambridge University Press, Cambridge

Zwebner B and Shofnos C (1989) *The Healing Visit: Insights into the mitzvah of Bikur Cholim*. Targum Press, Michigan

ABOUT AGE CONCERN

Culture, Religion and Patient Care in a Multi-Ethnic Society is one of a wide range of publications produced by Age Concern England, the National Council on Ageing. Age Concern works on behalf of all older people and believes later life should be fulfilling and enjoyable. For too many this is impossible. As the leading charitable movement in the UK concerned with ageing and older people, Age Concern finds effective ways to change that situation.

Where possible, we enable older people to solve problems themselves, providing as much or as little support as they need. A network of local Age Concerns, supported by many thousands of volunteers, provides community-based services such as lunch clubs, day centres and home visiting.

Nationally, we take a lead role in campaigning, parliamentary work, policy analysis, research, specialist information and advice provision, and publishing. Innovative programmes promote healthier lifestyles and provide older people with opportunities to give the experience of a lifetime back to their communities.

Age Concern is dependent on donations, covenants and legacies.

Age Concern England
1268 London Road
London SW16 4ER
Tel: 020 8765 7200
Fax: 020 8765 7211
Website: www.ageconcern.org.uk

Age Concern Scotland
113 Rose Street
Edinburgh EH2 3DT
Tel: 0131 220 3345
Fax: 0131 220 2779
Website: ageconcernscotland.org.uk

Age Concern Cymru
4th Floor
1 Cathedral Road
Cardiff CF1 9SD
Tel: 029 2037 1566
Fax: 029 2039 9562
Website: www.accymru.org.uk

Age Concern Northern Ireland
3 Lower Crescent
Belfast BT7 1NR
Tel: 028 9024 5729
Fax: 028 9023 5497
Website: www.ageconcernni.org

PUBLICATIONS FROM
AGE CONCERN BOOKS

ETHNIC ELDERS

Caring for Ethnic Minority Elders: a guide
Yasmin Alibhai-Brown

Addressing the delivery of care to older people from ethnic minority groups, this book highlights the impact of varying cultural tradition and stresses their significance in the design of individual care packages. Designed to help those planning the delivery of services and those working with ethnic minority elders, the book provides key guidance on developing and maintaining high standards in good practice and care.

£14.99   0-86242-188-8

POLICY

Baby Boomers: ageing in the 21st century
Edited by Maria Evandrou

Accessible and stimulating, *Baby Boomers* looks ahead to the next century and examines the kind of world the baby boom generations will experience, including prospects for employment and training, financial resources, health care, social care and housing. Future policy options are explored and a series of recommendations are made, making this essential reading for policy makers, managers, health and social care planners, politicians, students, researchers and anyone else concerned with retirement in the future.

£14.95   0-86242-153-5

Elder Abuse: critical issues in policy and practice
Edited by Phil Slater and Mervyn Eastman

The problem of elder abuse constitutes a challenge at the very heart of a would-be civilised society. There are no simple solutions, and the health and care professions face increasing demands to identify, combat and prevent elder abuse. The contributing authors are drawn evenly from the words of service provision and academic research, to provide a sound framework for exploring good practice and supporting the recognition, management and prevention of elder abuse.

£14.99   0-86242-248-5

HEALTH

Know Your Medicines
Pat Blair

This handy guide answers many of the common questions that older people – and those who care for them – often have about the medicines they use and how they work. While stressing safety throughout, the book includes information about dosage and strength, brands, storage and disposal of medicines.

£7.99   0-86242-226-4

HIV & AIDS and Older People
Tara Kaufman

About one person in ten with AIDS in the UK is aged over 50. Providing information, support and practical advice for older people facing the challenge of HIV and AIDS in their lives, this book is aimed at those who have HIV or AIDS themselves, for their families and those who are caring for someone who is affected. It is a source of guidance on the treatments available, how best to care for someone at home and sources of further help.

£9.95   0-86242-181-0

PROFESSIONAL

Working with Family Carers: a handbook
Jacqui Wood with Phill Watson

A multi-disciplinary handbook designed to enable care and health professions to view family carers as perhaps their greatest resource and work in partnership with them. There is clear and detailed information of the various aspects of working with carers, both practically and emotionally.

£14.99   0-86242-230-2

Promoting Mobility for People with Dementia
Rosemary Oddy

People with dementia must be enabled to move and given the opportunity to do so frequently, with or without help, if they are to remain mobile. The commonsense approaches described in this book should ease the task of retaining optimum levels of mobility for people with dementia for as long as possible, without jeopardising the health and safety of those who care for them – whether physiotherapists, occupational therapists, nurses or carers.

£14.99   0-86242-242-6

Dementia Care: a handbook for residential and day care
Alan Chapman, Mary Marshall and Alan Jacques

A comprehensive, practical guide to the delivery of care to people with dementia, this book has been designed for use by those working in both residential and day care settings. Stressing the importance of maintaining respect for people with dementia and upholding their rights as individuals, the handbook provides sound advice on good practice and offers reassurance and support.

£11.99 0-86242-128-4

If you would like to order any of these titles, please write to the address below, enclosing a cheque or money order for the appropriate amount (plus £1.99 p&p for one book; for additional books please add 75p per book up to a maximum of £7.50) made payable to Age Concern England. Credit card orders may be made on 0870 44 22 120. Books can also be ordered online at www.ageconcern.org.uk/shop

Age Concern Books
Units 5 & 6
Industrial Estate
Brecon
Powys LD3 8LA

Information Line

Age Concern produces over 40 comprehensive factsheets designed to answer many of the questions older people – or those advising them – may have, on topics such as:

- finding and paying for residential and nursing home care
- money benefits
- finding help at home
- legal affairs
- making a Will
- help with heating
- raising income from your home
- transfer of assets

Age Concern offers a factsheet subscription service that presents all the factsheets in a folder, together with regular updates throughout the year. The first year's subscription currently costs £65. Single copies, up to a maximum of five, are available free on receipt of an sae.

To order your FREE factsheet list, phone 0800 00 99 66 (a free call) or write to:

Age Concern
FREEPOST (SWB 30375)
Ashburton
Devon TQ13 7ZZ

INDEX

In order to avoid promoting generalisations and stereotyping, the index refers mainly to Parts One to Four of this book. It is important to understand the broad principles of providing care in a multi-ethnic society before considering specific factors that may (or may not) be relevant to individual patients and families of different cultural and religious groups. We have not given detailed references to Part Five, because it is important to read each of these chapters as a whole, and not to pick out and use one or two 'facts' in isolation.

Where more than one page number is given, those in *italic* indicate the main discussions.